Lorenz Büchler • Marius J.B. Keel
Editors

Fractures of the Hip

Springer

Editors
Lorenz Büchler
Department of Orthopaedic Surgery
Kantonsspital Aarau
Aarau
Switzerland

Marius J.B. Keel
Trauma Center Hirslanden
Clinic Hirslanden
Zürich
Switzerland

ISSN 2364-3250 ISSN 2364-3269 (electronic)
Fracture Management Joint by Joint
ISBN 978-3-030-18840-5 ISBN 978-3-030-18838-2 (eBook)
https://doi.org/10.1007/978-3-030-18838-2

This Springer imprint is published by the registered company Springer Nature Switzerland AG
The registered company address is: Gewerbestrasse 11, 6330 Cham, Switzerland

Fracture Management Joint by Joint

Series editors

Filippo Castoldi
Department of Orthopaedics
CTO Hospital Turin
Torino
Italy

Davide Edoardo Bonasia
University of Torino
AO Ordine Mauriziano
Torino
Italy

This book series aims to provide orthopedic surgeons with up-to-date practical guidance on the assessment, preoperative work-up, and surgical management of intra-articular fractures involving different joints, including the shoulder, knee, hip, elbow, ankle, and wrist. Complex articular fractures are difficult to treat and sometimes require specific surgical skills appropriate to the involved joint. In addition, arthroscopic-assisted fracture reduction is increasing in popularity, but trauma surgeons are generally not trained in arthroscopic techniques. For these reasons, articular fractures are often referred by the trauma team to surgeons experienced in the management of injuries to the joint in question. Therefore, across the world it is becoming common for orthopedic surgeons to specialize in treating fractures of only one joint. This series is designed to fill a gap in the literature by presenting the shared experience of surgeons skilled in the use of arthroscopic and open techniques on individual joints.

More information about this series at http://www.springer.com/series/13619

Foreword

This book series aims to provide orthopaedic surgeons with up-to-date practical guidance on the assessment, preoperative work-up and surgical management of intra-articular fractures involving different joints. Complex articular fractures are difficult to treat and sometimes require specific surgical skills appropriate to the involved joint. In addition, arthroscopic-assisted fracture reduction is increasing in popularity, but trauma surgeons are generally not trained in arthroscopic techniques. For these reasons, articular fractures are often referred by the trauma team to surgeons experienced in the management of injuries to the joint in question. Therefore, across the world it is becoming common for orthopaedic surgeons to specialize in treating fractures of only one joint. This series is designed to fill a gap in the literature by presenting the shared experience of surgeons skilled in the use of arthroscopic and open techniques on individual joints.

In this specific book, Dr. Büchler and Dr. Keel, world renowned experts in this field, developed a comprehensive table of contents regarding hip fractures. Surgical anatomy and relevant radiology are described together with different surgical approaches, including those that many surgeons are not very familiar with. Then, acetabulum and proximal femur fracture management is described in detail including conservative and surgical treatments. The management (open and arthroscopic) of some common complications (malunion, nonunion, loose bodies, etc.) is included as well. Experts from all over the world were invited to participate in this project. The result is a practical reference guide for the hip surgeon, trauma surgeons and orthopaedic resident approaching simple and complex fractures around the hip.

Torino, Italy — Filippo Castoldi
Torino, Italy — Davide Edoardo Bonasia

Preface

The series "Fracture Management Joint by Joint", to which this volume belongs, has introduced a new concept of up-to-date literature emphasizing the importance to assess articular fractures in the context of the entire anatomical region. Thus, the book is intended to be useful to the specialized orthopaedic surgeon and general trauma surgeon alike.

A wide variety of approaches and surgical techniques are used to treat hip fractures, and the selection of the best therapy is challenging. The purpose of this book is to support the reader towards a broad understanding of the traumatized hip, including anatomy, biomechanics, diagnosis and surgical treatment. As a result, the surgeon should be confident to choose the appropriate treatment for a specific fracture in an individual patient, may this be conservative, by osteosynthesis or through total hip arthroplasty.

We have assembled a group of renowned trauma surgeons from around the world to present a comprehensive, up-to-date overview over their respective field of expertise. The book is divided into three sections: Principles, including anatomy, biomechanics, radiology and initial management, chapters on surgical approaches and chapters on specific fracture types, pathological fractures and complications.

It has been a tremendous pleasure to interact with such an excellent faculty, and we thank the authors for having dedicated their time and expertise. We have learned a lot ourselves. Also, we would like to thank the editorial staff at Springer. Without their great assistance and support, this project would not have been possible.

We hope that the entire series, and this book in particular, will serve as a valuable tool in the reader's clinical practice.

Bern, Switzerland — Lorenz Büchler
Zürich, Switzerland — Marius J.B. Keel

Contents

Anatomy of the Hip Joint

1

Michael Wyatt, Carl Freeman, and Martin Beck

Abstract

The normal hip is often described as a synovial ball and socket joint but this hardly does it justice. The hip represents a remarkable coexistence of stability married to versatility in motion. Furthermore this biomechanical phenomenon is built to sustain the demands of a lifetime and today such demands are ever increasing. In broad terms the bony anatomy with concave socket articulating with the femoral head creates an incredibly stable joint challenged only in the most part by high-energy trauma. Its complex intra-articular structures and lubrication system create a mobile and durable couple, the secrets of which have not yet fully been elucidated. The intricate arterial anastomoses supplying the joint have only been revealed in recent years. The application of this anatomical knowledge has permitted surgeons to not only understand hip pathology but also to intervene safely with procedures such as surgical hip dislocations. In this chapter we will explore both acetabulum and proximal femur from their development to final morphology. We shall delve into what is known about the labrum and other articular structures. Finally we shall scrutinize the complex blood supply to the hip for this is paramount to the prognosis of non-arthroplasty treatment of intra-articular hip fractures and preventing complications.

Keywords

Hip · Anatomy · Embryology · Surface anatomy · Blood supply

1.1 Landmarks of the Hip Joint

The most readily identifiable landmarks for the hip and acetabulum are the greater trochanter and the anterior superior iliac spine (ASIS). The ASIS lies superiorly and just laterally to the acetabulum in the coronal plane and indicates the location of the anterior column, the anterior wall, and the iliac crest. The lateral femoral cutaneous nerve lies between two and four centimeters medial from the ASIS [1]. The anterior inferior iliac spine (AIIS) lies directly anterior and superior to the acetabulum (Fig. 1.1). The iliopectineal eminence, which develops from the pubic

M. Wyatt (✉)
Department of Trauma and Orthopaedics, MidCentral District Health Board, Palmerston North Hospital and Massey University, Palmerston North, Manawatu, New Zealand
e-mail: mike.wyatt@midcentraldhb.govt.nz

C. Freeman
Jacksonville Orthopaedic Institute, Jacksonville, FL, USA

M. Beck
Clinic for Orthopaedic and Trauma Surgery, Luzerner Kantonsspital, Luzern, Switzerland

L. Büchler, M. J.B. Keel (eds.), *Fractures of the Hip*, Fracture Management Joint by Joint,
https://doi.org/10.1007/978-3-030-18838-2_1

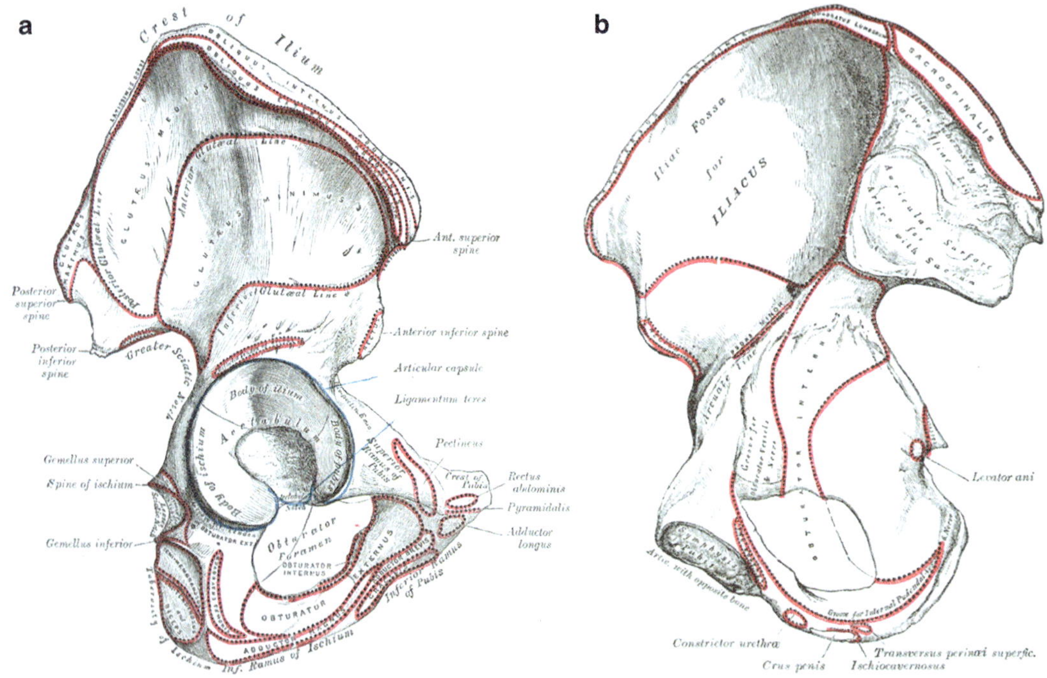

Fig. 1.1 (**a**, **b**) Anatomy of the bony pelvis including muscular attachments. Reproduced with permission and copyright © of Acta Orthop Scand suppl. [2]

extension of the triradiate cartilage, is an internal landmark marking both the medial border of the acetabulum in the coronal plane [3] and the iliopectineal bursa. The infracotyloid notch, which is a notch on the posterior ischium, just posterosuperior to the ischial tuberosity and hamstring origin is an internal landmark. It denotes an area of bone adjacent to the inferior acetabular rim. The ischial spine is a radiological landmark. Its spur like appearance is formed by the sacrospinous ligament and separates the greater and lesser sciatic notches. When visible on orthograde anteroposterior radiographs of the pelvis it may indicate retroversion of the acetabulum [4].

1.2 Development of the Hip

1.2.1 Embryology of the Hip

The embryological development of the hip begins at the fourth week and is essentially complete by the sixteenth (Fig. 1.2) [5, 6]. The hip anlage forms from scleroblastema arranged in two layers. The inner component is a spherical cluster of primitive chondroblasts, which will form the femoral head. The outer component consists of three discoid masses which will form the ilium, ischium, and pubis [5, 6]. The region of the future joint space is characterized by a crescent of densely packed cells between these two regions. By the end of the eighth week, the hip blood supply is established [5]. From weeks six to twelve, the hip increases in size via interstitial growth, and by the twelfth week the joint space has formed via apoptosis of cells between the anlage acetabulum and the femoral head. Both the ligamentum capitis femoris, which forms in the region of the cotyloid notch, and the limbus, which gives rise to the brim of the acetabulum and labrum, form at this time. By the sixteenth week, the centers of ossification of the ilium, ischium, and pubis emerge, and the triradiate cartilage is created [5].

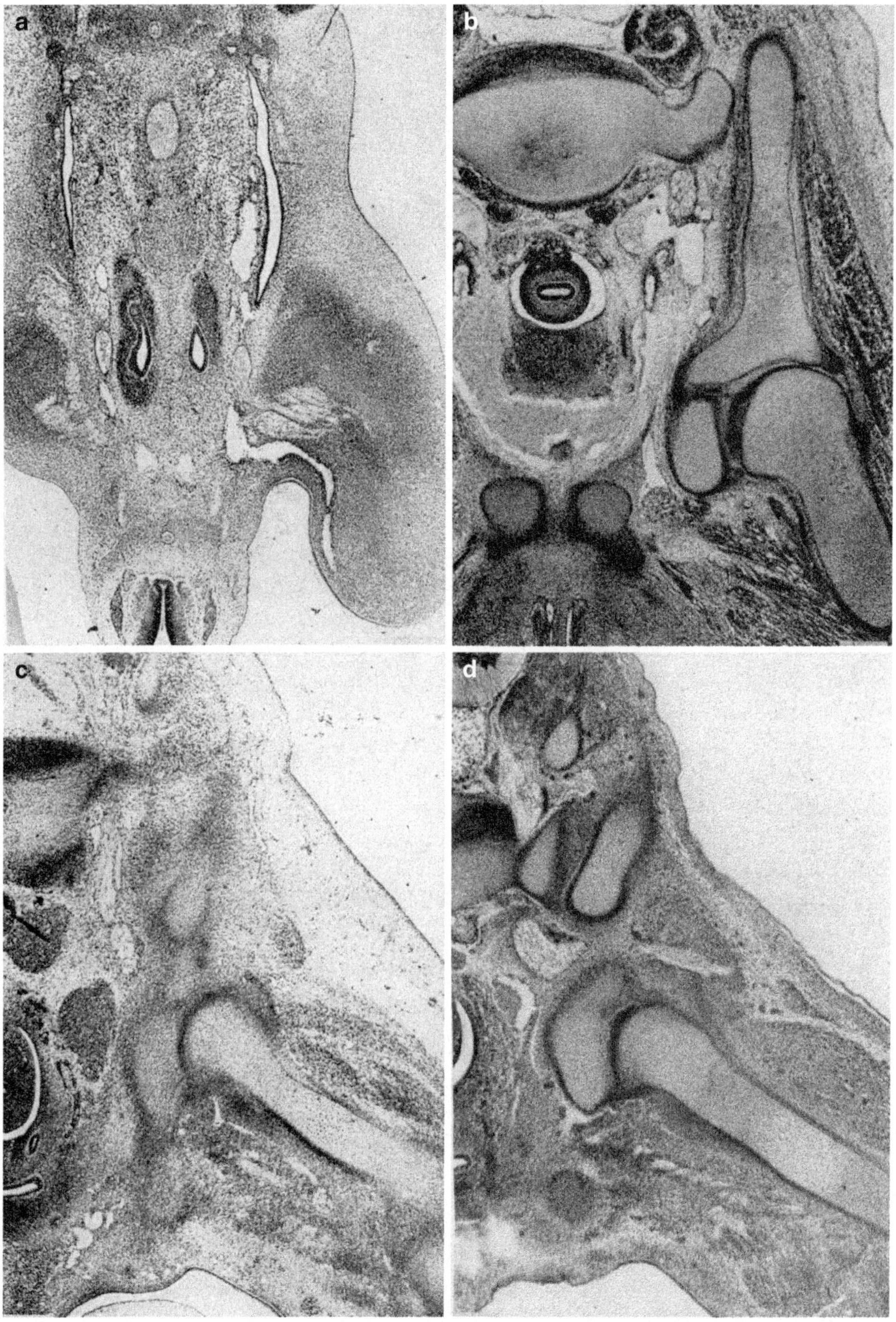

Fig. 1.2 (**a**) Around the sixth week, the hip begins to form as a densely packed group of cells called a sclero-blastema, from which forms the acetabular anlage and the femoral head. (**b**) The region of the future joint space is marked by a crescent of densely packed cells, which will eventually undergo apoptosis to form a joint space, and formally separate the acetabulum from the head. (**c**) From weeks six to twelve the acetabular anlage and femoral head increase in size via interstitial growth, and the joint space begins to form. (**d**) By the twelfth week, the hip has formed the following: a joint space, the ligamentum capitis femoris, the cotyloid fossa, and the limbus. Reproduced with permission and copyright © Clinical Orthopaedics and related research [5, 6]

1.2.2 Development of the Acetabulum After Birth

The acetabulum and labrum develop much of their final morphological features during childhood [7]. Between the innominate bones lies the triradiate cartilage, which is responsible for the formation of the anterior wall, posterior wall, and the dome of the acetabulum. It is the triradiate cartilage that is most responsible for the final depth of the acetabulum. Laterally, the triradiate cartilage gives rise to a circumferential lip composed of hyaline cartilage centrally and fibrocartilage on the periphery. This cartilaginous cup is the structure that will form the majority of the mature acetabulum when growth is complete, and is the location where the acetabular epiphyses form, all under the constantly shaping stimulus of the femoral head. The ilium and ischium contribute significantly to the final morphology of the dome and the posterior wall of the hip, respectively. The pubis contributes very little to the final structure of the mature acetabulum. This is because the anterior wall is almost completely formed by the *os acetabuli*, an epiphysis that forms adjacent to the pubis. The *os acetabuli* forms after age seven and has completed growth and closed before the age of nine. The triradiate cartilage closes at 14–16 years old but the acetabular epiphyses can remain open as late as 18 years [8].

1.2.3 Development of the Proximal Femur After Birth

At birth the greater trochanter and femoral head share a common physis. During growth the medial part of the physis evolves into the physis of the femoral head and the lateral part becomes the physis of the greater trochanter (Fig. 1.3). The separation of the common physis into two distinct ones occurs at the age of four. The physis of the femoral head is responsible for the development of the femoral neck. The growth of the neck occurs on the metaphyseal side of the physis contributing to most of the length of the femoral neck. This is in contrast to the greater trochanter, where appositional growth at the periphery contributes to the size of the greater trochanter. Incomplete separation of the common physis may lead to widening of the femoral neck in the anterosuperior area that eventually may predispose to cam-type femoroacetabular impingement [9]. The center of ossification in the femoral head appears in females at the age of 4–7 months and in males later at the age of 5–8 months. The ossification center of the greater trochanter develops generally at the age of 4 years. The ossification center in the lesser trochanter appears only much later at 12–14 years of age. Closure of the femoral head physis occurs at an age of approximately 18 years, the physis of the greater trochanter closes earlier at the age of 16–18 years.

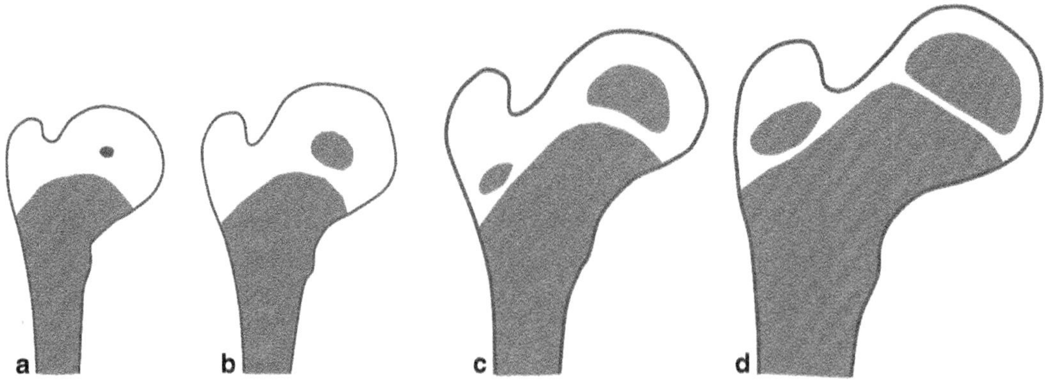

Fig. 1.3 Development of the center of ossification and the physis of the proximal femur. (**a**) age 4 months; (**b**) age 1 year; (**c**) age 4 years; (**d**) Modified and reproduced with permission and copyright © Acta Orthop Scand suppl. [2]

1.3 Osteology

1.3.1 The Acetabulum

The bony acetabulum forms a concentric dome over the femoral head. Its coverage of the femoral head is approximately 170°. The outer rim topography is independent of gender, but the male articular surface is larger than the female, where the acetabular fossa is wider. The average diameter of the native acetabulum is 52 mm ± 4 mm [10].

It is conventional to refer to points around the lateral acetabulum and labrum as positions on a clock face (Fig. 1.4). Using this nomenclature, 6:00 refers to the midpoint of the fossa inferiorly, and 12:00 refers to the superior part of the acetabulum directly across from the midpoint of the fossa. The 3:00 position refers to the anterior acetabulum on both right and left hips. The 3:00 position can be identified by the superior margin of the anterior labral sulcus, or "psoas-u" [11]. The 9:00 position refers to the midpoint of the posterior wall on both left and right hips. Four major regions of the bony acetabulum contribute to coverage of the femoral head: the anterior wall, the posterior wall, the medial wall, and the dome or *tectum* (latin for roof). The anterior wall is directly connected to the pubis, and the superior pubic ramus extends anteriorly from its

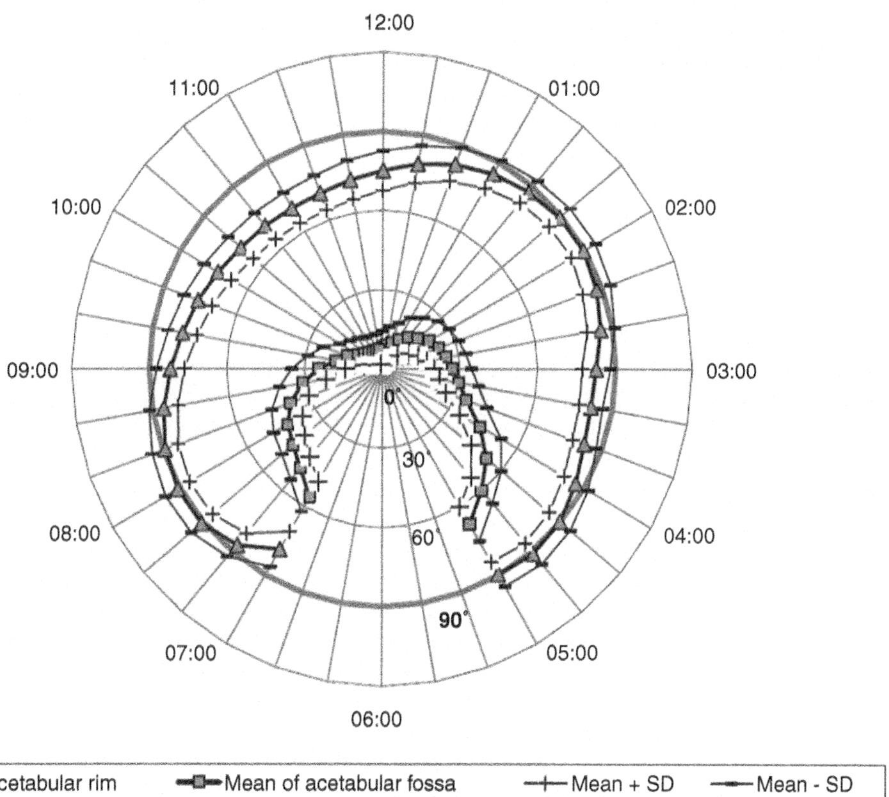

Fig. 1.4 This figure shows mean and standard deviation of rim and fossa values as a function of its geographical reconstruction. 0° is at the pole of the acetabular hemisphere, 30°, 60°, and 90° are indicating the depth of the cup (latitude). The circle at 90° marks the equatorial level of the hemisphere. The rim, fossa, and articular surface locations are indicated in a clockwise distribution, with the acetabular notch as the caudal landmark for 6:00 (longitude). 3:00 represents a point directly anterior on the anterior wall in both right and left hips. The three prominent areas are anterosuperior, anteroinferior, and posteroinferior. The two depressions along the anterior and posterosuperior wall can clearly be distinguished. Modified and reproduced with permission and copyright © Clinical Orthopaedics and Related Research [10]

medial border. The anterior wall and anterior rim of the acetabulum have a variable morphology. Most acetabula have a prominence that extends from the anterior rim from about 12:30 to 3:00 [10]. Proceeding medially along the anterior wall, the "psoas-u" is an indentation in the anterior wall adjacent to a prominent groove on the pelvic rim. This groove, just lateral to the iliopectineal eminence, provides a track for the iliopsoas, and represents the most medial aspect of the anterior wall easily accessible with an arthroscope. The iliopectineal eminence lies just anterior to the inferior half of the anterior wall on the pubic brim.

The posterior wall is larger and projects more laterally than the anterior wall. Its lateral edge has a nearly vertical but curved route, with few prominences or grooves, and little variation between individuals [3, 12]. The posterior wall is a major bony contributor to the stability of the hip. Trauma research has shown that hip stability depends most on an intact posterior wall, and to lesser extent on an intact capsule. In a cadaver study of hip stability, varying amounts of posterior wall bone were osteotomized. Hundred percent of hips were stable with as much as 25% of posterior wall disrupted, but with 33% of the posterior wall disrupted only 75% of hips were stable. When 50% of the posterior wall was disrupted all specimens were found to be unstable [13].

Surrounding the acetabulum are two columns of bone, the anterior and posterior column, which connect the acetabulum to the rest of the pelvis and provide significant structural support [14]. The acetabulum, which lies in the "concavity of the arch" created by the two columns, transmits the load superiorly via this arch.

The two columns in combination with the anterior and posterior walls allow for dynamic deformation of the acetabulum with differential load bearing [15]. At lower loads, only the anterior and posterior walls transmit force, and the dome does not contact the head. However, as loading increases, the two columns increasingly separate and allow the walls to deform, thus permitting the acetabular dome to receive force transmission. The anterior wall is considerably more rigid than the more flexible posterior wall. Consequently, when loaded the posterior wall deforms substantially more than the anterior wall [16]. This differential deformation is far more pronounced at lower loads (30% body weight), where the posterior wall deforms 40 times more than the anterior wall, and less pronounced at higher loads where the ratio approaches 3–1. When carrying peak physiologic loads such as with gait, nearly full contact and global transmission of force occurs [15]. Thus, the acetabulum including the anterior and posterior columns progressively deform, increasing contact area during joint loading. The transverse ligament, connecting anterior and posterior acetabular border, serves as a security chain against extreme deformation and is supported by a connecting plate of bone, the quadrilateral plate, extending proximally forming a tension band between the two columns. The quadrilateral plate is formed by the convergence of the three innominate bones and is the location of the center of the closed triradiate cartilage.

1.3.2 Fossa

The medial part of the acetabulum has a central cavity, where no articulation occurs. This, the acetabular fossa, is filled with a fat pad called the pulvinar, and the ligamentum capitis femoris. The bony fossa and the fat pad both appear to be involved in evenly distributing forces across the articular contact surfaces [17]. Its shape is variable between individuals, from semicircular to cloverleaf in shape [3, 10]. Multiple foramina serve as access for the small arterioles of the acetabular branch of the obturator artery which runs through the fat pad to both walls and to the dome area [18]. The ligamentum capitis femoris (ligamentum teres) is a small, synovial enclosed ligament averaging 30–35 mm in length, with a broad band at the distal border of the acetabular fossa. Connecting the inferior acetabulum to the fovea capitis femoris just inferior to the center of the femoral head, it originates on both the pubic and ischial sides of the inferior fossa in the form of two bands. In between these bands, the ligamentum blends with the transverse ligament, and attaches at a small section of the posteroinferior fossa. The ligamentum has been theorized to be involved in hip pain generation, stability, and synovial fluid circulation [19, 20]. Furthermore the ligamentum has a role in providing blood supply to the femoral head during growth. However this role is temporary, for there is no avascular necrosis (AVN) should the femoral head be surgically dislocated (as described in Sect. 1.6.2).

1.3.3 Acetabular Orientation

A description of the spatial orientation of the acetabulum in relation to the pelvis and body requires parameters which are difficult to describe, and to some extent, difficult to measure. In short, the most important spatial relationships of the acetabulum to the pelvis are version and inclination, also called abduction. Version is described as the angle between either a central horizontal line connecting the anterior and posterior walls or the averaged opening plane of the acetabulum and the sagittal plane [10]. Inclination is defined as the angle between either a central vertical line connecting the superior-lateral acetabulum to the inferior-medial fossa or the opening plane of the acetabulum and the transverse plane. Average anteversion has been reported to be from 16° to 21° [10, 12]. Males tend to have less anteversion than females, 12° to 20° versus 15° to 24°. The average inclination has been reported to be 48°, with minimal differences between sexes.

Acetabular orientation and its corresponding descriptive angles are affected by many variables, such as pelvic tilt or rotation, acetabular tilt, and the reference planes of the body. Version and inclination can vary substantially when accounting for differing degrees of pelvic tilt (Fig. 1.5) [10, 21, 22].

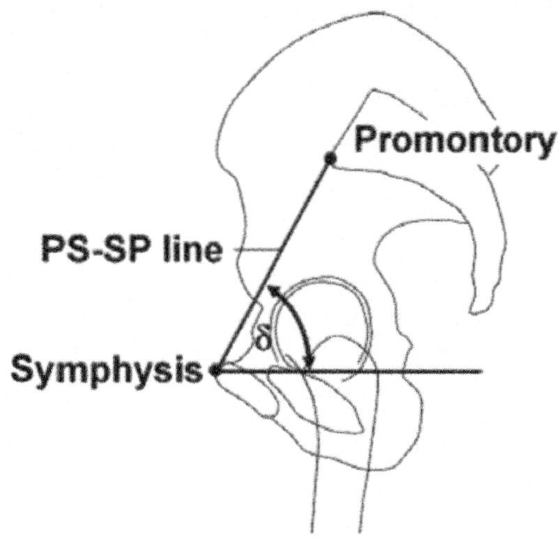

Fig. 1.5 Pelvic tilt, δ, is defined as the angle between a horizontal line and a line connecting the upper border of the symphysis with the sacral promontory (PS-SP line). Reproduced with permission and copyright © Skeletal Radiol. [21]

1.3.4 The Proximal Femur

1.3.4.1 Antetorsion

The femoral neck antetorsion is the inclination of the axis of the femoral neck with reference to a line placed on the posterior contour of the femoral condyles. If the axis of the neck inclines anteriorly, the angle of torsion is called antetorsion. Similarly, if it points posteriorly, it is called retrotorsion. Differences in both techniques of examination, and populations may explain contrasting values that have been reported [23, 24]. On average, femoral anteversion ranges from 30° to 40° at birth and decreases progressively throughout growth. According to Svenningsen et al. femoral antetorsion has a regression rate of about 1.5° (range 0.2°–3.1°) per year [24]. In the adult, mean femoral antetorsion is 10.5° ± 9.22°. Antetorsion increases the range of motion in flexion and internal rotation, and decreases external rotation in extension. Both increased femoral antetorsion and retrotorsion can cause femoroacetabular impingement and have been associated with early degenerative joint disease [25–27].

1.3.4.2 Neck-Shaft Angle

The neck-shaft angle is normally measured on anteroposterior radiographs as the angle formed by the axis of the femur and the axis of the neck going through the center of the femoral head. Projected values are largely influenced by the rotation of the femur. The normal neck-shaft angle measures 125° with values ranging between 121.4° and 137.5°. The average location of the tip of the greater trochanter is 3.4 ± 0.9 mm superior to the center of rotation (range from 20 mm superior to 10 mm inferior to the femoral head center).

1.3.4.3 Lesser Trochanter

The lesser trochanter is positioned at a retrotorsion angle (α) of −31.5° with a standard deviation of ±11.8°. In the same study an average antetorsion of the femoral neck (β) of 10.5° ± 9,22 was found. There was a high correlation between the antetorsion of the neck and the retrotorsion of the lesser trochanter [28].

1.3.4.4 Shape of the Femoral Neck

The femoral neck has an oval shape. The orientation of the greatest diameter of the femoral neck relative to the mechanical long axis of the femur is defined with the angle ρ (rho). Angle ρ was reported to measure in a normal hip 21° ± 9° and in hips with an aspheric head neck junction 25° ± 8°, the difference is not significant [29]. As a consequence of the oval cross section the modified alpha angle is reduced in the anterosuperior area of the head-neck junction and can add to cam-type femoroacetabular impingement. A gender difference was observed, with males having a significantly more prominent head neck junction anterosuperiorly [24] (Fig. 1.6).

1.3.4.5 Alpha Angle

The alpha angle was first described by Nötzli et al. as an indicator of femoral head neck asphericity [24]. The alpha angle is the acute angle between the neck axis and a line connecting the center of rotation with the point where the femoral head exits a circle around the femoral head. The alpha angle measures the anterior asphericity; however, the individual maximum value can be best determined with radial cuts of an MRI. Likewise although of less importance, the beta angle is measured posteriorly, the gamma angle superiorly, and the delta angle inferiorly (Fig. 1.7). The position of the femoral head on the femoral neck is defined by the AP and lateral physeal angles (Fig. 1.8). Based on several studies the normal alpha angle is between 43° and 50°, but normal values up to 60° are discussed [31–33].

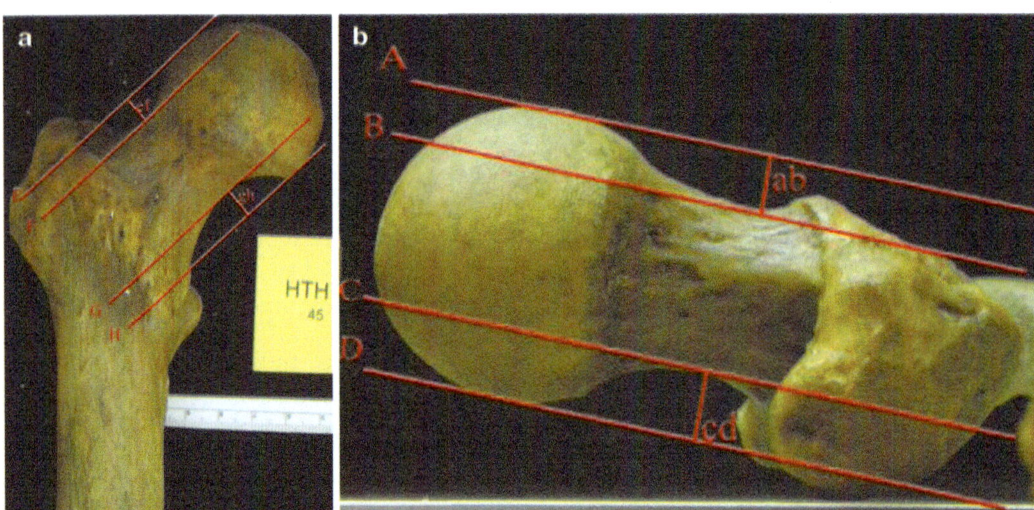

Fig. 1.6 Femoral head offset. (**a**) Shows the construction of the superior and inferior offset. (**b**) The construction of the anterior and inferior offset. Reproduced with permission and copyright © Clinical Orthopaedics and Related Research [30]

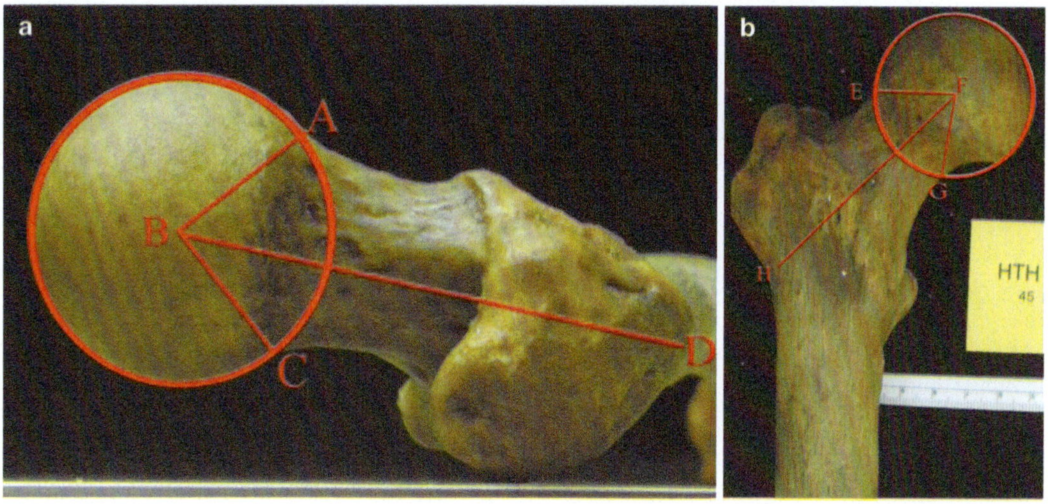

Fig. 1.7 Measurement of the asphericity of the head neck junction. (**a**) Shows the construction of the alpha anteriorly and beta angle posteriorly. Correspondingly, (**b**) shows the gamma angle superiorly and delta angle inferiorly. Reproduced with permission and copyright © Clinical Orthopaedics and Related Research [30]

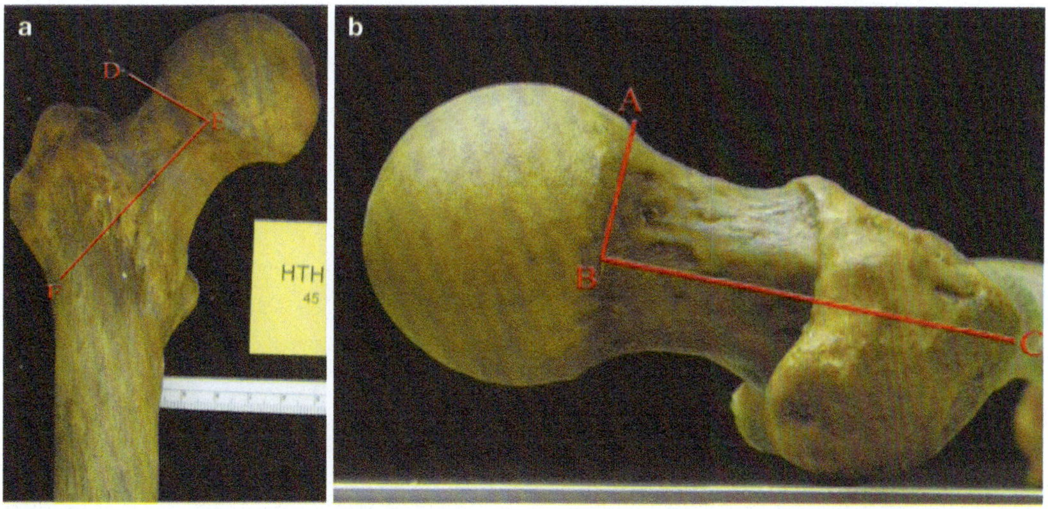

Fig. 1.8 Definition of the position of the femoral head on the neck. (**a**) Shows the AP physeal angle. (**b**) Shows the lateral physeal angle. Reproduced with permission and copyright © Clinical Orthopaedics and Related Research [30]

1.4 Cartilage

The acetabular socket is covered by a cartilaginous surface. This surface has a crescent shape, as cartilage covers the anterior and posterior walls and the majority of the dome, but is absent medially and inferiorly. Mathematic investigation has shown that the shape of the acetabular cartilage surface results in the optimal distribution of articular contact forces and the elimination of peak stress areas [17]. The acetabular cartilage surface is composed almost exclusively of hyaline cartilage, and averages about 1.5 mm in depth. However, the cartilaginous depth is not uniform throughout the acetabulum. The region of greatest cartilage depth is the anterosuperior quadrant, where depth can exceed 3 mm. Cartilage is thinnest at the region surrounding the acetabular fossa and inferiorly. In the most superior part of the dome, the cartilage surface often will have a round imprint. This area has been named the "stellate crease," and can be appreciated most easily arthroscopically [34]. It is composed of both hyaline and fibrocartilage, and is present in 90% of the population [16]. Between the stellate crease and the fossa is the supra-acetabular fossa. This is not covered by hyaline cartilage until maturity [35].

1.5 Labrum

The labrum is a ring of connective tissue continuous with the transverse acetabular ligament that surrounds the outer edge of the acetabulum [36]. It is composed of three distinct layers (Fig. 1.9) [37]. The first layer, adjacent to the articular surface of the acetabulum, is composed of a delicate network of fibrocartilage with interposed chondrocytes. This thin, superficial layer contains type II collagen in addition to I and III collagen, and is usually continuous with the acetabular chondral surface at the labral-chondral junction. The second layer is composed of intersecting "lamellar-like collagen fibril bundles." Finally, the third and most peripheral layer is composed of collagen fibrils which are oriented in a circumferential direction. This layer is much thicker than the other two, consisting of more than 90% of the labrum, and is continuous with the transverse acetabular ligament. Both the second and third layers are composed of only type I and III collagen.

The labrum deepens the acetabular socket to the extent that it contributes 33% of the combined acetabular and labral volume [36]. Additionally, the labrum increases the articular contact surface by 22%, but controversy exists in regard to

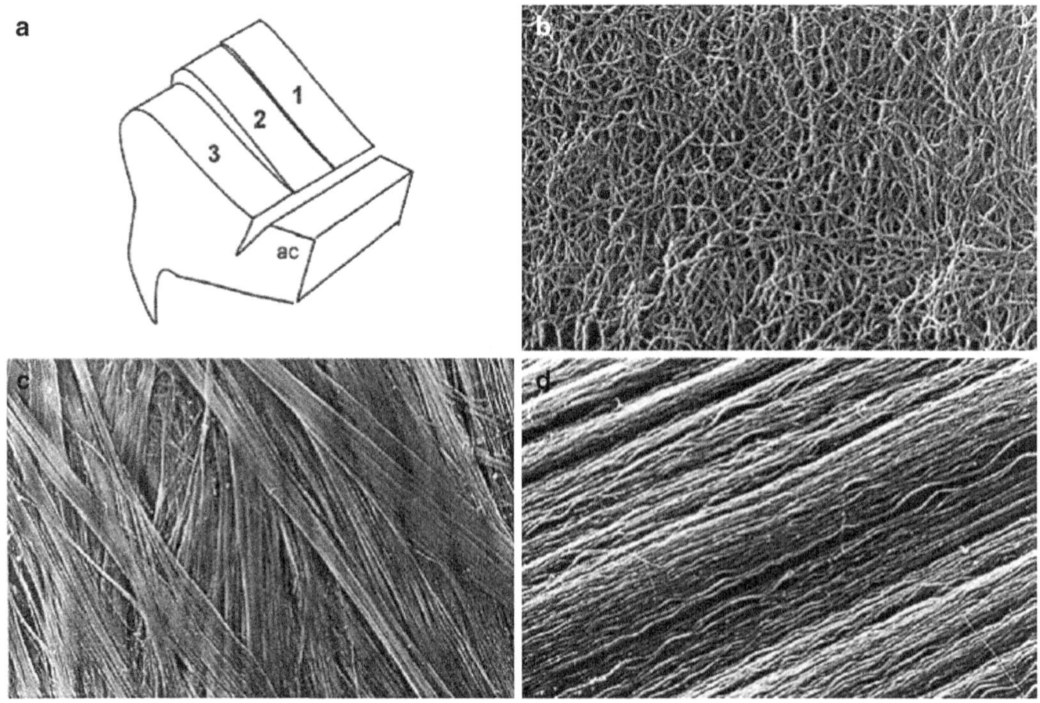

Fig. 1.9 (**a**) The labrum has three layers. (**b**) Layer 1 consists of a delicate network of fibrocartilage. (**c**) Layer 2 consists of intersecting "lamellar-like collagen fibril bundles." (**d**) Layer 3 is the thickest layer, and is composed of circumferential fibrils continuous with the transverse acetabular ligament. Reproduced with permission and copyright © Arch Orthop Trauma Surg [37]

whether the labrum participates in load sharing of contact forces. The labrum varies in its size around its circumference. It is widest anteriorly and thickest superiorly. Inferiorly, the labrum is indistinguishable from the transverse ligament. On its outer, superficial side, the labrum does not connect with the joint capsule, but rather a synovial-lined recess 6–8 mm in depth is formed as the capsule inserts directly onto the proximal portion of bony acetabulum.

The labrum merges with the acetabular hyaline cartilage over a 1–2 mm transition zone. Anteriorly, the labrum often has a cleft or recess separating it from the articular surface of the acetabulum, and the collagen fibers in this area run parallel to the chondro-labral junction [7]. This cleft has been reported in 20–75% of the population [37, 38]. Posteriorly, there is a "gradual and interdigitated" connection at the chondro-labral junction, and collagen fibers in this area run perpendicular to the transition zone [7]. The labrum is connected to the bony acetabulum over the area of a bony "tongue" that extends into the labrum from the acetabular brim [36]. On the articular-sided surface of this tongue the labrum attaches to the acetabular bone via a zone of calcified cartilage with a clear tidemark. However, on the outer surface of this tongue, the labrum inserts without either calcified cartilage zone or a tidemark.

The labrum has two immediately discernible biomechanical functions. The first function is that of a "suction seal" effect where the labrum maintains and promotes negative pressure within the joint when distracted to increase stability [39]. This role has been supported by research showing that venting and tearing of the labrum results in increased motion of the femur relative to the acetabulum, and reduced force required to displace the femur. The second and more important function is to seal the pressurized central compartment to prevent synovial fluid from retreating to the peripheral compartment. This pressurization effect within the joint likely results in a more uniform fluid boundary across the articular surface, increasing the lubrication and low friction properties of the hip joint [39, 40]. Additionally, this high pressure probably promotes an environment of readily available nutrition via maximal absorption of synovial fluid and water into cartilage surfaces [39]. Finally, the labrum contains nerve endings similar to the round ligament suggesting that the bumper effect may be less mechanical but represents more an alarm system to alert the musculature when joint motion exceeds physiological limits [41].

1.6 Blood Supply

1.6.1 The Blood Supply of the Acetabulum

The acetabulum receives a large anastomotic arterial network. The principal vessel is the nutrient artery of the ilium, a branch of the iliolumbar artery [18]. This ancillary vascular network is composed of the superior gluteal, inferior gluteal, and medial femoral circumflex arteries laterally, and the iliolumbar, obturator, and fourth lumbar arteries medially (Fig. 1.10).

The iliolumbar artery originates from either the posterior trunk of the internal iliac artery or the obturator artery [18]. It divides into a superficial and a deep branch, the largest rami of which forms the nutrient artery to the ilium. In half of patients, the nutrient artery enters the ilium anterior to the iliosacral joint and lateral to the pelvic brim. In the other half, the nutrient artery enters the ilium medial to the pelvic brim. This anatomical variance is important to note because this artery is not readily accessible when medial to the pelvic brim and can be quite large at times, producing moderate bleeding when disrupted.

The obturator artery supplies a few branches to the quadrilateral plate and superior pubic ramus before coursing through the obturator canal [18]. Together with branches from the medial femoral circumflex artery, it provides an acetabular branch which enters the joint deep to the transverse ligament. This vessel may be the final supply to the acetabulum if both the medial and lateral contributors are compromised. Thus, it should be protected when dissecting medial to the quadrilateral plate by strictly following a subperiosteal plane.

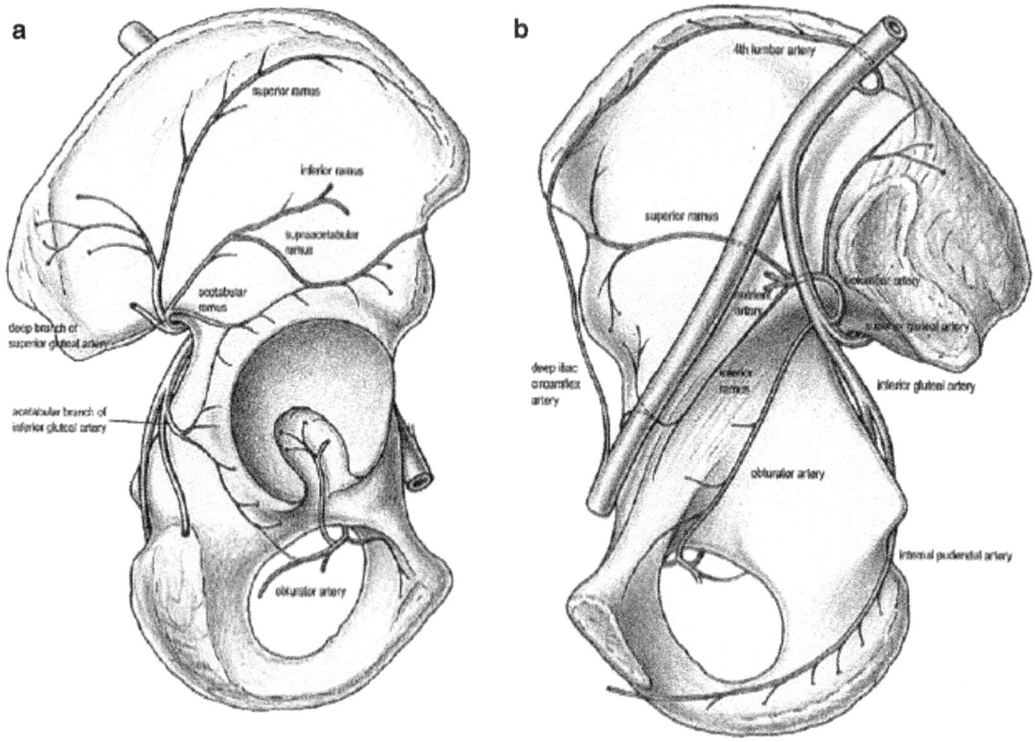

Fig. 1.10 The blood supply of the acetabulum and labrum is provided by a network of vessels composed of the superior gluteal, inferior gluteal, and medial femoral circumflex arteries laterally (**a**), and the iliolumbar, obturator, and fourth lumbar arteries medially (**b**). Reproduced with permission and copyright © Surgical and Radiologic Anatomy [18]

The superior gluteal artery is the most important lateral contributor to the acetabular blood supply. Initially, it divides into deep and superficial branches. The deep branch has four rami, the superior, inferior, supra-acetabular, and acetabular. The superior ramus forms the anastomotic network superiorly with the deep and superficial circumflex iliac vessels and the iliolumbar. The supra-acetabular ramus runs deep to and/or within the gluteus minimus near its origin along its way to supply the acetabular roof [18]. The acetabular ramus runs inferior to the gluteus minimus to supply the posterior-superior acetabulum and acetabular roof. The acetabular and supra-acetabular vessels then join, and the consolidated vasculature continues to the interspinous crest to anastomose with the iliolumbar artery and the ascending branch of the lateral femoral circumflex artery. Thus, the superior gluteal artery and its branches along with the iliolumbar and circumflex iliac vessels create an anastomotic ring around the ilium at the level of the interspinous crest and sciatic notch.

The inferior gluteal artery has two acetabular branches. One runs deep to the short external rotators to supply the posterior wall via several smaller vessels [42]. The other, distal acetabular branch runs between the inferior gemellus and the quadratus femoris to supply the posterior acetabulum and anastomose with the medial femoral circumflex artery (MFCA). The acetabular branches of the gluteal vessels create a periosteal anastomotic ring of around the lateral acetabulum, providing blood supply to the labrum (Fig. 1.11). The labrum also receives a significant arterial supply from capsular vessels. The labrum itself is poorly vascularized. Only the peripheral one third of the labrum is penetrated by blood vessels, the largest of which run adjacent to the outer brim of acetabular bone [36, 37]. The deep

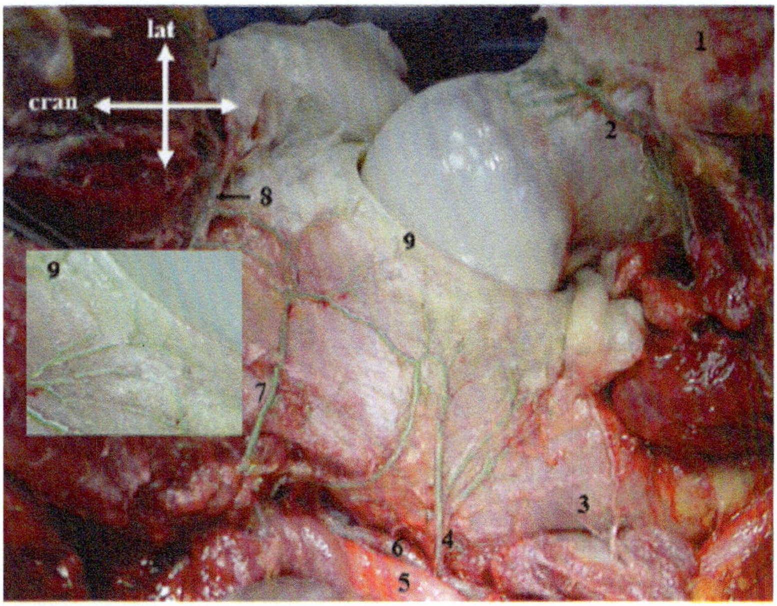

Fig. 1.11 Posterior aspect of the acetabulum and the hip joint after capsulotomy to show the acetabular branches of the gluteal arteries and anastomoses between them. 1 = greater trochanter (osteotomized), 2 = deep branch of the medial femoral circumflex artery (intra-capsular part and retinacular arteries), 3 = lesser sciatic notch, 4 = acetabular branch of the interior gluteal artery, 5 = sciatic nerve, 6 = inferior gluteal artery, 7 = acetabular branch of the superior gluteal artery, 8 = supra-acetabular branch of the superior gluteal artery, 9 = terminal vessel supplying the labrum, cran = cranial, lat = lateral. Reproduced with permission and copyright © Surgical and Radiologic Anatomy [18]

branch of the MFCA contributes a couple of branches to the anterior-inferior acetabulum in addition to its anastomotic relationship with this network.

1.6.2 The Blood Supply of the Proximal Femur

In the adult the vascular blood supply of the femoral head is secured through the retinacular arteries from the deep branch of the MFCA [43]. The evolution of the blood supply to the femoral head and proximal femur depends largely on the development of the growth plates and growth of femoral neck and greater trochanter. The blood supply of the growing proximal femur [44, 45] covering the entire growth period until the end of adolescence is now discussed. In the initial stages of growth, before the development of the ossification nuclei and growth plate, the femoral head mainly is perfused by metaphyseal blood vessels. With the development of the femoral head physis, the lateral epiphyseal vessels of the MFCA increasingly contribute to the blood supply of the femoral epiphysis. At birth, the major part of the common proximal femoral physis is extraarticular. The lateral femoral circumflex artery (LFCA) supplies the anterolateral physis, the majority of the greater trochanter, and anteromedial parts of the femoral head.

The MFCA supplies the anteromedial physis, the posteromedial epiphysis, and the posterior parts of the greater trochanter. By the age of 18 months the blood supply of the femoral epiphysis mainly is provided through the lateral epiphyseal vessels of the MFCA. At birth there is an inconsistent anastomosis between the MFCA and LFCA in the area of the greater trochanter. During growth of the femoral neck the LFCA loses its contribution to the blood supply of the femoral epiphysis and physis and reduces its contribution to the greater trochanter and anterior femoral neck. At the age of three the blood supply of the entire epiphysis and physis comes through the lateral and inferior retinacular vessels of the MFCA. Blood vessels in the ligamentum capitis femoris are observed at the age of four, but this contribution to the femoral head perfusion remains inconstant throughout growth and rarely contributes significantly to the perfusion of the epiphysis.

1.6.3 Blood Supply to the Adult Femoral Head

Numerous publications investigated the blood supply of the femoral head and the contribution of the intraosseous terminations of the MFCA, LCFA, the artery of the round ligament, the vessels of the medial synovial fold (Ligament of Weitbrecht), and the intramedullary blood vessels [44].

The deep branch of the MFCA is the most important contributor to the blood supply of the femoral head. The extra-capsular course of the medial femoral circumflex artery was investigated in a cadaveric injection study [43]. After its origin from the deep femoral artery and the division of the ascending and superficial branches, the deep branch of the MFCA runs dorsally between the iliopsoas and the pectineus muscles and continues proximal to the lesser trochanter at the base of the femoral neck along the inferior border of the obturator externus muscle. The vessel runs anterior and cranial to the quadratus femoris muscle toward the intertrochanteric crest and emerges between the quadratus femoris and the obturator externus muscle adjacent to their insertion at the proximal femur. At this point, one or two branches are given off to the greater trochanter, the trochanteric branches. The main vessel continues proximally along the intertrochanteric crest and crosses the tendon of the obturator externus posteriorly and the tendon of inferior gemellus, internal obturator, and superior gemellus anteriorly. It obliquely perforates the capsule just cranial to the insertion of the tendon of the superior gemellus and caudal to the tendon of the piriformis, where it ramifies into 2–4 subsynovial terminal branches, the lateral retinacular arteries (Fig. 1.12). In addition to the work of Gautier et al. [43] who described inconstant inferior retinacular arteries, Kalhor et al. [42] found a constant branch of the MFCA, which perforated the capsule inferomedially, entered the joint, and continued as an inferior retinacular artery, and was identified in all hips. This arterial branch ran toward the femoral head in the ligament of Weitbrecht [42]. An important anastomosis exists between the MFCA and a branch of the inferior gluteal artery, which runs along the inferior border of the piriformis, crosses posterior to the triceps coxae, and meets the deep branch in the interval between quadratus and obturator externus muscle. Its size correlates inversely to the size of the deep branch. Kalhor et al. [42]

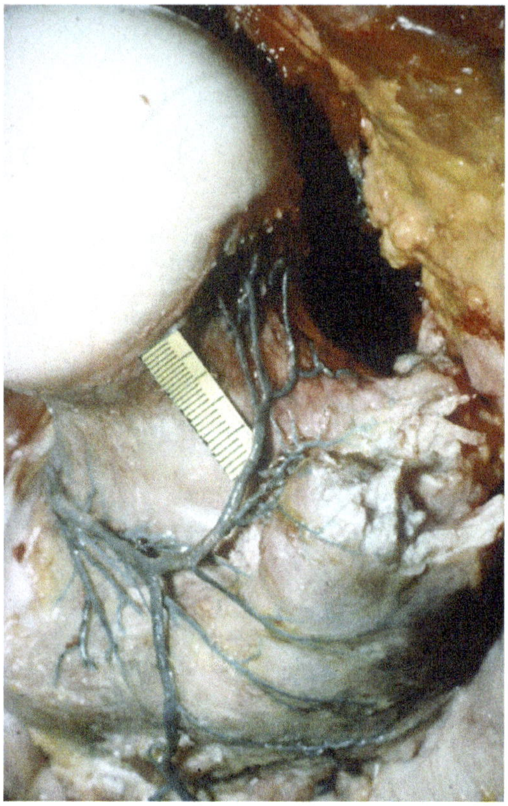

Fig. 1.12 Course of the deep branch of the MFCA. Reproduced with permission and copyright © Surgical and Radiologic Anatomy [18]

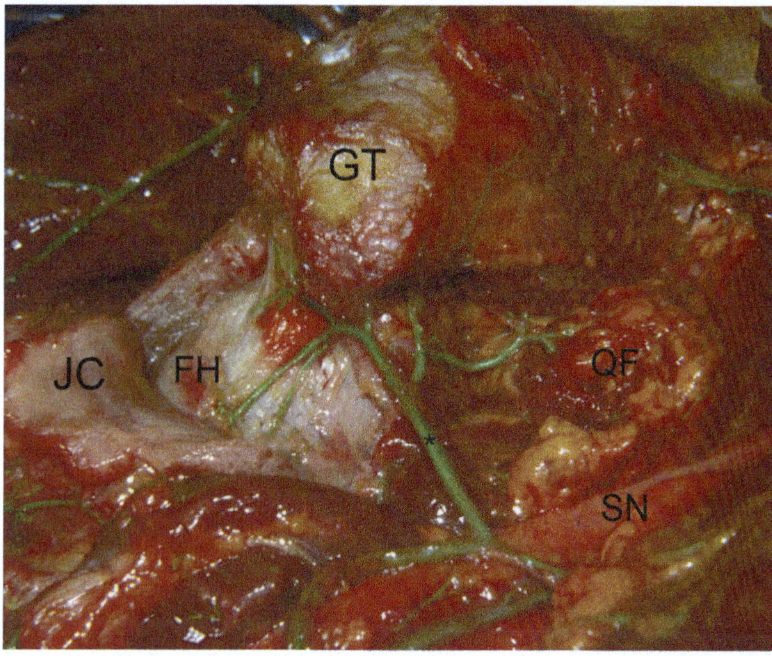

Fig. 1.13 Superior view on a left hip showing a direct anastomosis (*) from the inferior gluteal artery supplying the femoral head. *JC* joint capsule, *FH* femoral head, *GT* greater trochanter, *QF* quadratus femoris muscle, *SN* sciatic nerve. Reproduced with permission and copyright © Surgical and Radiologic Anatomy [18]

described another anastomosis between the inferior gluteal artery and the deep branch of the MFCA at the level of the inferior sciatic notch (Fig. 1.13). In two of 20 specimens this anastomosis had replaced the deep branch. When present, this branch of the inferior gluteal artery occupied the more common position of the MFCA at the level of the greater trochanter [42, 46]. The artery of the ligamentum capitis femoris usually originates from the obturator artery, though occasionally it arises as a branch of the MFCA. Its contribution in adults is restricted to the perifoveal area [45–47]. The intraosseous branches of the first perforating artery and the intraosseous vascular system supply the proximal part of the shaft and the neck of the femur. They anastomose with vessels within the femoral head, particularly in the caudal part of the head, but their primary contribution is limited to the femoral neck. The combined contribution from epiphyseal and metaphyseal vessels that cross the physis after closure has been postulated by various authors [45, 47–49]. In the nonarthritic femoral head there is no relevant metaphyseal contribution to the femoral blood supply [50].

1.7 Surgical Implications

By understanding the anatomy of the MFCA, it is possible to dislocate the hip with an osteotomy of the greater trochanter without risking AVN [50]. That the blood supply can be preserved by this technique was demonstrated by continuous laser Doppler flowmetry measurement [51]. Tension on the retinacular arteries may obstruct the perfusion to the femoral head. The knowledge of the course of the MFCA with respect to the tendons of the external rotators and the distance to the intertrochanteric crest are prerequisites to perform this type of surgery. This technique can be used to treat a variety of articular pathologies, including femoroacetabular impingement (FAI), cartilage pathologies, intra-articular deformities, tumors and fractures of the acetabulum and femoral head [52, 53]. Techniques such as femoral neck osteotomies, femoral head reduction osteotomies, and subcapital reorientation can be performed safely without risk of AVN [54]. However, the extra-capsular portion of the MFCA can be damaged during a posterior approach. Detaching the short external rotators close to their insertion carries a high risk of iatrogenic damage to the deep branch of the MFCA. It is recommended to divide the external rotators about 1.5 cm from their trochanteric insertion, sparing completely the tendon of the obturator externus [43]. AVN of the femoral head in adolescence after antegrade intramedullary nailing of the femur is a rare complication and most likely secondary to injury to retinacular vessels of the deep branch of the MFCA at the time of insertion of the nail. Because of the smaller diameter of the femoral neck, the insertion of the nail in the piriformis fossa puts this vessel at risk. As a consequence, either antegrade femoral nailing should be avoided in the adolescent or nail designs with the entry point at the tip of the greater trochanter should be used [55, 56].

1.8 Innervation

Most publications report that the hip is innervated by the femoral nerve, obturator nerve, sacral plexus via the nerve to quadratus femoris, and sometimes by the accessory obturator nerve or directly by the sacral or sciatic plexuses [57]. However, it is not clear which nerves are most significant in regard to the innervation of the acetabular bone or fossa, as it has not been thoroughly investigated yet. Much controversy remains on this subject. Dee, who researched the topic most closely, found three "primary articular nerves," the posterior articular nerve, the medial articular nerve, and the nerve to the ligamentum capitis femoris [58]. The posterior articular nerve group included several short branches from the nerve to the quadratus femoris muscle. They follow the ischium and the obturator internus tendon to enter the posterior capsule. Once inside the joint, they run superiorly along the acetabular rim. The medial articular nerve stems as a single branch from the anterior division of the obturator nerve near the obturator foramen. This nerve then forms multiple branches, which innervate the anterior-medial, and inferior areas of the joint capsule, and presumably the acetabulum as well. The nerve to the ligamentum capitis femoris exits from the posterior division of the obturator nerve near the obturator foramen. It then enters the acetabular notch where it innervates the contents of the acetabular fossa, including the ligamentum. The contents of the acetabular fossa have also been described as being innervated via branches from the sciatic nerve [59].

The type of nerve endings, their location, and their relative densities have been elucidated in regard to the contents of the fossa. The ligamentum capitis femoris contains only Type IVa nerves and free nerve endings [20, 60]. Thus, the ligamentum is not involved in mechanoreception or proprioception, but rather senses only pain and inflammatory stimuli. The fatty contents of the acetabular fossa have nerves located within the perivascular tissues. These nerve fibers contain the neuropeptides substance P and calcitonin gene-related peptide, suggesting that they also perform a pain nociception function [60]. The labrum has a wealth of innervation. Eighty percent of the nerves in the labrum lie in the superficial zone, alongside blood vessels. Free nerve endings are numerous in the labrum, especially in the anterior and superior areas, which suggests that the labrum is a powerful pain generator of the hip. This may explain the early pain associated with pincer impingement compared with that of cam impingement where labral involvement is late in the disease process [61]. Additionally, histologic examination has found nerve end organs responsible for deep sensation, pressure, tactile sensation, and temperature within the labrum suggesting that the labrum also plays a role in proprioception of the hip. Furthermore nerve endings within the hip capsule provide important proprioceptive feedback crucial for hip stability.

References

1. Ray B, D'Souza AS, Kumar B, et al. Variations in the course and microanatomical study of the lateral femoral cutaneous nerve and its clinical importance. Clin Anat. 2010;23:978–84. https://doi.org/10.1002/ca.21043.
2. Gray H, Lewis WH. Anatomy of the human body. Philadelphia: Lea & Febiger; 1918. https://doi.org/10.5962/bhl.title.20311.
3. Govsa F, Ozer MA, Ozgur Z. Morphologic features of the acetabulum. Arch Orthop Trauma Surg. 2005;125:453–61. https://doi.org/10.1007/s00402-005-0020-6.

4. Kalberer F, Sierra RJ, Madan SS, et al. Ischial spine projection into the pelvis. Clin Orthop Relat Res. 2008;466:677–83. https://doi.org/10.1007/s11999-007-0058-6.
5. Watanabe RS. Embryology of the human hip. Clin Orthop Relat Res. 1974;98:8–26. https://doi.org/10.1097/00003086-197401000-00003.
6. Strayer LM. Embryology of the human hip joint. Clin Orthop Relat Res. 1971;74:221–40. https://doi.org/10.1097/00003086-197101000-00029.
7. Cashin M, Uhthoff H, O'Neill M, Beaule PE. Embryology of the acetabular labral-chondral complex. J Bone Joint Surg Br Vol. 2008;90-B:1019–24. https://doi.org/10.1302/0301-620x.90b8.20161.
8. Liporace FA, Ong B, Mohaideen A, et al. Development and injury of the triradiate cartilage with its effects on acetabular development. J Trauma. 2003;54:1245–9. https://doi.org/10.1097/01.ta.0000029212.19179.4a.
9. Siebenrock KA, Wahab KHA, Werlen S, et al. Abnormal extension of the femoral head epiphysis as a cause of cam impingement. Clin Orthop Relat Res. 2004;418:54–60. https://doi.org/10.1097/00003086-200401000-00010.
10. Köhnlein W, Ganz R, Impellizzeri FM, Leunig M. Acetabular morphology: implications for joint-preserving surgery. Clin Orthop Relat Res. 2009;467:682–91. https://doi.org/10.1007/s11999-008-0682-9.
11. Philippon MJ, Michalski MP, Campbell KJ, et al. An anatomical study of the acetabulum with clinical applications to hip arthroscopy. J Bone Joint Surg Am. 2014;96:1673–82. https://doi.org/10.2106/JBJS.M.01502.
12. Maruyama M, Feinberg JR, Capello WN, Antonio JAD. Morphologic features of the acetabulum and femur. Clin Orthop Relat Res. 2001;393:52–65. https://doi.org/10.1097/00003086-200112000-00006.
13. Vailas JC, Hurwitz S, Wiesel SW. Posterior acetabular fracture-dislocations. J Trauma. 1989;29:1494–6. https://doi.org/10.1097/00005373-198911000-00007.
14. Letournel E, Judet R. Fractures of the acetabulum. Berlin: Springer; 1993. https://doi.org/10.1007/978-3-642-75435-7.
15. Greenwald AS, O'Connor JJ. The transmission of load through the human hip joint. J Biomech. 1971;4:507–28. https://doi.org/10.1016/0021-9290(71)90041-8.
16. Lazennec JY, Laudet CG, Guérin-Surville H, et al. Dynamic anatomy of the acetabulum: an experimental approach and surgical implications. Surg Radiol Anat. 1997;19:23–30. https://doi.org/10.1007/s00276-997-0023-9.
17. Daniel M, IgliC A, Kralj-IgliC V. The shape of acetabular cartilage optimizes hip contact stress distribution. J Anat. 2005;207:85–91. https://doi.org/10.1111/j.1469-7580.2005.00425.x.
18. Beck M, Leunig M, Ellis T, et al. The acetabular blood supply: implications for periacetabular osteotomies. Surg Radiol Anat. 2003;25:361–7. https://doi.org/10.1007/s00276-003-0149-3.
19. Bardakos NV, Villar RN. The ligamentum teres of the adult hip. J Bone Joint Surg Br Vol. 2009;91-B:8–15. https://doi.org/10.1302/0301-620x.91b1.21421.
20. Leunig M, Beck M, Stauffer E, et al. Free nerve endings in the ligamentum capitis femoris. Acta Orthop Scand. 2000;71:452–4. https://doi.org/10.1080/000164700317381117.
21. Tannast M, Murphy SB, Langlotz F, et al. Estimation of pelvic tilt on anteroposterior X-rays—a comparison of six parameters. Skelet Radiol. 2005;35:149–55. https://doi.org/10.1007/s00256-005-0050-8.
22. Zilber S, Lazennec JY, Gorin M, Saillant G. Variations of caudal, central, and cranial acetabular anteversion according to the tilt of the pelvis. Surg Radiol Anat. 2004;26:462–5. https://doi.org/10.1007/s00276-004-0254-y.
23. Jain AK, Maheshwari AV, Nath S, et al. Anteversion of the femoral neck in Indian dry femora. J Orthop Sci. 2003;8:334–40. https://doi.org/10.1007/s10776-003-0648-5.
24. Nakahara I, Takao M, Sakai T, et al. Gender differences in 3D morphology and bony impingement of human hips. J Orthop Res. 2010;29:333–9. https://doi.org/10.1002/jor.21265.
25. Terjesen T, Benum P, Anda S, Svenningsen S. Increased femoral anteversion and osteoarthritis of the hip joint. Acta Orthop Scand. 1982;53:571–5. https://doi.org/10.3109/17453678208992260.
26. Tönnis D, Heinecke A. Diminished femoral antetorsion syndrome: a cause of pain and osteoarthritis. J Pediatr Orthop. 1991;11:419–31. https://doi.org/10.1097/01241398-199107000-00001.
27. Reikerås O, Høiseth A. Femoral neck angles in osteoarthritis of the hip. Acta Orthop Scand. 1982;53:781–4. https://doi.org/10.3109/17453678208992292.
28. Herzberg W, Meitz R, Halata Z. Antetorsion of the femur neck. A variable of the trochanter minor? Unfallchirurg. 1991;94:168–71.
29. Meyer DC, Beck M, Ellis T, et al. Comparison of six radiographic projections to assess femoral head/neck asphericity. Clin Orthop Relat Res. 2006;445:181–5. https://doi.org/10.1097/01.blo.0000201168.72388.24.
30. Toogood PA, Skalak A, Cooperman DR. Proximal femoral anatomy in the normal human population. Clin Orthop Relat Res. 2008;467:876–85. https://doi.org/10.1007/s11999-008-0473-3.
31. Nötzli HP, Wyss TF, Stoecklin CH, et al. The contour of the femoral head-neck junction as a predictor for the risk of anterior impingement. J Bone Joint Surg. 2002;84:556–60. https://doi.org/10.1302/0301-620x.84b4.12014.
32. Bealule P, Zaragoza E, Motamedi K, et al. Three-dimensional computed tomography of the hip in the assessment of femoroacetabular impingement. J Orthop Res. 2005;23:1286–92. https://doi.org/10.1016/j.orthres.2005.03.011.
33. Neumann M, Cui Q, Siebenrock KA, Beck M. Impingement-free hip motion: the "normal" angle alpha after osteochondroplasty. Clin Orthop Relat

Res. 2008;467:699–703. https://doi.org/10.1007/s11999-008-0616-6.
34. Keene GS, Villar RN. Arthroscopic anatomy of the hip: an in vivo study. Arthroscopy. 1994;10:392–9. https://doi.org/10.1016/s0749-8063(05)80189-6.
35. Byrd JWT. Portal anatomy. In: Operative hip arthroscopy. New York: Springer; 2005. p. 110–6. https://doi.org/10.1007/0-387-27047-7_7.
36. Seldes RM, Tan V, Hunt J, et al. Anatomy, histologic features, and vascularity of the adult acetabular labrum. Clin Orthop Relat Res. 2001;382:232–40. https://doi.org/10.1097/00003086-200101000-00031.
37. Petersen W, Petersen F, Tillmann B. Structure and vascularization of the acetabular labrum with regard to the pathogenesis and healing of labral lesions. Arch Orthop Trauma Surg. 2003;123:283–8. https://doi.org/10.1007/s00402-003-0527-7.
38. McCarthy J, Noble P, Aluisio FV, et al. Anatomy, pathologic features, and treatment of acetabular labral tears. Clin Orthop Relat Res. 2003;406:38–47. https://doi.org/10.1097/00003086-200301000-00008.
39. Safran MR. The acetabular labrum: anatomic and functional characteristics and rationale for surgical intervention. J Am Acad Orthop Surg. 2010;18:338–45. https://doi.org/10.5435/00124635-201006000-00006.
40. Ferguson SJ, Bryant JT, Ganz R, Ito K. An in vitro investigation of the acetabular labral seal in hip joint mechanics. J Biomech. 2003;36:171–8. https://doi.org/10.1016/s0021-9290(02)00365-2.
41. Kim YT, Azuma H. The nerve endings of the acetabular labrum. Clin Orthop Relat Res. 1995;320:176–81. https://doi.org/10.1097/00003086-199511000-00029.
42. Kalhor M. Capsular and pericapsular contributions to acetabular and femoral head perfusion. J Bone Joint Surg Am. 2009;91:409. https://doi.org/10.2106/jbjs.g.01679.
43. Gautier E, Ganz K, Krügel N, et al. Anatomy of the medial femoral circumflex artery and its surgical implications. J Bone Joint Surg. 2000;82:679–83. https://doi.org/10.1302/0301-620x.82b5.10426.
44. Lauritzen J. The arterial supply to the femoral head in children. Acta Orthop Scand. 1974;45:724–36. https://doi.org/10.3109/17453677408989681.
45. Trueta J. Vascular pattern of the femoral head during growth. In: Studies of the development and decay of the human frame. Philadelphia: JB Lippincott; 1968. p. 135–42. https://doi.org/10.1016/b978-1-4831-6802-9.50024-9.
46. Grose AW, Gardner MJ, Sussmann PS, et al. The surgical anatomy of the blood supply to the femoral head: description of the anastomosis between the medial femoral circumflex and inferior gluteal arteries at the hip. J Bone Joint Surg Br Vol. 2008;90-B:1298–303. https://doi.org/10.1302/0301-620x.90b10.20983.
47. Letournel E, Judet R. Surgical anatomy. In: Fractures of the acetabulum. Berlin: Springer; 1981. p. 1–6. https://doi.org/10.1007/978-3-662-02325-9_1.
48. Freeman MAR. Some anatomical and mechanical considerations relevant to the surface replacement of the femoral head. Clin Orthop Relat Res. 1978;134:19–24. https://doi.org/10.1097/00003086-197807000-00004.
49. Hulth A. Circulatory disturbances in osteoarthritis of the hip: a venographic study. Acta Orthop Scand. 1958;28:81–9. https://doi.org/10.3109/17453675808988610.
50. Ganz R, Gill TJ, Gautier E, et al. Surgical dislocation of the adult hip. J Bone Joint Surg. 2001;83:1119–24. https://doi.org/10.1302/0301-620x.83b8.11964.
51. Nötzli HP, Siebenrock KA, Hempfing A, et al. Perfusion of the femoral head during surgical dislocation of the hip: monitoring by laser doppler flowmetry. J Bone Joint Surg. 2002;84:300–4. https://doi.org/10.1302/0301-620x.84b2.12146.
52. Ellis TJ, Beck M. Trochanteric osteotomy for acetabular fractures and proximal femur fractures. Orthop Clin N Am. 2004;35:457–61. https://doi.org/10.1016/j.ocl.2004.05.002.
53. Tannast M, Kruger A, Mack PW, et al. Surgical dislocation of the hip for the fixation of acetabular fractures. J Bone Joint Surg Br Vol. 2010;92-B:842–52. https://doi.org/10.1302/0301-620x.92b6.22994.
54. Leunig M, Slongo T, Kleinschmidt M, Ganz R. Subkapitale Korrekturosteotomie bei der Epiphyseolysis capitis femoris mittels chirurgischer Hüftluxation. Oper Orthop Traumatol. 2007;19:389–410. https://doi.org/10.1007/s00064-007-1213-7.
55. Orler R, Hersche O, Helfet DL, et al. Avascular necrosis of the femoral head as a serious complication following femoral nailing in children and adolescents. Unfallchirurg. 1998;101:495–9. https://doi.org/10.1007/s001130050301.
56. Buford D, Christensen K, Weatherall P. Intramedullary nailing of femoral fractures in adolescents. Clin Orthop Relat Res. 1998;350:85–9. https://doi.org/10.1097/00003086-199805000-00012.
57. Gardner E. The innervation of the hip joint. Anat Rec. 1948;101:353–71. https://doi.org/10.1002/ar.1091010309.
58. Dee R. Structure and function of hip joint innervation. Ann R Coll Surg Engl. 1969;45:357–74.
59. Saxler G, Löer F, Skumavc M, et al. Localization of SP- and CGRP-immunopositive nerve fibers in the hip joint of patients with painful osteoarthritis and of patients with painless failed total hip arthroplasties. Eur J Pain. 2007;11:67–74. https://doi.org/10.1016/j.ejpain.2005.12.011.
60. Sarban S, Baba F, Kocabey Y, et al. Free nerve endings and morphological features of the ligamentum capitis femoris in developmental dysplasia of the hip. J Pediatr Orthop B. 2007;16:351–6. https://doi.org/10.1097/01.bpb.0000243830.99681.3e.
61. Gerhardt M, Johnson K, Atkinson R, et al. Characterisation and classification of the neural anatomy in the human hip joint. Hip Int. 2018;22:75–81. https://doi.org/10.5301/HIP.2012.9042.

2 Radiology of the Hip Joint

Florian Schmaranzer, Till D. Lerch, Inga A. S. Todorski, Moritz Tannast, and Simon Steppacher

Abstract

The aim of this chapter is to describe the different imaging modalities of the hip in the trauma setting; this includes the conventional radiography, which is still an essential modality for fracture evaluation due to fast acquisition, cost effectiveness, and the good overview on hip morphology. However, the acquisition technique has a direct implication on radiographic anatomy of the hip and, therefore, this chapter also aims to demonstrate the different technical principles and views of conventional imaging of the hip. In the trauma setting computed tomography (CT) has emerged as an indispensable tool for detailed preoperative planning with the possibility of 3D-reconstruction and multiplanar reformatting. Magnetic resonance imaging (MRI) of the hip is of minor significance in acute hip trauma but is very helpful to detect occult fractures, assess soft tissue injuries, or evaluate posttraumatic deformities.

F. Schmaranzer (✉) · T. D. Lerch · I. A. S. Todorski · M. Tannast · S. Steppacher
Department of Orthopaedic Surgery and Traumatology, Inselspital, Bern University Hospital, Bern, Switzerland
e-mail: florian.schmaranzer@insel.ch

Keywords

Hip fracture · Acetabular fracture · Femur fracture · Trauma imaging · Conventional imaging · Computed tomography · Magnetic resonance imaging

2.1 Conventional Radiography

Despite the continuously increasing availability of multidetector CT, plain radiographs are still the standard imaging modality for assessment of the hip joint in the trauma setting. Conventional imaging is widely available, cost-effective and the acquisition is very fast. In addition, it gives a good overview on the radiographic morphology of the hip and allows fracture detection in the early evaluation of trauma. Serial radiographic imaging of the hip allows detection of secondary displacement or confirmation of healing of a hip fracture. Furthermore, it serves as the basis for preoperative planning of total hip arthroplasty or correction osteotomy of posttraumatic deformities [1, 2].

The acquisition technique and the different views have a direct implication on the radiographic anatomy of the hip. Therefore, the technical principles including film-tube distance, centering and direction of the central X-ray beam, and pelvic orientation during acquisition are described in detail. The anteroposterior (AP) pelvic view and an axial view serve as the basis of conventional imaging; additional views include Judet views [3, 4].

L. Büchler, M. J.B. Keel (eds.), *Fractures of the Hip*, Fracture Management Joint by Joint,
https://doi.org/10.1007/978-3-030-18838-2_2

2.1.1 Technical Principles of Conventional Radiography

Technical principles with implications on the radiographic anatomy of the hip include: film-tube distance, centering of the central X-ray beam, direction of the central X-ray beam, and pelvic orientation [5].

2.1.1.1 Film-Tube Distance

In contrast to CT scans, radiographs are based on a conical projection that originates from a point-shaped X-ray source. The more anterior an anatomic structure is located, the more lateral it will be projected on the film. For example, with increasing film-tube distance the acetabulum will appear more anteverted (Fig. 2.1) [5]. Therefore,

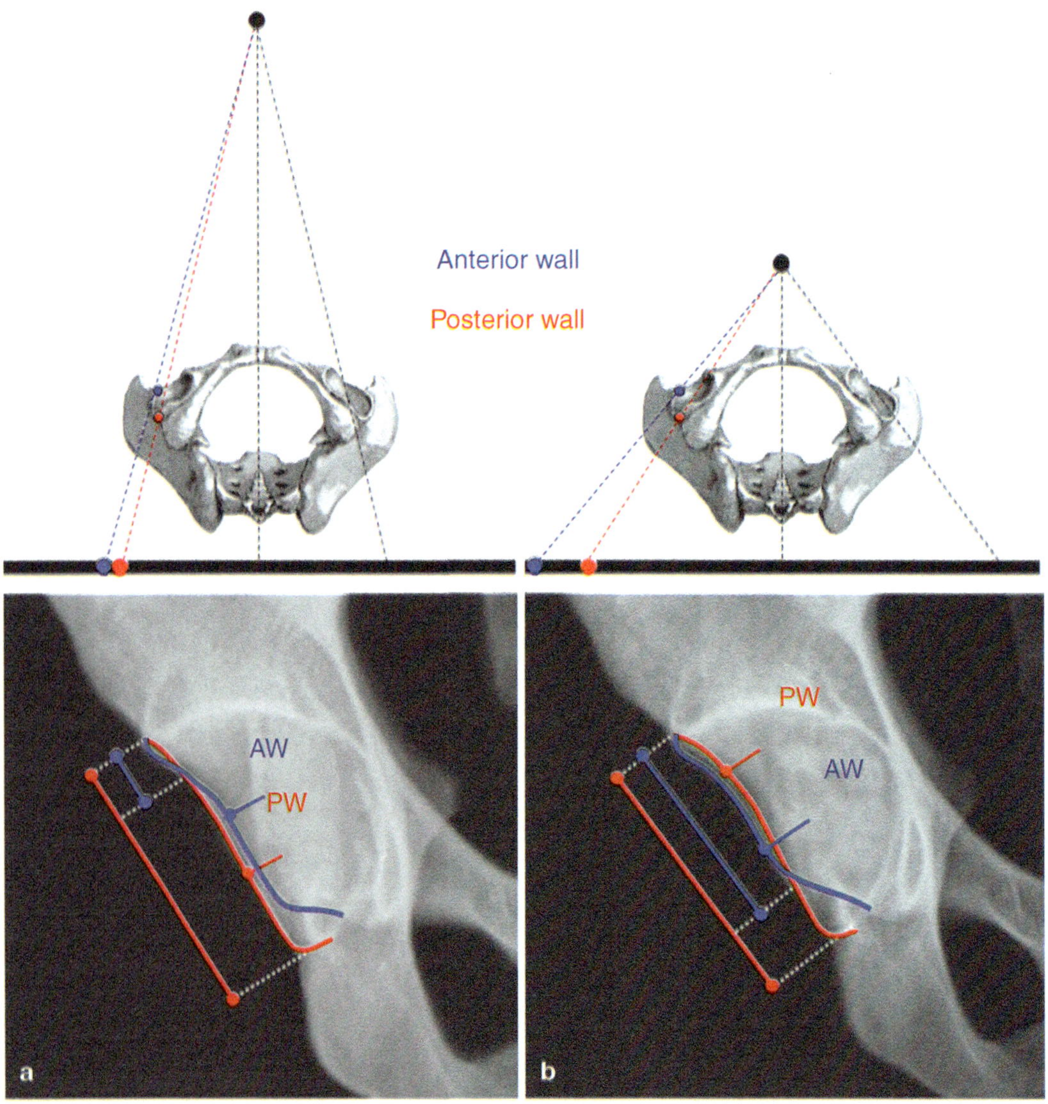

Fig. 2.1 Impact of film-tube distance on pelvic anatomy. (**a**) Compared to the regular film-tube distance (**b**) a decrease in the distance leads to a decrease in apparent acetabular anteversion, respectively, an increase in acetabular retroversion. This is indicated by a more distal overlap of the crossover sign (anterior wall [AW] projecting more laterally than the posterior wall [PW]). (**a**, **b**) Schematic drawing shows that structures that are located more anteriorly are visualized more laterally on the film than posterior anatomic structures

standardization of the film-tube distance is important. In the countries with the metric system the standard film-tube distance usually is 120 cm and 40 inches (101.6 cm) in the countries with the imperial system.

2.1.1.2 Centering of the Central X-Ray Beam

The centering of the central beam has a major influence on the projected anatomy of the hip joint. On a standard AP pelvic view the central beam should point at the midpoint between the upper border of the symphysis and a line which connects the superior anterior iliac spines. Lowering of the central beam, which is often used for planning of total hip arthroplasty, leads to an increase in acetabular anteversion (Fig. 2.2) [5]. Similarly, centering the central beam over one hip leads to a decrease of acetabular anteversion compared to the pelvic-centered view (Fig. 2.3) [5]. Furthermore, the acetabular socket appears deeper in hip-centered views (Fig. 2.3) [5]. The depth of the acetabular socket can vary and has to be considered since safety zones for screw placement in acetabular fractures depend on acetabular morphology. For definite preoperative assessment of safe zones, CT is very helpful (Fig. 2.4).

2.1.1.3 Pelvic Orientation

Pelvic orientation can vary regarding obliqueness, rotation, and pelvic tilt [2]. For correction of measurement errors due to pelvic obliqueness, anatomic reference lines such as the teardrop line

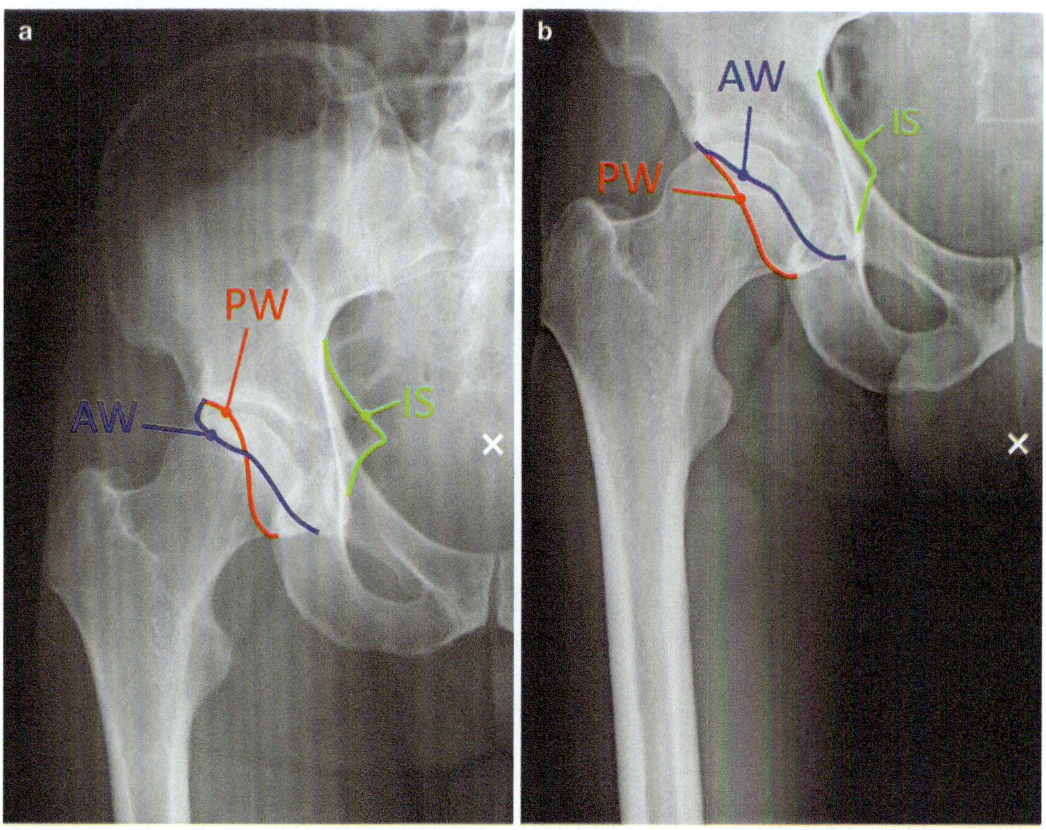

Fig. 2.2 Impact of the level of centration of the central beam (white cross) on the projected hip anatomy. (**a**) AP pelvic radiograph centered over the pelvis shows a retroverted acetabulum indicated by a more lateral projection of the anterior wall (AW) compared to the posterior wall (PW) and a prominent projection of the ischial spine (IS) into the pelvic inlet. (**b**) On the low-centered AP pelvic view, the apparent acetabular anteversion increases as the ischial-spine sign and the crossover between the anterior and posterior acetabular disappears

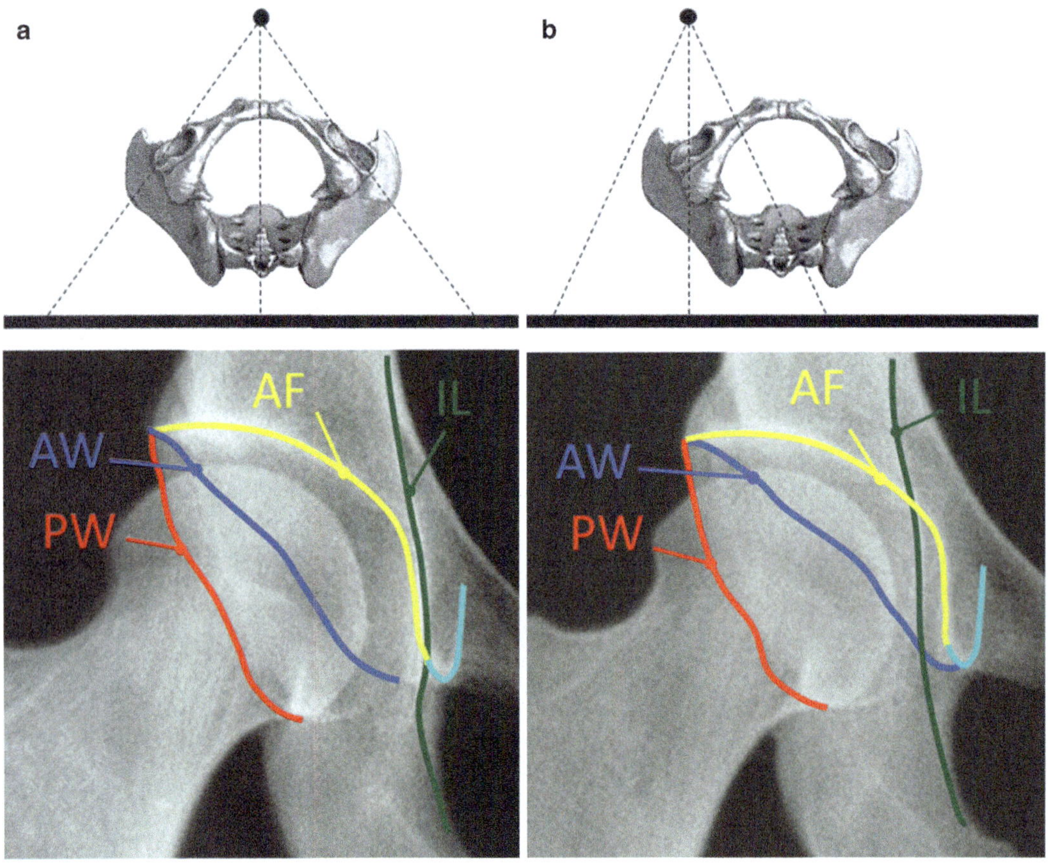

Fig. 2.3 Impact of the centration of the central beam on the projected hip anatomy. (**a**) Compared to the film centered over the midpoint of the pelvis, (**b**) the hip-centered view shows more apparent acetabular anteversion as the distance between the anterior (AW) and posterior wall (PW) is greater. Furthermore in (**b**) the femoral head and the acetabular fossa are projected more medially toward the ilioischial line (IL) compared to the pelvic-centered view

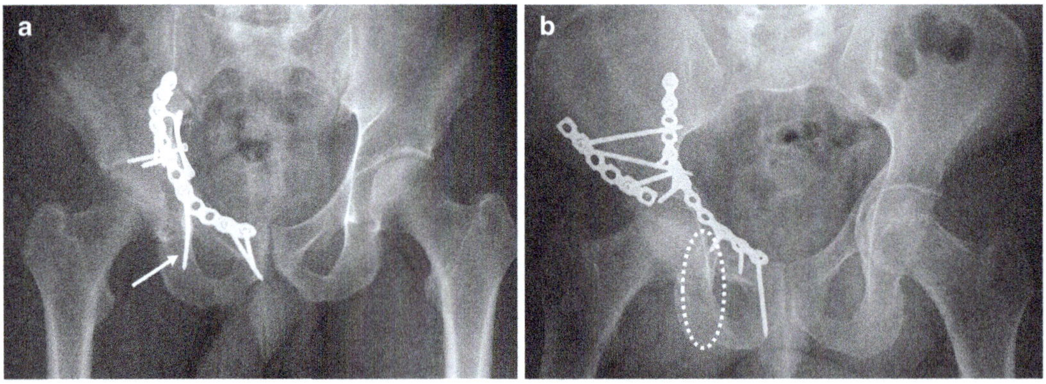

Fig. 2.4 Impact of acetabular depth on safety zones for screw placement after pelvic trauma. (**a**) An infraacetabular screw was used for fixation in a hip with normal acetabular depth. (**b**) By contrast in this patient with bilateral protrusio acetabuli (overlap between he femoral head and the ilioischial line) no infraacetabular screw was used for fixation (dashed lines). Axial CT scans show that in severely overcovered hips (**d**) the acetabular walls, especially the medial acetabular facet is much thinner than in hips with normal coverage (**c**)

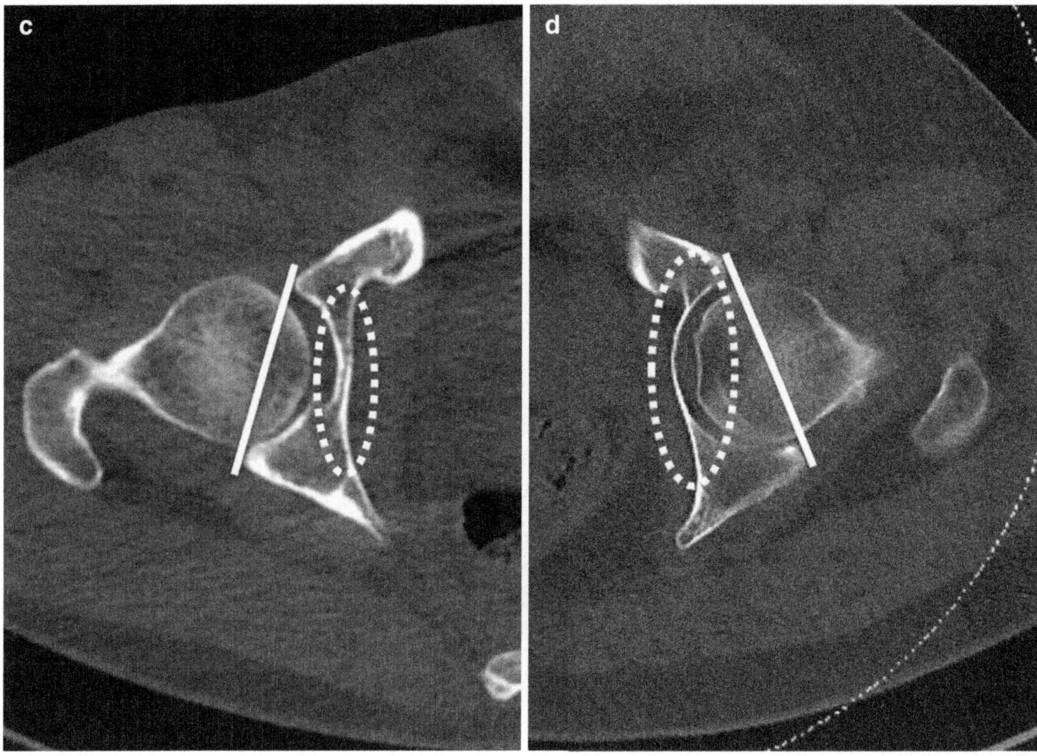

Fig. 2.4 (continued)

can be drawn. Malrotation of the pelvis affects acetabular anteversion and is present if the sacrococcygeal joint is not aligned with the center of the symphysis. Rotation to one side leads to an ipsilateral decrease in acetabular anteversion. Pelvic tilt can be indirectly assessed with the distance between the sacrococcygeal joint and the upper border of the symphysis. Anterior pelvic tilt, i.e. an increase in the sacrococcygeal-symphyseal distance leads to an decrease in acetabular version, and vice versa [2].

2.1.2 Different Views of Conventional Imaging

The different views of conventional imaging of the hip in the trauma setting and their applications are described in detail.

2.1.2.1 AP Pelvic View

AP pelvic views are part of the initial screening for detection of femoral and acetabular fractures. Knowledge of the key radiographic landmarks of the hip is the prerequisite for accurate image interpretation and includes: the anterior acetabular wall, the posterior acetabular wall, the acetabular roof, the teardrop, the iliopectineal line, and the ilioischial line (Fig. 2.5). On radiographs the iliopectineal line corresponds to the anterior column of the pelvis, which is defined as the bony structure that runs from the sacroiliac joint down to the ipsilateral pubic ramus. The anterior column includes the superior pubic ramus, anterosuperior/-inferior iliac spines, the anterior half of the acetabulum, and the anterior iliac crest [6]. The ilioischial line corresponds to the radiographic projection of the anatomic posterior column and runs from the posterosuperior iliac spine down to the ischial tuberosity. The posterior column includes the part of the ischium which extends from the ischiopubic junction to the greater sciatic notch and the posterior half of the acetabulum [6].

For acquisition of AP pelvic views, patients are positioned supine with both legs 15° inter-

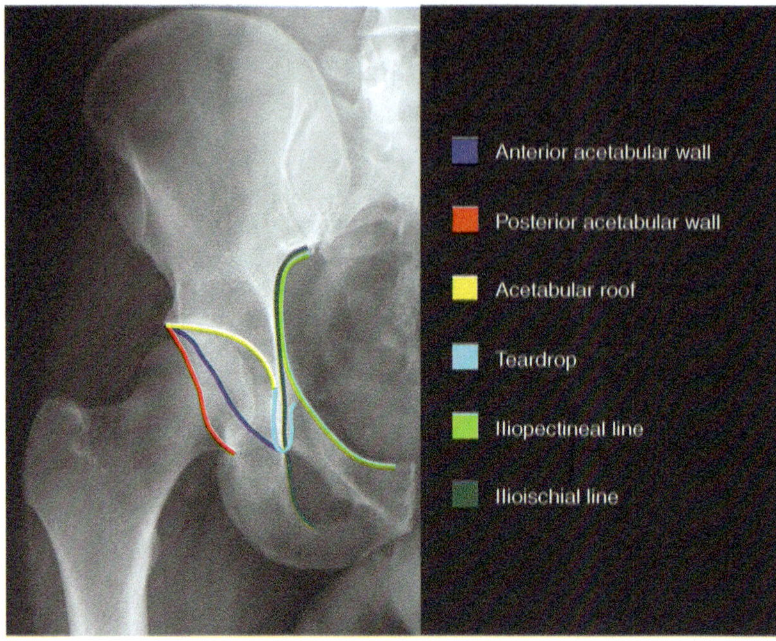

Fig. 2.5 Six lines according to Letournel in a normal hip joint

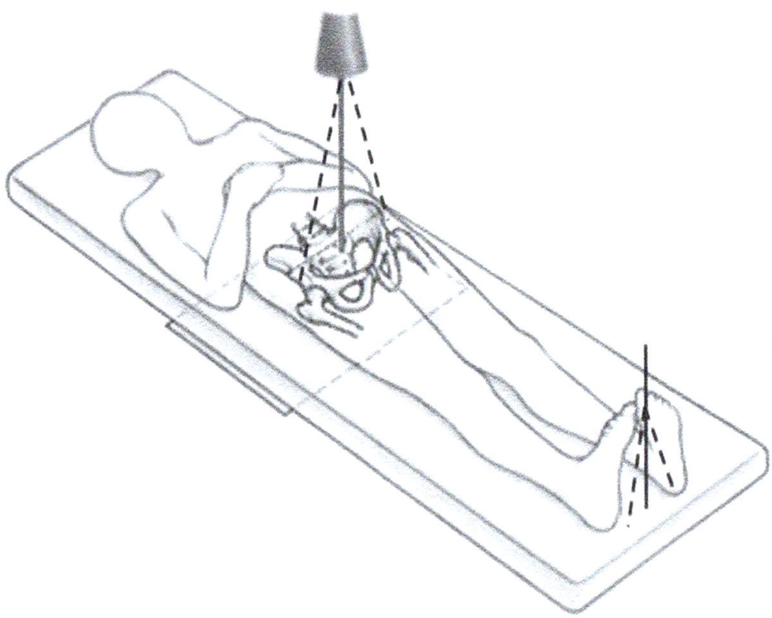

Fig. 2.6 Acquisition of AP pelvic views. Patients are positioned supine, with both legs 15° internally rotated. The tube-film distance is 1.2 m and the central beam points at the midpoint between the upper border of the symphysis and a line which connects the left and right superior anterior iliac spine

nally rotated. The tube-film distance is 120 cm and the central beam points at the midpoint between the upper border of the symphysis and a line which connects the left and right superior anterior iliac spine (Fig. 2.6) [2].

2.1.2.2 Lateral Views: Axial Cross-Table View

A secondary view of the hip is mandatory for evaluation of hip. For femoral fractures this is done with an axial view. Different techniques exist

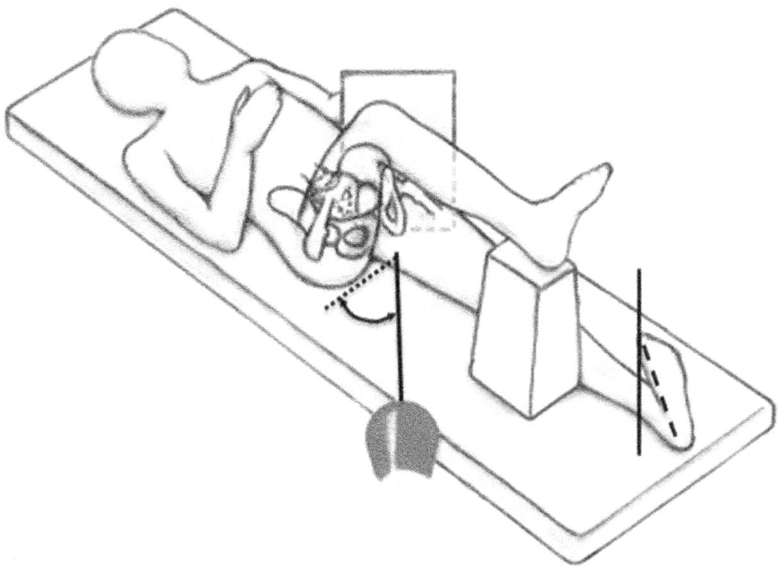

Fig. 2.7 Acquisition of axial crosstable views. Patients are positioned supine, with the ipsilateral leg 15° internally rotated to compensate for femoral torsion. The central beamed is angled 45° and points to the inguinal fold

which include the cross-table axial, Dunn view, Lauenstein view, or frog-leg lateral view. For the acetabulum and its fracture evaluation the Judet views have been described (see Sect. 2.1.2.3).

The axial cross-table view enables visualization of the anterior and posterior contour of the femoral head and neck and is invaluable for preliminary conformation and further assessment of displacement of a suspected fracture visible on AP pelvic views. Patients are positioned supine, with the ipsilateral leg 15° internally rotated to compensate for femoral torsion. The central beam is angled 45° and points to the inguinal fold (Fig. 2.7). Alternatives of axial views include the Dunn view (AP view with 90° of flexion and 20° abduction in the hips), the modified Dunn view (45° of flexion instead of 90°), Lauenstein view (45° of flexion and 34° of abduction in the hip) or Frog-Leg lateral views (bilateral Lauenstein view) can be obtained [7]. Among all these views only the axial cross-table view enables assessment in a true secondary plane of the acetabulum while the remaining views are all based on an AP projection.

2.1.2.3 Judet Views

Before the advent of CT, Judet views, i.e. right posterior oblique (RPO) (also known as: "ala view," right iliac oblique or left obturator oblique) and left posterior oblique (LPO) (also known as: "obturator view," left iliac oblique or right obturator oblique) projections were the basis of radiographic classification of acetabular fractures [6].

Based on these views, the Letournel classification was developed which differentiates between ten types of acetabular fractures [8]. Among these, three elementary fractures can be identified: Wall fractures, column fractures, and transverse fractures. The iliac oblique view shows the ipsilateral ilioischial line, the entire iliac wing, and the anterior wall of the acetabulum. The obturator oblique view shows the ipsilateral iliopectineal line and the posterior wall.

For acquisition of right posterior oblique and left posterior oblique views, the patient is positioned supine at 45° of rotation to the right and to the left on the radiographic table (Fig. 2.8). The central beam is centered over the hip. We recommend the standard acquisition of CT scans with subsequent 3D reconstruction of the pelvis and femur and acquisition of Judet views to get an overview of pelvic anatomy and for postoperative comparison.

2.1.3 Fluoroscopy

Fluoroscopy is an important intra-operative modality in the trauma setting. In contrast to

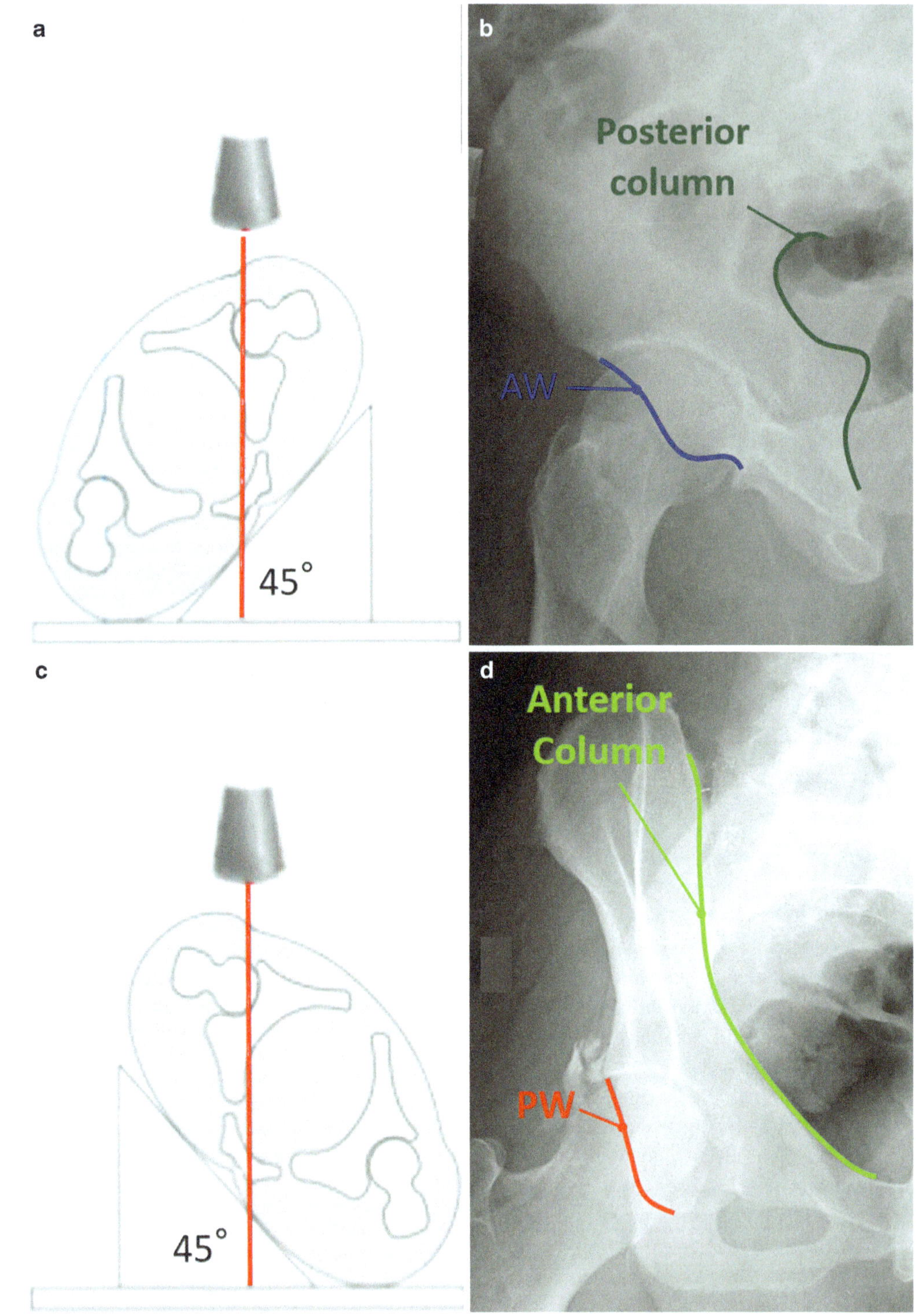

Fig. 2.8 (**a**, **b**) Right posterior oblique view of the right hip ("ala view," right iliac oblique view) and (**c**, **d**) left posterior oblique view of the right hip ("obturator view," right obturator oblique view) of a 54-year-old patient. (**a**) Schematic drawing shows patient rotated 45° to the right side. (**b**) Ipsilateral posterior column and the anterior acetabular wall (AW) are nicely outlined. (**c**) Schematic drawing shows patient rotated 45° to the left side. (**d**) Ipsilateral anterior acetabular column and the posterior acetabular wall (PW) fracture are nicely outlined

standard pelvic views it is based on a postero-anterior projection and is centered over one hip. One has to be aware of the fact that this leads to an increase in the projected acetabular anteversion while resulting measurements for acetabular coverage do not change [9].

2.2 Computed Tomography (CT)

Although conventional radiographs are the diagnostic basis in hip trauma, CT imaging has emerged as an indispensable tool for detailed preoperative planning with the possibility of 3D-reconstruction and multiplanar reformatting. In fractures of the femur, CT imaging can be performed for detailed evaluation of the fracture pattern and to aid in choosing the implant for osteosynthesis. Multiplanar and 3D-reconstruction is very helpful for the surgeon to plan the steps needed for reduction and osteosynthesis of the fracture. This is especially true in comminuted fractures or when surgery is performed through a minimal invasive approach. For fractures of the acetabulum, CT imaging is performed routinely. The complex anatomy of the acetabulum and pelvis and the very different courses of acetabular fractures make it difficult for evaluation of the fracture using conventional imaging only (Fig. 2.4). Postoperative CT imaging can be performed to verify anatomic reduction of the fracture and correct placement of screws. Since a non-anatomic reduction in articular fractures of the hip is associated with increased risk of secondary osteoarthritis of the joint, CT imaging can be indicated following surgery [10].

Integration of a whole-body CT (non-contrast head, contrast-enhanced: spine, chest, abdomen, and pelvis) into the acute trauma care algorithm enables fast recognition or exclusion of life-threatening injuries and facilitates treatment planning. An early whole-body CT in polytraumatized patients reportedly increases the survival rate [11, 12].

Due to its almost universal availability and the possibilities of fast acquisition of multiplanar reformatted 2D images, 3D reconstructions of the pelvis and the reconstruction of virtual radiographs using special software, CT has become a standard tool for surgical decision making and treatment planning in hip and pelvic trauma. The reliability of the Letournel classification was improved based on the evaluation of CT images [3, 13].

2.3 Magnetic Resonance Imaging (MRI)

Conventional radiographs and especially CT are the primary diagnostic tools for assessment of hip in trauma setting. In the elderly patient, a hip fracture may not be visible in 3–5% of cases with conventional radiographs. MRI is the modality of choice to exclude undislocated femoral fractures (Fig. 2.9) in patients with high clinical suspicion and negative radiographs or CT scans [14, 15]. Furthermore the excellent soft tissue contrast of MRI enables assessment of other pathologies such as muscular injuries (for instance, hamstring injuries) which may explain the symptoms. The standard trauma MRI protocol of the pelvis includes [1]: coronal and axial: T1-/T2-weighted turbo/fast spin-echo without fat saturation (T1-w TSE, T2-w TSE), and fluid-sensitive sequences (T2-w/PD-w with fat saturation or short-tau inversion recovery) over the entire pelvis. On MRI a fracture appears as a hypointense ("dark") line on all pulse sequences which is surrounded by a hyperintense ("bright") bone marrow edema on the fluid-sensitive sequences, respectively, with low intensity on T1-w images (Fig. 2.9). Only rarely application of contrast is needed for inconclusive cases with a suspect hip fracture to further improve visualization of the non-vascularized fracture line [1].

In the setting of an acute traumatic posterior hip dislocation, MRI can be used to assess the integrity of the external obturator muscle which is the anatomic landmark for the deep branch of the medial femoral circumflex artery. This vessel maintains vascularization of the femoral head. Hence an intact external obturator muscle is a morphologic MRI predictor for a preserved blood supply to the femoral head [16] (Fig. 2.10).

In young patients with femoral and acetabular fractures, traumatic sequelae have to be considered

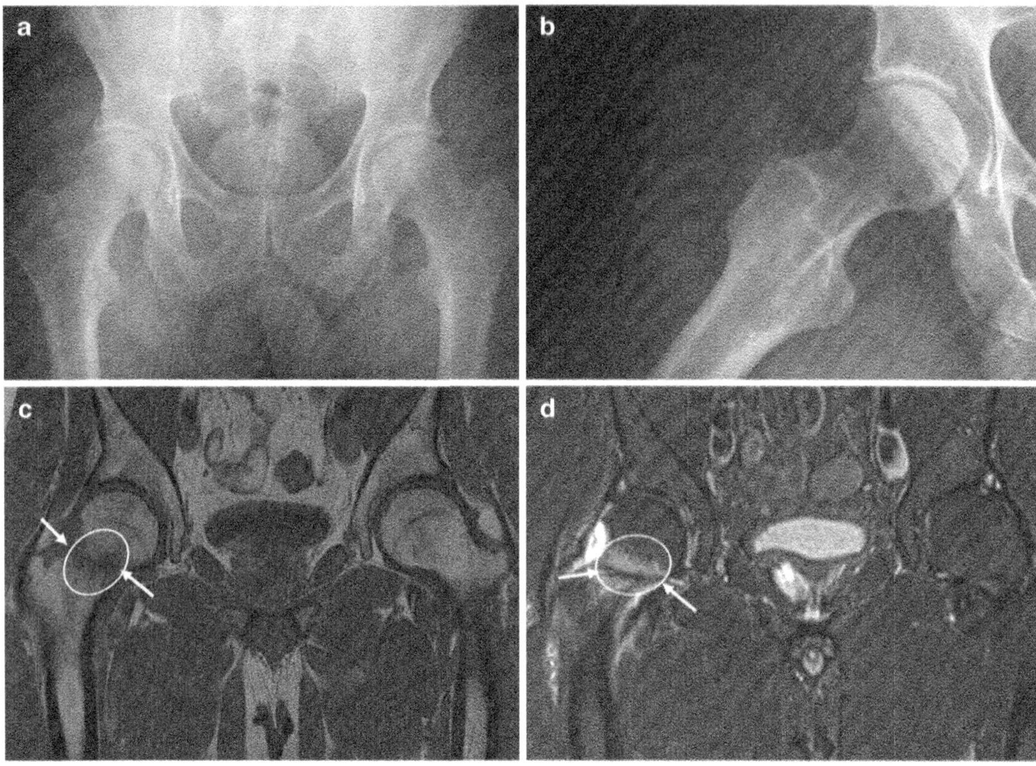

Fig. 2.9 (**a**) AP pelvic- and (**b**) modified Dunn views of a 48-year-old man with recurrent groin pain 4 weeks after arthroscopic offset correction for correction of a cam deformity without a history of trauma. (**a**, **b**) Plain radiographs show no apparent fractures. (**c**) Coronal T1-w TSE image without fat saturation and (**d**) coronal STIR image show a hypointense fracture line (arrows) and adjacent bone marrow edema (arrows) corresponding to a stress fracture of the femoral neck

in primary fixation and/or in the follow-up after primary surgery (Fig. 2.11). Posttraumatic deformities can lead to femoroacetabular Impingement (FAI) and eventually to the development of osteoarthritis [17]. MR imaging in the posttraumatic setting includes the assessment of the proximal-femoral neck junction, femoral torsion, labrum tears (Fig. 2.12), intraarticular loose bodies, osteochondral injuries, and ligamentum teres lesions (Fig. 2.13) [18]. Accurate identification and localization of these lesions and the underlying bony pathomorphologies is important to refer these patients to surgical treatment. This may be either hip arthroscopy for more focal, anterior lesions or surgical hip dislocation for more complex corrections and reconstructions related to femoral malalignment [2, 19, 20].

Assessment of FAI and intraarticular lesions requires a different imaging approach than the trauma MR protocol. Direct MR arthrography is the current modality of choice for assessment of chondrolabral lesions and superior to non-contrast MRI [21, 22]. Direct MR arthrography can be further combined with axial traction to achieve a distinct visualization of the cartilage layers and the ligamentum teres [23–26]. Based on the institutional preferences T1-w or PD-w images with or without fat-saturation in coronal, axial/axial-oblique, and sagittal planes are acquired using a small field of view (16–20 cm) [18]. Since radial slices which rotate around the femoral neck axis are the gold-standard for imaging of the cam deformity, either 2D radial images or radial reformats from gradient-echo sequences (GRE) should be acquired [27]. The availability of high-field scanners at 3 T, high performance

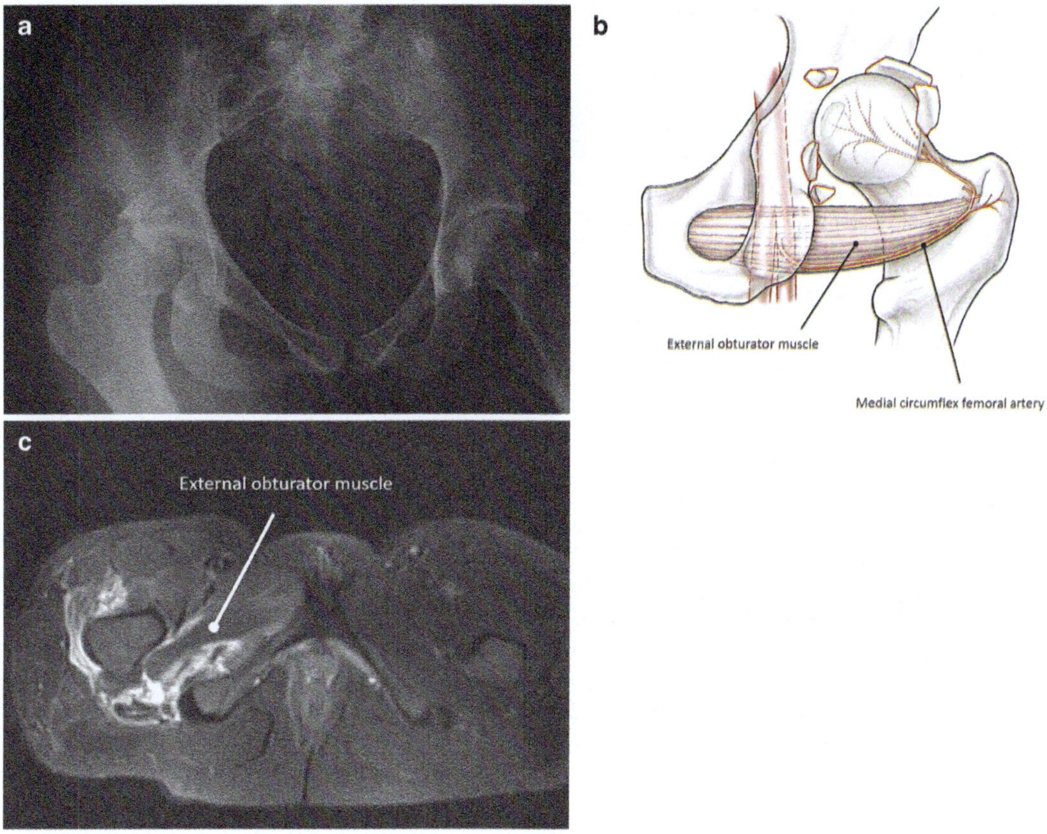

Fig. 2.10 (**a**) AP pelvic view of a 45-year-old woman who had a traumatic posterior dislocation and a resulting acetabular fracture. (**b**) Schematic drawing shows the course of the medial circumflex femoral artery which passes through the obturator foramen, runs on the external obturator muscle, and maintains the blood supply to the femoral head. (**c**) MRI was performed to assess the vitality of the femoral head. Axial STIR image of the pelvis shows hyperintense signal indicating edema and hemorrhagia of the periarticular musculature. The obturator extensor muscle is intact. The patient did not develop avascular necrosis of the femoral head

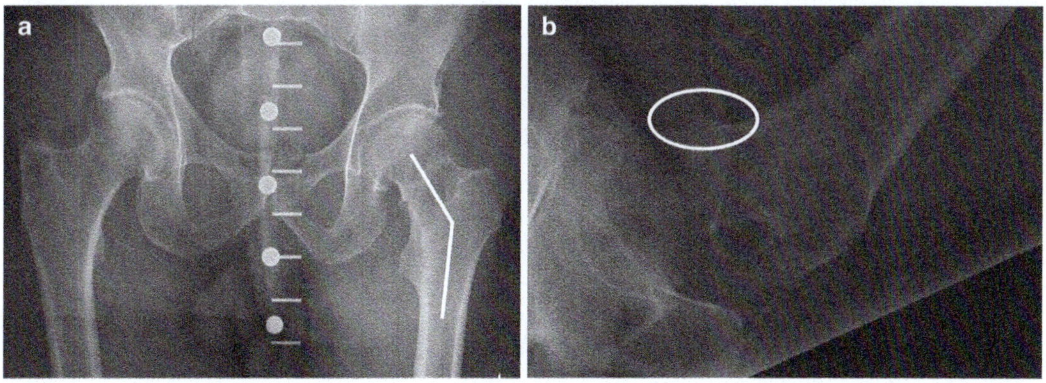

Fig. 2.11 (**a**) AP pelvic view of a 45-year-old patient with a posteriorly displaced, valgus-impacted medial femoral neck fracture. (**b**) Axial view shows a resulting bony spur (circle) in the anterior femoral neck. (**c**) Open reduction and fixation with an angular stable plate and (**d**) offset correction to prevent secondary posttraumatic FAI

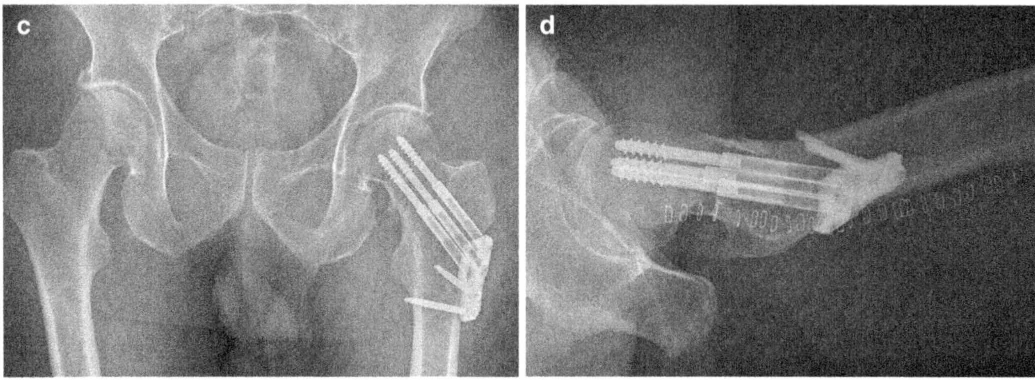

Fig. 2.11 (continued)

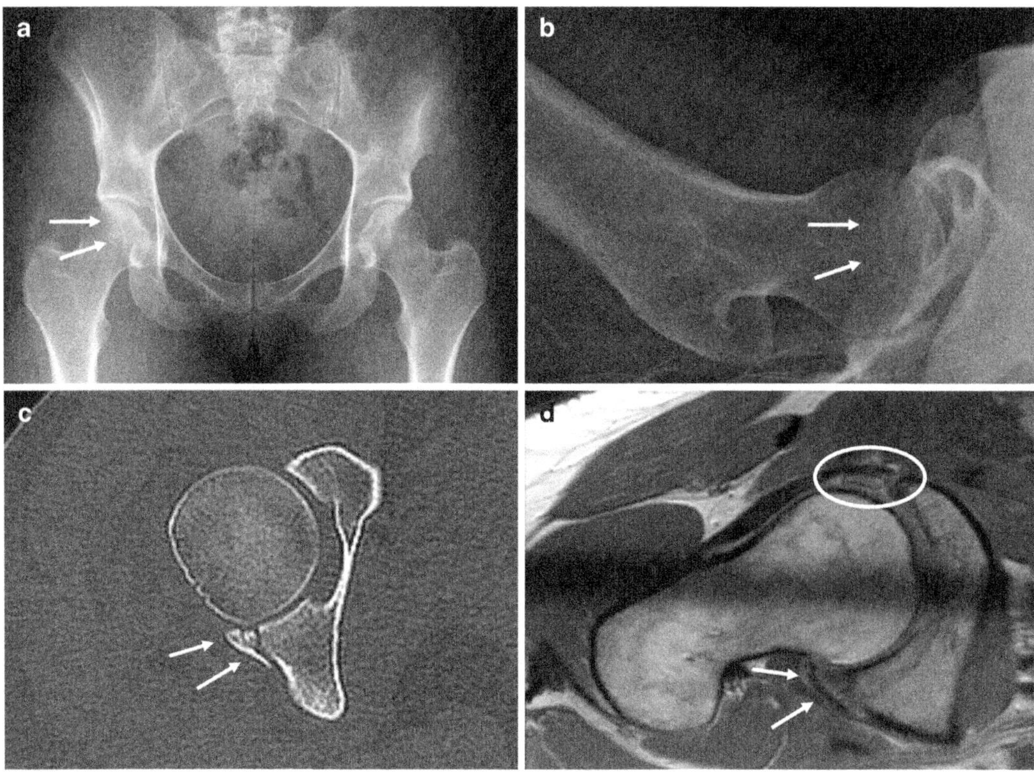

Fig. 2.12 A 28-year-old woman who sustained a hyperextension and external rotation trauma. (**a–c**) AP pelvic-, crosstable lateral-view, and an axial CT scan show a non-displaced fracture of the posterior acetabular wall (arrows). (**d**) Three months after the injury patient presented with groin pain with prolonged sitting and standing. Radial direct MR arthrograms show anterior partial tear of the labrum with intrasubstance degeneration (circle) and the posterior fracture of the acetabular wall

gradients, dedicated multi-channel coils have paved the way for the routine acquisition of 3D GRE sequences. These sequences enable thin, multiplanar image reformation with comparable or higher resolution to CT scans within reasonable imaging time. Using this 3D volume multiplanar reformation according to patient-specific anatomy is possible. This enables

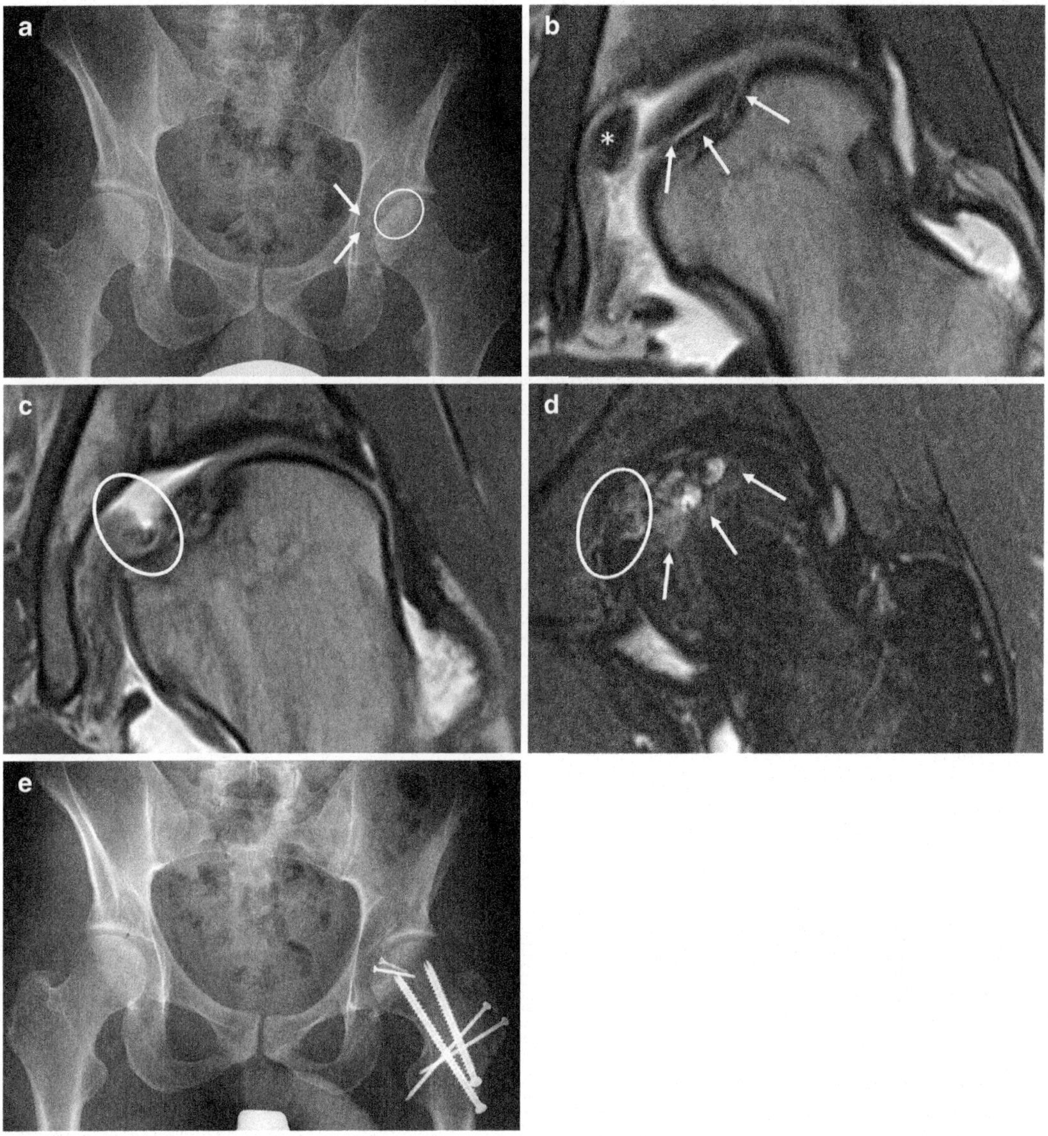

Fig. 2.13 (**a**) AP pelvic view of a 25-year-old man with excessive femoral antetorsion who sustained a hip subluxation of the left hip via a hyperextension-adduction trauma. A radiolucent structure in the acetabular fossa is suggestive for a loose body (arrows), the opposing femoral head appears deformed and with subtle inhomogeneous radiolucency. (**b**) Coronal proton density-weighted (PD-w) turbo spin-echo (TSE) images show an osteochondral loose body in the acetabular fossa (asterisk) and a perifoveal osteochondral fragment still partly attached to the femoral head. (**c**) Consecutive coronal PD-w TSE image shows complete rupture of one bundle of the ligamentum teres (circle). (**d**) Coronal TIRM image shows hyperintense signal suggesting partial rupture of the second bundle of the ligamentum teres (circle) and bone marrow edema in the fovea capitis (arrows). (**e**) Postoperative AP pelvic view following an extension wedge-osteotomy of the femoral neck via a surgical hip dislocation and fixation of the central osteochondral fragment

reduction of out-of-plane artifacts and partial volume averaging [28]. Furthermore preliminary in-house data shows excellent correlation between the mean surface distance (<1 mm) of manual MRI and manual CT segmentations. The increasing use of machine learning applications will probably allow fully automated MR segmentation in the future.

References

1. Karantanas AH. What's new in the use of MRI in the orthopaedic trauma patient? Injury. 2014;45:923–33.
2. Tannast M, Siebenrock KA, Anderson SE. Femoroacetabular impingement: radiographic diagnosis–what the radiologist should know. AJR Am J Roentgenol. 2007;188:1540–52.
3. Clarke-Jenssen J, Øvre SA, Røise O, Madsen JE. Acetabular fracture assessment in four different pelvic trauma centers: have the Judet views become superfluous? Arch Orthop Trauma Surg. 2015;135:913–8.
4. Ricci WM, Mamczak C, Tynan M, Streubel P, Gardner M. Pelvic inlet and outlet radiographs redefined. J Bone Joint Surg Am. 2010;92:1947–53.
5. Steppacher SD, Albers CE, Tannast M, Siebenrock KA. Plain radiographic evaluation of the hip. In: Nho S, Leunig M, Kelly B, Bedi A, Larson C, editors. Hip arthroscopy and hip joint preservation surgery. New York: Springer; 2014. p. 1–22.
6. Lawrence DA, Menn K, Baumgaertner M, Haims AH. Acetabular fractures: anatomic and clinical considerations. Am J Roentgenol. 2013;201:W425–36.
7. Meyer DC, Beck M, Ellis T, Ganz R, Leunig M. Comparison of six radiographic projections to assess femoral head/neck asphericity. Clin Orthop Relat Res. 2006;445:181–5.
8. Letournel E. Acetabulum fractures: classification and management. Clin Orthop Relat Res. 1980;151:81–106.
9. Büchler L, Schwab JM, Whitlock PW, Beck M, Tannast M. Intraoperative evaluation of acetabular morphology in hip arthroscopy comparing standard radiography versus fluoroscopy: a cadaver study. Arthroscopy. 2016;32:1030–7.
10. Tannast M, Najibi S, Matta JM. Two to twenty-year survivorship of the hip in 810 patients with operatively treated acetabular fractures. J Bone Joint Surg Am. 2012;94:1559–67.
11. Huber-Wagner S, Lefering R, Qvick L-M, Körner M, Kay MV, Pfeifer K-J, Reiser M, Mutschler W, Kanz K-G, Working Group on Polytrauma of the German Trauma Society. Effect of whole-body CT during trauma resuscitation on survival: a retrospective, multicentre study. Lancet. 2009;373:1455–61.
12. Huber-Wagner S, Mand C, Ruchholtz S, Kühne CA, Holzapfel K, Kanz K-G, van Griensven M, Biberthaler P, Lefering R, Trauma Register DGU. Effect of the localisation of the CT scanner during trauma resuscitation on survival – a retrospective, multicentre study. Injury. 2014;45(Suppl 3):S76–82.
13. Ohashi K, El-Khoury GY, Abu-Zahra KW, Berbaum KS. Interobserver agreement for letournel acetabular fracture classification with multidetector ct: are standard judet radiographs necessary? Radiology. 2006;241:386–91.
14. Collin D, Geijer M, Göthlin JH. Computed tomography compared to magnetic resonance imaging in occult or suspect hip fractures. A retrospective study in 44 patients. Eur Radiol. 2016;26:3932–8.
15. Haubro M, Stougaard C, Torfing T, Overgaard S. Sensitivity and specificity of CT- and MRI-scanning in evaluation of occult fracture of the proximal femur. Injury. 2015;46:1557–61.
16. Tannast M, Pleus F, Bonel H, Galloway H, Siebenrock KA, Anderson SE. Magnetic resonance imaging in traumatic posterior hip dislocation. J Orthop Trauma. 2010;24:723–31.
17. Leunig M, Beaulé PE, Ganz R. The concept of femoroacetabular impingement: current status and future perspectives. Clin Orthop Relat Res. 2009;467:616–22.
18. Schmaranzer F, Todorski IAS, Lerch TD, Schwab J, Cullmann-Bastian J, Tannast M. Intra-articular lesions: imaging and surgical correlation. Semin Musculoskelet Radiol. 2017;21:487–506.
19. Steppacher S, Schwab J, Siebenrock K, Tannast M. Actual management of femoroacetabular impingement. Minerva Ortopedica e Traumatologica. 2012;63:365–78.
20. Lerch TD, Todorski IAS, Steppacher SD, Schmaranzer F, Werlen SF, Siebenrock KA, Tannast M. Prevalence of femoral and acetabular version abnormalities in patients with symptomatic hip disease: a controlled study of 538 hips. Am J Sports Med. 2018;46:122–34.
21. Saied AM, Redant C, El-Batouty M, El-Lakkany MR, El-Adl WA, Anthonissen J, Verdonk R, Audenaert EA. Accuracy of magnetic resonance studies in the detection of chondral and labral lesions in femoroacetabular impingement: systematic review and meta-analysis. BMC Musculoskelet Disord. 2017;18:83.
22. Smith TO, Hilton G, Toms AP, Donell ST, Hing CB. The diagnostic accuracy of acetabular labral tears using magnetic resonance imaging and magnetic resonance arthrography: a meta-analysis. Eur Radiol. 2011;21:863–74.
23. Schmaranzer F, Klauser A, Kogler M, Henninger B, Forstner T, Reichkendler M, Schmaranzer E. Improving visualization of the central compartment of the hip with direct MR arthrography under axial leg traction: a feasibility study. Acad Radiol. 2014;21:1240–7.
24. Schmaranzer F, Klauser A, Kogler M, Henninger B, Forstner T, Reichkendler M, Schmaranzer E. Diagnostic performance of direct traction MR arthrography of the hip: detection of chondral and labral lesions with arthroscopic comparison. Eur Radiol. 2015;25:1721–30.
25. Schmaranzer F, Klauser A, Kogler M, Henninger B, Forstner T, Reichkendler M, Schmaranzer E. MR arthrography of the hip with and without leg traction: assessing the diagnostic performance in detection of ligamentum teres lesions with arthroscopic correlation. Eur J Radiol. 2016;85:489–97.
26. Schmaranzer F, Lerch TD, Strasser U, Vavron P, Schmaranzer E, Tannast M. Usefulness of MR arthrography of the hip with and without leg traction in detection of intra-articular bodies. Acad Radiol. 2018. https://doi.org/10.1016/j.acra.2018.10.008.
27. Agten CA, Sutter R, Buck FM, Pfirrmann CWA. Hip imaging in athletes: sports imaging series. Radiology. 2016;280:351–69.
28. Naraghi A, White LM. Three-dimensional MRI of the musculoskeletal system. AJR Am J Roentgenol. 2012;199:W283–93.

Initial Management of Hip Fractures Prior to Surgical Intervention

3

Mark Haimes and Michael Blankstein

Abstract

Initial deliberate management of hip fractures is imperative to set the stage for a successful hospital course and surgical treatment. The hip fracture population can be separated into two groups: elderly patients that sustained low energy osteoporotic fractures and young patients following high-energy trauma. Low energy hip fracture patients require a focus on medical comorbidities with consultation of the appropriate services for perioperative optimization. The primary goal is early operative intervention in order to mobilize patients as quickly as possible. Regional nerve blocks may be beneficial, but traction is not. High-energy hip fracture management differs with a focus on resuscitation, identification of concomitant injuries, and emergent reduction. In both groups, attention should be paid to appropriate anticoagulation.

Keywords

Hip fracture · Emergency · Initial management · Preoperative · Low energy · High energy

M. Haimes (✉) · M. Blankstein
Department of Orthopaedic Surgery, University of Vermont Medical Center, Burlington, VT, USA
e-mail: mark.haimes@uvmhealth.org

3.1 Introduction

This chapter will focus on the initial management of patients with hip fractures. Hip fractures should be separated into two populations, elderly patients following a low energy fall and young patients who sustained high energy trauma, each with different management strategies.

When evaluating the low-energy osteoporotic hip fractures, the focus should be on a thorough history, physical exam, and metabolic/nutritional workup, with early involvement of family, physical therapy, social work, nutrition, and medicine/geriatric co-management teams. The ultimate goal is surgery within 24–48 h to allow early mobilization.

The high-energy hip fractures usually occur in a younger population and are associated with other concomitant trauma requiring emergent attention and resuscitation. The initial focus is the history, thorough physical and acute stabilization by the general surgery/trauma teams. The orthopedic goals are to stabilize the patient and surgically treat when safe to proceed. Principles of damage control orthopedics should be applied. Ultimately, the patient should undergo urgent operative intervention if the joint is concentrically reduced, but emergent surgery otherwise.

L. Büchler, M. J.B. Keel (eds.), *Fractures of the Hip*, Fracture Management Joint by Joint,
https://doi.org/10.1007/978-3-030-18838-2_3

3.2 Low Energy Elderly Osteoporotic Hip Fractures

3.2.1 Presentation

The osteoporotic hip fracture patient presents most often after a fall from standing height. It is important to assess for concomitant injuries and differentiate the nature of the fall: mechanical, neurological, or cardiopulmonary. It is also important to inquire about antecedent hip pain, which could be a clue of a pathologic fracture.

3.2.2 History and Physical

The medical history is extremely important with this elderly population. Due to the high prevalence of medical comorbidities [1], the osteoporotic hip fracture population is relatively difficult to manage and has a variable prognosis. Worldwide, the 1-year mortality rate of this population can be up to 30%, with even more experiencing significant functional deficits [1]. Along with the medical history and other medical comorbidities, it is also important to gauge the patient's functional status and social history, specifically ambulatory status, living situation, level of function, and activities of daily living (ADLs). Support from family and other healthcare professionals is extremely important to help guide the decision for surgery.

All medications, allergies, past medical/surgical/family history should be reviewed, including any anticoagulation, complications with anesthesia, or family history of hematological or cardiopulmonary disorders. Prior to admission, it is important to discuss code status with these patients, as well as the code status specifically surrounding the perioperative period. The patient's code status addresses their wishes should they undergo cardiopulmonary arrest and possibly require resuscitation or other long-term life-sustaining measures. It is best to involve family early regarding the gathering of history and direction of management, especially in those patients that cannot provide a thorough and detailed history themselves.

On physical exam, the affected extremity is classically shortened and externally rotated, but this may not always be the case. It is important to logroll the unaffected and affected side to help confirm the diagnosis. A Stinchfield exam (resisted straight leg raise) is a more sensitive test to help determine intra-articular pathology [2]. With subtle intra-articular hip pathologies and osteoarthritis, the Stinchfield test is less sensitive [3], but in a hip fracture population it approaches 100% sensitivity. A good cardiopulmonary exam is important as well, as many of these patients have multiple cardiopulmonary medical comorbidities that need to be identified to assist the internal medicine and anesthesia colleagues [1]. In demented patients especially, or those that cannot provide a thorough history, it is important to examine the head, chest, abdomen, and all extremities in the usual head-to-toe fashion to detect other injuries. Finally, a good dermatologic exam should be performed in all patients, ideally with the help of nursing, to identify skin lesions or tears, and pressure ulcers as they are a significant cause of morbidity and can be prevalent in 10–60% of patients [4–6].

3.2.3 Diagnostic Testing

Radiographs are the predominant imaging modality of choice. An anteroposterior (AP) pelvis, isolated hip AP and cross table lateral, and completion images of the entire femur are important for surgical planning. A standardized marker should be used to correct for magnification error and subsequent calibration for implant sizing. A traction view can be useful, as it assists in identification of fracture pattern. A traction view is performed by obtaining an AP radiograph of the hip while the operator pulls axial traction and internal rotation through the affected lower extremity. An assistant will need to hold counter-traction by the axillae during the X-ray. An AP chest X-ray may be obtained at this point if clinically relevant based on history and preoperative planning for the anesthesia or medicine teams.

In rare instances, a patient's history and physical exam correlates with a hip fracture, however, there may be no findings on plain radiographs. In this case, an MRI of the hip can assist in ruling out an occult hip fracture. This is in concordance with the American Academy of Orthopedic Surgeons (AAOS) guidelines that provide moderate support for using MRI to assist in the diagnosis [7]. Management is controversial regarding the occult fracture, however, both operative and non-operative intervention may be appropriate after an in-depth conversation and informed decision making with the patient and families (Case 1).

Laboratory data is obtained to assess overall medical condition and comorbidities, as well as nutritional deficits and endocrinopathies. Standard laboratory orders include a complete blood count (CBC), basic metabolic profile (BMP), prothrombin time, INR, and partial thromboplastin time. For osteoporotic hip fracture patients, calcium, magnesium, phosphorus, alkaline phosphatase, albumin, prealbumin, parathyroid hormone (PTH), vitamin D, and hemoglobin A1c should be used to assist with nutrition and endocrine status. An electrocardiogram and urinalysis are ordered due to the high prevalence of abnormal cardiac pathologies and high risk of urinary tract infections. In the USA, nasal swab to detect methicillin-resistant Staphylococcus aureus (MRSA) is also performed, as MRSA colonization could compromise the surgical recovery, increase cost, and contribute to potential postoperative infection [1, 8–11].

3.2.4 Consulting Additional Services

Internal medicine co-management services have shown to improve outcomes, including, but not limited to, in-hospital mortality, long-term mortality, and length of stay [1, 12]. Economic cost-effective analyses demonstrate reduction of costs with a dedicated elderly hip fracture team, consisting of orthopedic, internal medicine, physical therapy, and social work [13]. Due to the benefit of early surgical management [7, 14], the focus should be to expedite optimization of the patient for surgery with appropriate risk stratification. Anesthesia may be consulted early if there is a concern for difficulty providing anesthesia with the patient's medical comorbidities, depending on the institution's anesthesia preoperative protocol.

3.3 Management of Low Energy Hip Fractures in the Emergency Department

After the patient has been evaluated, further optimization can be performed in the emergency department. A Foley catheter is recommended due to the significant pain and immobilization that will occur until surgery. Two peripheral IVs are placed to assist with fluids and medication and minimize delay in the operative room. Traction is rarely applied for osteoporotic hip fracture patients. A prospective randomized control trial of 100 consecutive elderly patients with femoral neck and intertrochanteric femur fractures compared use of cutaneous traction with five pounds versus no traction and only placement of a pillow. The authors concluded that preoperative skin traction in patients with hip fractures does not provide significant pain relief, as compared with pillow placement under the injured extremity, and thus should not be routinely performed [15]. A 2011 Cochrane Review, including 11 trials and 1654 patients compared skin traction to no traction in elderly patients with hip fractures. There was no difference of relief of pain, ease of fracture reduction, or quality of fracture reduction at the time of surgery [16]. Furthermore, a digital subtraction angiography study of nine patients with femoral neck fractures demonstrated a decrease in femoral head perfusion when placed in 3 kg of traction compared to the contralateral side. Perfusion was further decreased with 5 kg of traction, which suggests that traction decreases blood flow to the femoral head in patients with hip fractures [17]. Therefore, we advocate against the use of traction in the elderly hip fracture population. This is in concordance with the recommendations of the AAOS which states there is moderate evidence that does not support the use of routine preoperative traction in patients with a hip fracture [7].

Pain medication should be limited to non-narcotics, as narcotics in the elderly may be associated with adverse outcomes [18]. Acetaminophen, tramadol, and methocarbamol are the mainstays of treatment for pain at our institution. Anticoagulation should be provided to all patients with hip fractures and this can begin prior to surgery if surgery will be delayed. The American College of Chest Physicians recommends use of heparin or low molecular weight heparin if there is likely to be a delay to surgery [19]. If admitted patients are already on anticoagulants due to a history of atrial fibrillation or other indications, anticoagulation reversal should be initiated. INR <1.5 should be achieved by administering vitamin K or prothrombin complex concentrate [20]. Fresh frozen plasma is rarely used with vitamin K antagonist reversal due to its delay and incomplete reversal [20]. Other novel oral anticoagulants such as thrombin and direct factor Xa inhibitors should be held. New reversal agents have been developed to expedite surgery for patients on these medications, but it is unclear how long the surgeon should wait before considering safe surgical intervention. Aspirin and clopidogrel should not change hip fracture management protocols and delay a trip to the operating room. Studies and systematic review have shown no difference in bleeding complications, blood loss or transfusion requirements, overall mortality and hospital length of stay when comparing patients who underwent hip fracture surgery with antiplatelet therapy and those without [20, 21]. Furthermore, there is an increase in thromboembolic and infectious complications if surgery is delayed in the population on antiplatelet therapy. The American Society of Regional Anesthesia does not recommend neuroaxial anesthesia in this population, although there are cases of the use of platelet transfusion in patients on clopidogrel and aspirin leading to safe use of spinal anesthesia [20].

Regional nerve blocks have been shown to have some benefit in pain reduction and even a reduction in delirium in patients at moderate risk [22–26]. A prospective randomized control trial of 50 patients with femoral neck fractures treated with a bupivacaine femoral nerve block and IV morphine versus IV morphine alone, demonstrated faster time to lowest pain score, 2.88 h vs. 5.81 h, as well as requiring less morphine per hour than controls [22]. Results are similar with multiple fracture patterns and even superior when fascia iliaca compartment blocks (FICB) were used with fewer side effects of systemic anesthetics like opioids [23, 27–29]. Further studies show a decrease in delirium in moderate risk patients and even a decreased time to achieving spinal anesthesia [25, 26]. Overall, a regional anesthetic may be beneficial and should be considered part of the standard protocol for patients with hip fractures in the preoperative period. There is difficulty in implementing a hip fracture protocol which incorporates an FICB due to inadequate staff, other resumption of anesthetics, and misperception of benefit [27].

The discussion for surgery should happen early, and in the presence of family if possible. The risks, benefits, and non-operative treatment options should be discussed in detail. Surgical treatment is the preferred method of choice for most patients with the goal of giving patients the best chance at returning to their baseline functional status. Chlebeck et al. in a retrospective matched cohort study of 154 operative and 77 nonoperative patients with hip fractures, found significantly higher percent in-hospital (28.6 vs 3.9; $p<0.0001$), 30-day (63.6 vs. 11.0; <0.0001) and one-year (84.4 vs 36.4;$p<0.0001$) mortality. Their mean life expectancy after a hip fracture for the nonoperative cohort was significantly shorter than the operative group (221 vs. 1024 days; $p<0.0001$) [44]. According to the AAOS guidelines, it is important to get hip fracture patients to surgery within 24–48 h due to the significant improved outcomes [7]. A recent retrospective analysis of 42,230 patients with hip fractures demonstrated an increased risk of complications and even a higher 30-day mortality rate when wait times were greater than 24 h [14]. This newer evidence, although retrospective, attempted to match patients based on medical comorbidities and other known confounders. Furthermore, a linear relationship is demonstrated between 1-year-mortality rate and timing to surgery with a 5% increase per 10-h delay [30]. Assuming the patient is stable, a 24-h goal for surgery, and even an urgent time sensitive protocol similar to management of stroke and myocardial infarction may be appropriate.

3.4 High Energy Hip Fractures

3.4.1 Presentation

As with most orthopedic injuries, there is a bimodal distribution of age when referring to patients with fractures about the hip. The younger patients with hip fractures are more likely to be a result of high-energy mechanisms such as motor vehicle collisions or falls from extreme heights.

The first presentation of these patients should be addressed using the advanced traumatic life support (ATLS) algorithm. The orthopedic assessment can be extremely valuable but should not interfere with the ATLS treatment by the emergency and general surgery trauma teams. When assessing the patient's circulation, external hemorrhage from extremity trauma or intra-pelvic hemorrhage from pelvic trauma are extremely important to identify as early potential sites for volume loss.

3.4.2 History and Physical

Unlike the osteoporotic population, imaging may not be obtained prior to the orthopedic consultation and physical exam, so the physical exam is extremely important to identify injuries. Concomitantly with the general surgery trauma or emergency medical teams, a thorough orthopedic evaluation is performed as part of the secondary survey. The orthopedic surgeon should perform a head-to-toe evaluation. Special attention is given to all extremities, the back, perineum, and pelvis. The skin, major long bone deformities, and neurovascular status should be assessed for each extremity. All clothing, traction, and splints used for stabilization should be removed for the physical exam, as a significant portion is applied inappropriately and with minimal proven benefit in the poly-trauma patient [31]. The back and spine should be inspected to assess for any skin defects and palpated to assess for tenderness, bogginess, or step-offs. A rectal exam is performed to assess neurologic status and to identify pelvic/rectal injuries with gross blood after digital rectal exam. Assessing stability of the pelvis and a thorough hip exam should be performed.

3.4.3 Diagnostic Testing

After the physical exam, an AP chest radiograph and AP pelvis radiograph are obtained according to the ATLS protocol. A focused assessment with sonography for trauma (FAST) exam is performed followed by a CT scan of the cervical spine, chest, abdomen, and pelvis if indicated. Patients with a diaphyseal femur fracture have a 1–9% rate of having a concomitant femoral neck fracture, and historically up to one-third of these are missed or diagnosed on a delayed basis [32]. Therefore, a fine-cut CT of the pelvis should be considered with a high energy diaphyseal femur fracture [33, 34] (Case 2). Blood work is obtained with a CBC, BMP, coagulation studies, and type and screen.

3.5 Management of High Energy Hip Fractures in the Emergency Department

Once the patient is appropriately evaluated and injuries identified, a treatment plan should be implemented. In the high-energy traumatic injuries, fractures are more variable and dislocations have a much higher incidence. High-energy hip fractures include the intertrochanteric/sub trochanteric region, femoral neck, femoral head, acetabular fracture, and these may be associated with a dislocation or subluxation of the hip. These injuries may be also associated with injuries of the pelvic ring that may require a pelvic sheet or binder acutely.

All hip reductions should be addressed emergently to help preserve cartilage and blood supply to femoral head. If a suspected hip dislocation or subluxation is present, it should be confirmed with plain radiographs, and acute emergent intervention is necessary. These should be closed reduced gently under good sedation and post reduction radiographs should be obtained.

Traction assists in reduction of fractures or dislocations, helps maintain length and alignment, decreases muscle spasms, and allows tamponade of bleeding [35]. Isolated native hip dislocations have a wide range of treatment; however, traction has not been shown to have a clear benefit. A retrospective analysis of isolated native hip dislocations treated with skeletal traction versus early partial weight bearing shows no difference in outcomes with earlier return to work [36].

If there is an associated hip fracture, the use of skeletal traction may be indicated. Traction through the hip is thought to prevent pressure necrosis of the articular cartilage and viability of the femoral head and acetabulum [35].

Skeletal traction should be considered following a hip fracture dislocation. Skeletal traction may be placed in the distal femur or proximal tibia prior to the reduction to assist in stability immediately after reduction. A threaded pin is used as it decreased the likelihood of loosening, although is more likely to bend [37]. Skeletal traction may be used with 5–10 kg, and even reports of up to 15 kg for months of treatment. A proximal tibial or distal femoral traction pin may be used with a few exceptions. A proximal tibial traction pin should not be used in patients with injuries about the knee including suspected ligamentous knee injuries or proximal tibia fractures. A distal femoral traction pin is most often used. The disadvantage is the <1% risk of infection [38], and the placement of the pin may occupy the space for an intramedullary femoral nail if the pin is not anterior or posterior enough. The distal femoral traction pin is placed medial to lateral, >0.7 cm proximal to the adductor tubercle near the metaphyseal flare. and <2 cm proximal to the superior pole of the patella [45]. The goal is to avoid the femoral artery as it passes through the adductor hiatus and to avoid intra-articular placement of the pin within the knee [35]. A proximal tibial traction pin may be placed from lateral to medial, 2.5 cm distal and 2.5 cm posterior to the tibial tubercle, parallel to the joint line. The goal is to avoid the peroneal nerve [35].

If the joint is unable to be reduced or a fracture fragment remains in the incongruous joint, open reduction should be performed on an emergent basis [39]. Surgery may be delayed otherwise after initial stabilization, however, should be performed urgently within 24 h. A prospective cohort of 107 patients aged 18–55 with femoral neck fractures found that fracture displacement, quality of reduction, and nonunion were associated with a poor physical component outcome score [40]. Furthermore, in a systematic review of 1558 young femoral neck fractures, avascular necrosis (AVN) and nonunion were the most common complications leading to re-operation in about 20% of cases. This was associated with degree of fracture displacement [41]. These injuries are classically regarded as more urgent than the osteoporotic hip fractures. A survey of 540 orthopedic surgeons from the USA and Canada was performed regarding urgency of young femoral neck fractures. About one-quarter indicated their preference to operate within 8 h and about two-thirds indicated that fractures were typically treated within 8–24 h [42]. The young patient with a high-energy hip fracture is difficult to manage. They have a high incidence of concomitant injuries, AVN, nonunion, and need for re-operation [32, 43]. Their injuries are more urgent and there is a strong preference to operate within 24 h.

3.6 Conclusion

Hip fractures are very common injuries. It is important to utilize a collaborative approach when managing these injuries. The osteoporotic hip fracture management team consists of orthopedics, internal medicine, physical therapy, nutrition, and social work. In patients with high-energy hip fractures, the collaborative approach involves the general surgery trauma and emergency teams with initial stabilization as the primary goal. Other preoperative management includes a regional anesthetic block, FICB or femoral nerve, which has shown some benefit in pain and even delirium reduction. Traction should not be used in the osteoporotic hip fracture population, as it does not reduce pain compared to placement of a pillow. However, in the younger high-energy population, traction plays an important role in maintaining reduction and preserving cartilage. Anticoagulation is important in preventing DVT and anticoagulation reversal should be implemented in specific cases. Recent data suggests improved outcomes with operative treatment within 24 h.

Case 1

Occult intertrochanteric femur fracture: 90-year-old female with history of a ground level fall and persistent pain with weight bearing, pain with log roll on physical exam and pain with any hip range of motion. An MRI was obtained which showed an intertrochanteric femur fracture. After a long discussion, the patient was treated non-operatively with protected weight bearing and the fracture healed without further displacement (Fig. 3.1).

Case 2

Ipsilateral diaphyseal and femoral neck fracture: 26-year-old male who presented after a high-speed motor vehicle accident and sustained an ipsilateral diaphyseal and femoral neck fractures. A thin sliced 1 mm CT scan is shown, which better visualizes the femoral neck fracture (Fig. 3.2).

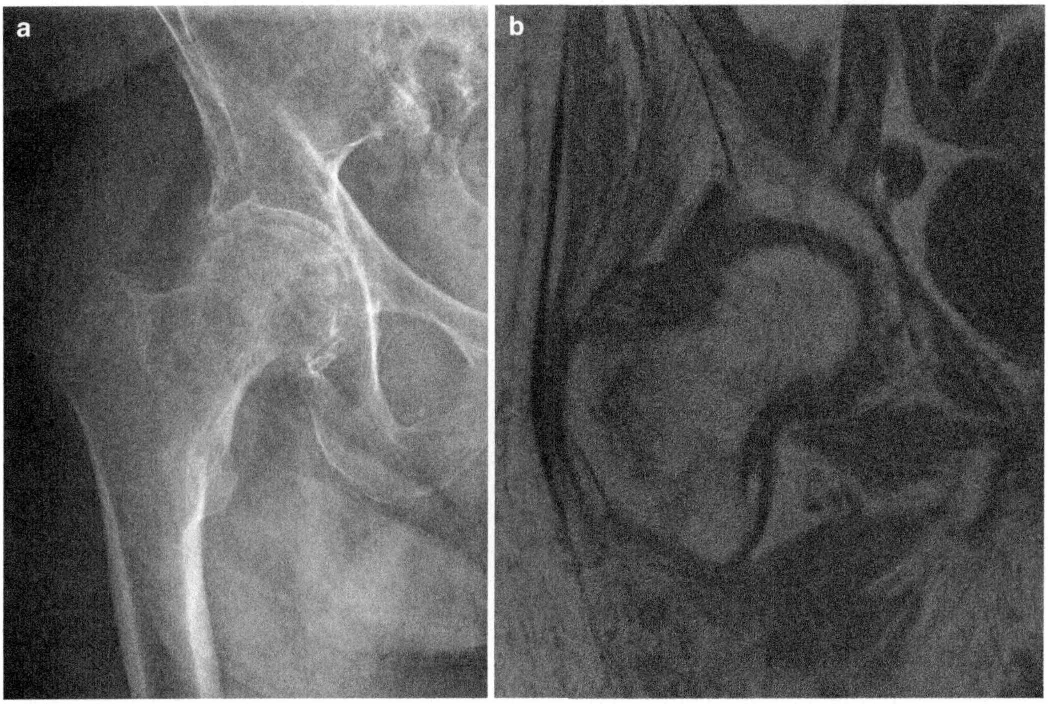

Fig. 3.1 (**a**) An AP radiograph of the right hip demonstrates degenerative changes with no fracture identified. (**b**) Coronal slice of T1-weighted MRI demonstrates hypointensity along the intertrochanteric line which confirms the diagnosis of a non-displaced, standard obliquity, intertrochanteric femur fracture

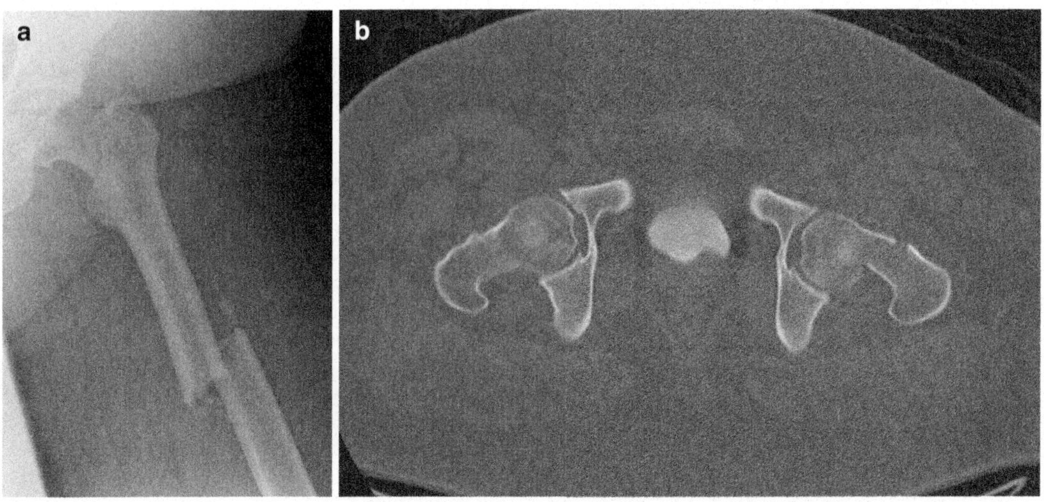

Fig. 3.2 (**a**) An AP radiograph of the left proximal femur demonstrates a completely displaced transverse diaphyseal femur fracture. The femoral neck is difficult to visualize. There is a radioluceny along the femoral neck. (**b**) Thin sliced axial CT of the femoral neck confirms left femoral neck fracture

References

1. Brauer CA, Coca-Perraillon M, Cutler DM, Rosen AB. Incidence and mortality of hip fractures in the United States. JAMA. 2009;302:1573–9.
2. Mcgrory BJ. Stinchfield resisted hip flexion test. Hosp Physician. 1999;35:41–2.
3. Maslowski E, Sullivan W, Harwood JF, et al. The diagnostic validity of hip provocation maneuvers to detect intra-articular hip pathology. PM R. 2010;2:174–81.
4. Beaupre LA, Allyson Jones C, Duncan Saunders L, Johnston DWC, Buckingham J, Majumdar SR. Best practices for elderly hip fracture patients. J Gen Intern Med. 2005;20:1019–25.
5. Houwing R, Rozendaal M, Wouters-Wesseling W, Beulens J, Buskens E, Haalboom J. A randomised, double-blind assessment of the effect of nutritional supplementation on the prevention of pressure ulcers in hip-fracture patients. Clin Nutr. 2003;22:401–5.
6. Baumgarten M, Margolis D, Berlin JA, et al. Risk factors for pressure ulcers among elderly hip fracture patients. Wound Repair Regen. 2003;11:96–103.
7. American Academy of Orthopaedic Surgeons. Management of Hip Fractures in the Elderly - Evidence Based Clinical Practice Guideline. https://www.aaos.org/research/guidelines/HipFxGuideline.pdf. Published September 5, 2014.
8. Thyagarajan D, Sunderamoorthy D, Haridas S, Beck S, Praveen P, Johansen A. Mrsa colonisation in patients admitted with hip fracture: implications for prevention of surgical site infection. Acta Orthop Belg. 2009;75:252–7.
9. Shukla S, Nixon M, Acharya M, Korim M, Pandey R. Incidence of MRSA surgical-site infection in MRSA carriers in an orthopaedic trauma unit. J Bone Joint Surg Br. 2009;91:225–8.
10. Nixon M, Jackson B, Varghese P, Jenkins D, Taylor G. Methicillin-resistant staphylococcus aureus on orthopaedic wards: incidence, spread, mortality, cost and control. J Bone Joint Surg Br. 2006;88:812–7.
11. Prokuski L. Prophylactic antibiotics in orthopaedic surgery. J Am Acad Orthop Surg. 2008;16:283–93.
12. Grigoryan KV, Javedan H, Rudolph V. Ortho-geriatric care models and outcomes in hip fracture patients: a systematic review and meta-analysis. J Orthop Trauma. 2014;28:E49.
13. Swart E, Vasudeva E, Makhni EC, Macaulay W, Bozic KJ. Dedicated perioperative hip fracture comanagement programs are cost-effective in high-volume centers: an economic analysis. Clin Orthop Relat Res. 2016;474:222–33.
14. Pincus D, Ravi B, Wasserstein D, et al. Association between wait time and 30-day mortality in adults undergoing hip fracture surgery. JAMA. 2017;318:1994–2003.
15. Rosen JE, Chen FS, Hiebert R, Koval KJ. Efficacy of preoperative skin traction in hip fracture patients: a prospective, randomized study. J Orthop Trauma. 2001;15:81–5.
16. Handoll HH, Queally JM, Parker MJ. Pre-operative traction for hip fractures in adults. Cochrane Libr. 2011;12:CD000168.
17. Lin J, Yang H. DSA observation of hemodynamic response of femoral head with femoral neck fracture during traction: can traction really increase the risk of osteonecrosis of the femoral head? J Orthop Trauma. 2012;26:E168.
18. Abou-Setta AM, Beaupre LA, Rashiq S, et al. Comparative effectiveness of pain management interventions for hip fracture: a systematic review. Ann Intern Med. 2011;155:234–45.
19. Geerts WH, Bergqvist D, Pineo GF, et al. Prevention of venous thromboembolism: American College of Chest Physicians evidence-based clinical practice guidelines. Chest. 2008;133:381s–453s.
20. Yassa R, Khalfaoui MY, Hujazi I, Sevenoaks H, Dunkow P. Management of anticoagulation in hip fractures: a pragmatic approach. EFORT Open Rev. 2017;2:394–402.
21. Soo CG, Della Torre PK, Yolland TJ, Shatwell MA. Clopidogrel and hip fractures, is it safe? A systematic review and meta-analysis. BMC Musculoskelet Disord. 2016;17:136.
22. Fletcher AK, Rigby AS, Heyes FL. Three-in-one femoral nerve block as analgesia for fractured neck of femur in the emergency department: a randomized, controlled trial. Ann Emerg Med. 2003;41:227–33.
23. Foss NB, Kristensen BB, Bundgaard M, et al. Fascia iliaca compartment blockade for acute pain control in hip fracture patientsa randomized, placebo-controlled trial. Anesthesiology. 2007;106:773–8.
24. Haddad F, Williams R. Femoral nerve block in extracapsular femoral neck fractures. Bone Joint Journal. 1995;77:922–3.
25. Mouzopoulos G, Vasiliadis G, Lasanianos N, Nikolaras G, Morakis E, Kaminaris M. Fascia iliaca block prophylaxis for hip fracture patients at risk for delirium: a randomized placebo-controlled study. J Orthop Traumatol. 2009;10:127–33.
26. Yun M, Kim Y, Han M, Kim J, Hwang J, Do S. Analgesia before a spinal block for femoral neck fracture: fascia iliaca compartment block. Acta Anaesthesiol Scand. 2009;53:1282–7.
27. Miller GW, Godrey JJ, Sagmeister ML, Lewis TL. Provision of fascia iliaca compartment block in the acute management of proximal femoral fractures: a national observational study of UK hospitals. Injury. 2016;47:2490–4.
28. Haines L, Dickman E, Ayvazyan S, et al. Ultrasound-guided fascia iliaca compartment block for hip fractures in the emergency department. J Emerg Med. 2012;43:692–7.
29. Pinson S. Fascia iliaca (Ficb) block in the emergency department for adults with neck of femur fractures: a review of the literature. Int Emerg Nurs. 2015;23:323–8.
30. Maheshwari K, Planchard J, You J, et al. Early surgery confers 1-year mortality benefit in hip-fracture patients. J Orthop Trauma. 2018;32:105–10.

31. Wood SP, Vrahas M, Wedel SK. Femur fracture immobilization with traction splints in multisystem trauma patients. Prehosp Emerg Care. 2003;7:241–3.
32. Hak DJ, Mauffrey C, Hake M, Hammerberg EM, Stahel PF. Ipsilateral femoral neck and shaft fractures: current diagnostic and treatment strategies. Orthopedics. 2015;38:247–51.
33. Zettas JP, Zettas P. Ipsilateral fractures of the femoral neck and shaft. Clin Orthop Relat Res. 1981;160:63–73.
34. Tornetta P III, Kain MSH, Creevy WR. Diagnosis of femoral neck fractures in patients with a femoral shaft fracture: improvement with a standard protocol. J Bone Joint Surg Am. 2007;89:39–43.
35. Matullo KS, Gangavalli A, Nwachuku C. Review of lower extremity traction in current orthopaedic trauma. J Am Acad Orthop Surg. 2016;24:600–6.
36. Schlickewei W, Elsässer B, Mullaji A, Kuner E. Hip dislocation without fracture: traction or mobilization after reduction? Injury. 1993;24:27–31.
37. Althausen PL, Hak DJ. Lower extremity traction pins: indications, technique, and complications. Am J Orthop (Belle Mead NJ). 2002;31:43–7.
38. Austin DC, Donegan D, Mehta S. Low complication rates associated with the application of lower extremity traction pins. J Orthop Trauma. 2015;29:E259–E65.
39. Stannard JP, Harris HW, Volgas DA, Alonso JE. Functional outcome of patients with femoral head fractures associated with hip dislocations. Clin Orthop Relat Res. 2000;377:44–56.
40. Slobogean GP, Stockton DJ, Zeng B, Wang D, Ma B-T, Pollak AN. Femoral neck fractures in adults treated with internal fixation: a prospective multicenter Chinese cohort. J Am Acad Orthop Surg. 2017;25:297–303.
41. Slobogean G, Sprague S, Scott T, Bhandari M. Complications following young femoral neck fractures. Injury. 2015;46:484–91.
42. Slobogean G, Sprague S, Scott T, Mckee M, Bhandari M. Management of young femoral neck fractures: is there a consensus? Injury. 2015;46:435–40.
43. Damany D, Parker MJ, Chojnowski A. Complications after intracapsular hip fractures in young adults: a meta-analysis of 18 published studies involving 564 fractures. Injury. 2005;36:131–41.
44. Chlebeck JD, Birch CE, Blankstein M, Kristiansen T, Bartlett CS, Schottel PC. Nonoperative Geriatric Hip Fracture Treatment is Associated with Increased Mortality: A Matched Cohort Study. J Orthop Trauma. 2019 Feb.
45. McElvany M, Benninger B, Smith S, Mirza A, Marshall L, Friess D. Are distal femoral traction pins intra-articular? A cadaveric study. J Orthop Trauma. 2013;27(11):e250–3.

4 Ilio-Inguinal Approach

Lorenz Büchler and Helen Anwander

Abstract

The ilio-inguinal approach is an anterior approach to the pelvis, introduced by Letournel in 1965. With its use, the results of surgical treatment of acetabular fractures with the main dislocation in the anterior column were greatly improved. The anatomical dissection leads to a low complication rate and fast recovery of the patient. Three anatomical windows are developed: The first exposes the anterior sacro-iliac joint and iliac fossa, the second exposes the anterior column, the anterior wall, and the quadrilateral surface, and the third exposes the superior pubic ramus. The main advantage of the ilio-inguinal approach is that by using all three windows, an extended direct view on the entire inner side of the pelvis can be achieved for fracture reduction and plate positioning. Main disadvantages are the lack of direct visualization of the acetabular surface, the impaired view on the posterior column, and the need to open the inguinal canal.

L. Büchler (✉)
Department of Orthopaedic Surgery, Kantonsspital Aarau, Aarau, Switzerland
e-mail: lorenz.buechler@ksa.ch

H. Anwander
Department of Orthopaedic Surgery and Traumatology, Inselspital, Bern University Hospital, Bern, Switzerland

Keywords

Acetabulum · Fractures · Ilio-inguinal · Anterior pelvic approach · Letournel

4.1 Introduction and History

Before the groundbreaking work from Letournel and Judet in the early 1960s, fractures of the acetabulum were mainly treated conservatively. Results were generally poor due to persisting dislocation, femoral head necrosis, and early progression to osteoarthritis. In his thesis under the supervision of Judet in 1961, Letournel classified the fractures of 75 cases and suggested surgical approaches according to the specific fracture patterns [1, 2]. The postero-lateral approach had been the one most frequently used. Two cases (transverse fracture, anterior column/post-hemitransverse fracture) were treated with a modification of the ilio-femoral approach developed by Smith-Petersen [3, 4]. It was however mentioned that the approach caused great difficulties, as the large vessels prevented access to the quadrilateral plate [2]. To improve the access, anatomical studies were performed for a new anterior approach where the distal part of the incision was curved upwards towards the midline and the entire internal iliac fossa as well as the pelvic brim was exposed. This research culminated in the *ilio-inguinal approach* to the pelvis, an anatomical

L. Büchler, M. J.B. Keel (eds.), *Fractures of the Hip*, Fracture Management Joint by Joint,
https://doi.org/10.1007/978-3-030-18838-2_4

muscle-sparing approach with extended visualization of the anterior column, ideally exposing the inner aspect of the ilium and pubic bone from the sacro-iliac joint to the pubic symphysis [5]. Since 1965, this new approach was frequently and successfully used by Judet and Letournel and has become the gold standard in the treatment of anterior column fractures [5–7]. The surgical exposure allows the development of three working windows: The first (lateral) window extends between the sacro-iliac joint and the iliopsoas, providing access to the sacro-iliac joint, the internal iliac fossa, and the proximal pelvic brim. The second (middle) window extends between the iliopsoas and the external iliac vessels, providing access to the distal pelvic brim, the quadrilateral surface, the acetabular roof, the greater sciatic notch, and the anterior acetabular wall. The third (medial) window extends between the iliac vessels and the symphysis, providing access to the space of Retzius, the pubic symphysis, the superior pubic ramus from the pubic tubercle to the pectineus recess and includes the spermatic cord (male) or round ligament (female) [8]. Limitations are the limited access to the posterior column and the inferior quadrilateral surface as well as the lack of direct visualization of the acetabular surface.

4.2 Indications

The ilio-inguinal approach is the gold standard for anterior wall and anterior column fractures as an excellent, direct visualization of the anterior column can be achieved [9]. The posterior column and the quadrilateral plate can be visualized indirectly through the second window; subsequently, this approach can also be used for more complex acetabular fractures with the main displacement in the anterior column, such as two column fractures, anterior column-posterior hemitransverse fractures as well as some t-type and transverse fractures. Articular reduction is done indirectly based on the extraarticular anatomy, as the joint cannot be directly visualized. Consequently, the quality of the articular reduction relies on the quality of cortical osseous reductions of the innominate bone and the confirmation provided by intraoperative fluoroscopy or CT. Acetabular fractures are mainly addressed using the second window, with extensions proximal or distal for plate fixation.

The direct anterior visualization of the sacro-iliac joint and the inner aspect of the ilium through the first window can be used for reduction and internal stabilization of sacro-iliac injuries such as sacro-iliac dislocation in a type C pelvic ring fracture, reposition and internal fixation of a transiliac fracture (crescent fracture) as well as a fracture of the wing of the ilium and treatments of infections of the sacro-iliac joint or abscesses and hematomas of the iliopsoas. Over the second window, a fracture of the quadrilateral surface can be reduced and fixated. This may occur in the case of an internal luxation of the hip or in an intrapelvic protrusion of the acetabular component following total hip prosthesis. Injuries to the anterior pelvic ring, such as transpubic fractures and disruptions of the symphysis can be addressed using the third window (Fig. 4.1).

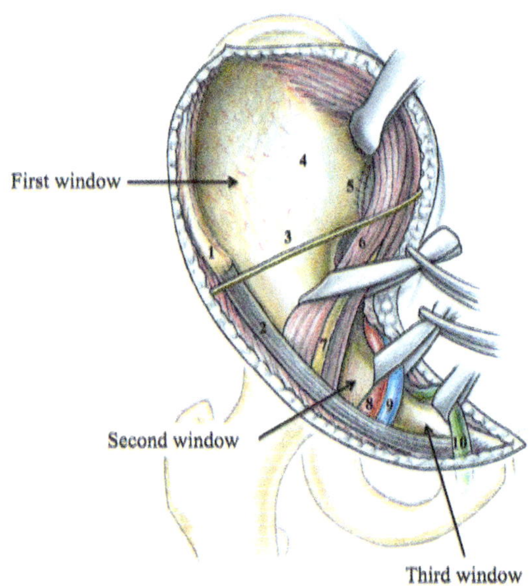

Fig. 4.1 Overview of the three windows of the ilio-inguinal approach with the relevant anatomical structures. (1) Anterior superior iliac spine, (2) Inguinal ligament, (3) N. cutaneus femoris lateralis, (4) Ala ossis ilii, (5) ilio-sacral joint, (6) M. iliopsoas, (7) N. femoralis, (8) A. femoralis communis, (9) V. femoralis communis, (10) Ductus spermaticus/Lig. rotundum. Adopted and reproduced with permission and copyright © of Der Unfallchirurg, Springer [9]

4.3 Technique

4.3.1 Preparation, Patient Positioning

The patient is put under general anesthesia with complete muscle relaxation. Due to the often prolonged operation time and wide exposures, temperature regulation is important to prevent a decrease of core temperature of the patient. Intraoperative blood salvage with the use of cell savers and reinfusion after processing should be considered. A urinary catheter should be inserted to empty the bladder. The patient is placed in supine position with the greater trochanter at the rim of a radiolucent table. The leg of the fractured side is draped freely to enable hip flexion during surgery for relaxation of the iliopsoas and traction via a subtrochanteric pin for fracture reduction. The fluoroscope is tested for unrestricted positioning for AP, ala- and obturator images as well as 3D reconstructions if available.

4.3.2 Incision

The landmarks are the crista iliaca, the anterior superior iliac spine (ASIS), and the pubic symphysis. The incision follows the crista iliaca to the ASIS, and then slightly curved medially following the inguinal ligament to the midline 2 cm proximal to the symphysis. After skin incision, the subcutaneous fat is dissected (Fig. 4.2).

4.3.3 Exposure of the First Window

After releasing the external oblique muscle insertion from the lateral iliac crest, the inner side of the ilium is exposed through subperiosteal elevation of the M. iliacus from the internal iliac fossa to the anterior sacro-iliac joint posteriorly and the pelvic brim inferiorly. Medial retraction of the M. iliopsoas requires placement of retractors on the quadrilateral surface and flexion of the hip to release muscle tension. Bleeding from the nutrient foramina can be controlled using bone wax and temporary packing the iliac fossa. The first window provides access to the sacro-iliac joint, the internal iliac fossa, and the proximal pelvic brim (Fig. 4.3).

4.3.4 Exposure of the Second Window

The aponeurosis of the external oblique is incised from the ASIS to the lateral border of the rectus

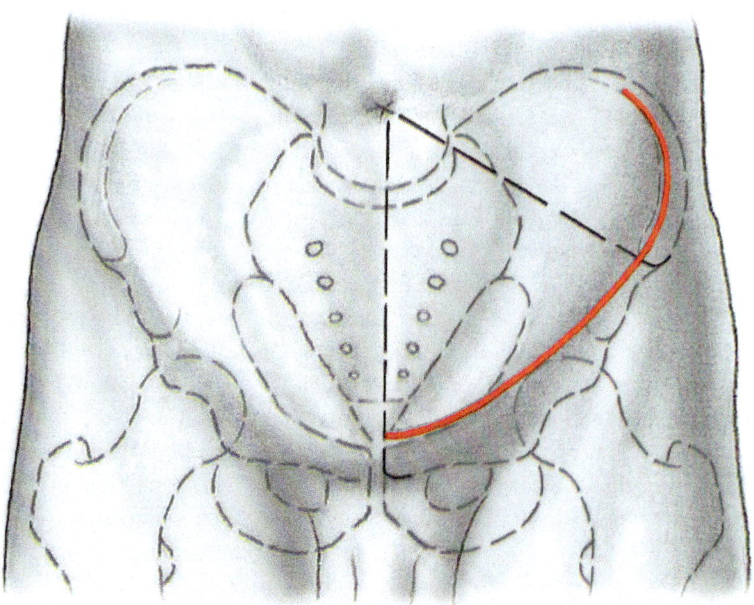

Fig. 4.2 Skin incision for the ilio-inguinal approach (red line). The incision begins cranially at the posterior superior iliac spine (PSIS) and follows the iliac crest to the anterior superior iliac spine (ASIS). The incision is then slightly curved medially towards the midline proximal of the symphysis. Adopted and reproduced with permission and copyright © of Der Unfallchirurg, Springer [9]

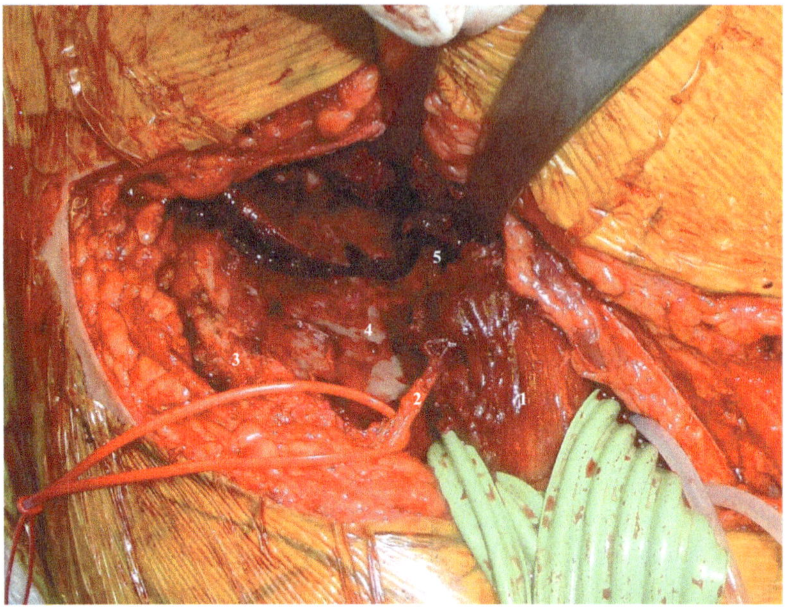

Fig. 4.3 Intraoperative view of the first ilio-inguinal window (right hip). (1) M. iliopsoas, (2) lateral femoral cutaneous nerve, (3) Spina iliaca, (4) Iliac fossa, (5) Pelvic brim

sheath, passing 1 cm cranial to the inguinal canal, identifying and protecting the lateral femoral cutaneous nerve, which usually lies on the lateral border of the iliacus muscle and passes 1–2 cm medial of the ASIS below the inguinal ligament into the compartment of the sartorius muscle. The conjoint tendon of the internal oblique and the transversus abdominis muscles is incised two to three millimeters cranial of the inguinal ligament and the ilio-inguinal nerve is identified. It emerges from the lateral border of the psoas major muscle, passes across the iliacus muscle, the anterior part of the iliac crest and the internal oblique muscle to follow the spermatic cord/round ligament. Next, the spermatic cord/the round ligament is identified and mobilized.

To develop the second window, the iliopectineal arch, a thickened band of fused iliac and psoas fascia that separates the inguinal canal, is incised (Fig. 4.4). On the lateral side, the lacuna musculorum contains the M. iliopsoas, the femoral nerve and the lateral femoral cutaneous nerve. On the medial side, the lacuna vasorum contains the external iliac artery and vein and the surrounding lymphatics. The M. iliopsoas and the femoral nerve are mobilized laterally, the external iliac vessels medially. The iliopectineal arch is divided distally and the fascia following the terminal line to the sacro-iliac joint is opened. This exposes the iliopectineal eminence, the acetabular roof, and the quadrilateral space (Fig. 4.5). To expose the greater sciatic notch and the entire quadrilateral space to the sciatic spine, the pectineus and the internal obturator muscles are elevated subperiosteally. Anteriorly, the anastomoses between the obturator vessels and either the inferior epigastric or external iliac vessels (the corona mortis) have to be ligated. If torn, they can lead to major bleeding.

4.3.5 Exposure of the Third Window

The plane between the pubic symphysis and the bladder (space of Retzius) is bluntly dissected. The bladder can be identified by palpating the urinary catheter bulb. In acute trauma, wound hematoma frequently dilates this space and is easily removed. In revision surgery significant adhesions have to be expected, which render the dissection more difficult with the risk of injuries to the bladder or peritoneum. Mobilizing the bladder cranially provides visualization of the space between the rectus and the spermatic cord/round ligament. Infrapectineal dissection carefully proceeds along

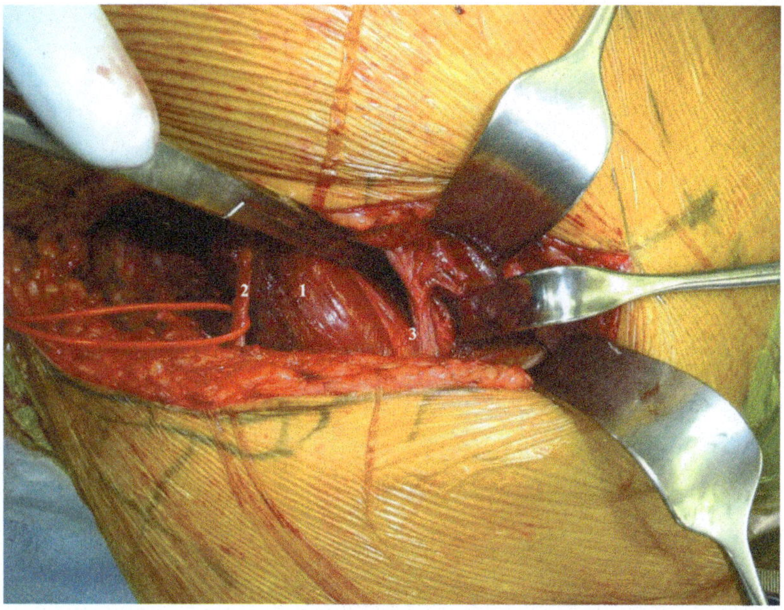

Fig. 4.4 Intraoperative view of the iliopectineal arch. The lateral femoral cutaneus nerve is identified and marked with a red rubber strap. (1) M. iliopsoas, (2) lateral femoral cutaneous nerve, (3) iliopectineal arch

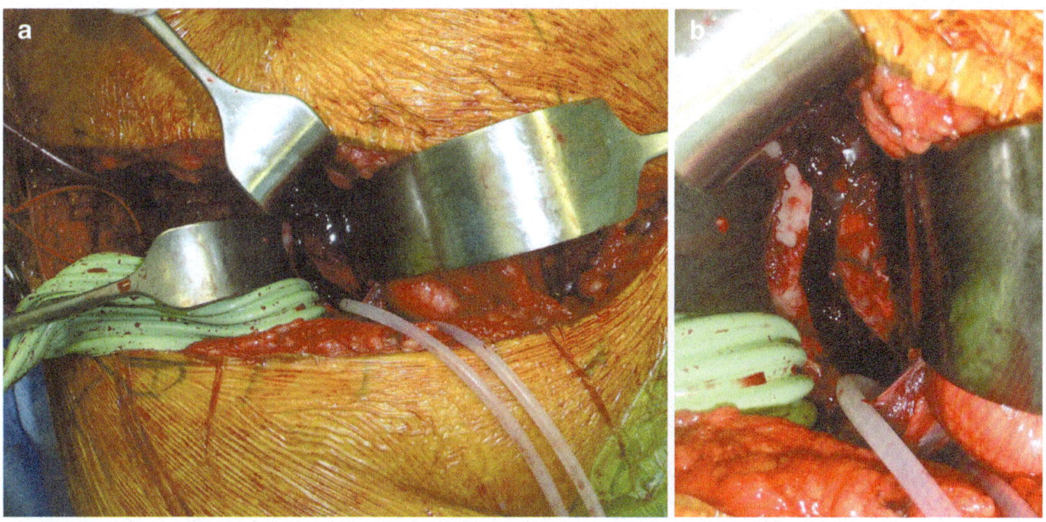

Fig. 4.5 (**a**) Intraoperative view of the second ilio-inguinal window. The M. iliacus and femoral nerve are retracted laterally and the inguinal vessels (marked with the transparent rubber strap) retracted medially to expose the quadrilateral plate. (**b**) close-up view of a dislocated fracture of the anterior column

the medial surface of the pubic ramus and posteriorly following the pelvic brim. The iliopectineal fascia has already been released allowing elevation of the external iliac vessels. The third window provides access to the space of Retzius, the pubic symphysis, the superior pubic ramus and includes the spermatic cord (male) or round ligament (female). The third window can be expanded to allow direct, intrapelvic access to the entire quadrilateral surface and the posterior column (Fig. 4.6).

If a visualization of the contralateral side of the symphysis is required, the ipsilateral rectus insertion is released or the linea alba between the two rectus heads is split in the midline similar to the Stoppa approach (fourth window) (Fig. 4.7).

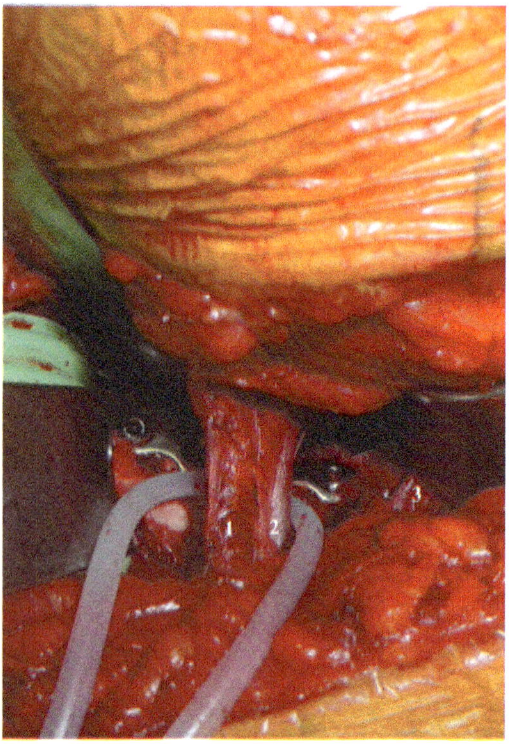

Fig. 4.6 Intraoperative view of the third ilio-inguinal window. (1) Inguinal artery (2) Inguinal vein, (3) spermatic cord

4.3.6 Fracture Reduction

Simultaneous exposure of all three windows is not possible. The iliopsoas with the femoral nerve, the external inguinal vessels with the surrounding lymphatics and the spermatic cord/round ligament are mobilized and retracted alternating. Fractures are reduced sequentially, usually working from dorsal to ventral using the appropriate clamps or ball spike pushers. In medially displaced fractures, lateral traction of the femur can be applied with the help of a pin inserted in the proximal femur or femoral neck. Preshaped plates can be inserted and fixed from anterior to posterior with the alternating use of the different windows. Anatomical reduction and correct screw placement is verified with the fluoroscope using different image settings.

4.3.7 Wound Closure

Before closure, drains are placed in the space of Retzius and along the quadrilateral surface.

Fig. 4.7 Far medial dissection of the ilio-inguinal approach (fourth window). The left and right portions of the M. rectus abdominis and the spermatic cord are retracted with Hohmann-retractors placed on the superior pubic ramus. The bladder is retracted cranially using a malleable retractor. In this case, a laminar spreader is placed in the symphysis to facilitate fracture reduction

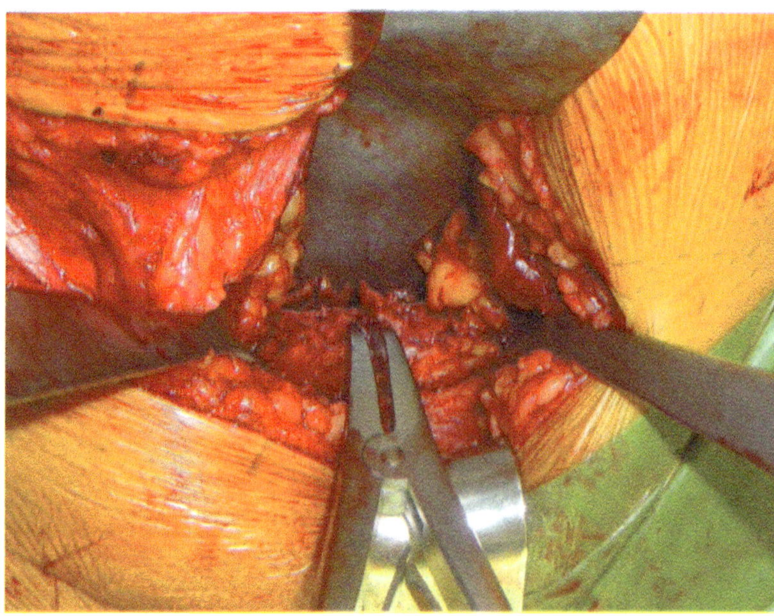

Closure of the different wound layers begins with reattachment of the conjoint tendon of the internal oblique and the transversus abdominis muscles to the inguinal ligament. The roof of the inguinal canal is repaired by closure of the aponeurosis of the external oblique muscle and the rectus sheath, followed by secure reattachment of the abdominal wall origin to the iliac crest. A hernia-free repair and avoidance of entrapment of the spermatic cord and the inguinal nerve should be achieved. The iliopectineal fascia is not repaired. Finally, closure of the subcutaneous tissue and skin is performed.

4.4 Structures at Risk and Complications

4.4.1 Nerves

The overall risk of an intervention-related nerve injury is 2–20% [10–12]. Damage to the lateral femoral cutaneous nerve is the most common complication of the ilio-inguinal approach. Transient neuropraxia can result from tension of the nerve with retractors. Due to its anatomical proximity, damage frequently occurs during the incision of the conjoint tendon or during closure of the aponeurosis of the internal oblique muscle due to its anatomical proximity, leading to various degree of dysesthesia or anesthesia in the lateral thigh. Damage to the femoral or obturator nerves are rare but can lead to significant impairment with weakened hip flexion and knee extension or weakened hip adduction and anesthesia of the medial thigh, respectively. The inguinal nerve follows the spermatic cord/round ligament and is mainly at risk when closing the inguinal canal.

4.4.2 Blood Vessels and Lymphatics

Dissection of the perivascular tissue around the inguinal vessels should be minimized. This limits the risk of vascular injury and also preserves the path of the primary lymphatic trunk to the lower extremity, which passes medial to the vein. Damage to the iliac vessels or corona mortis can lead to severe bleeding and ischemia of the leg. Prolonged excessive retraction of the vessels should be avoided to prevent thrombosis and pulmonary embolism [11].

4.4.3 Spermatic Cord

The spermatic cord contains the vas deferens and the testicular artery. Damage can cause testicular ischemia or infertility.

4.4.4 Heterotopic Ossification

There is a strong association between the operative approach and the prevalence and severity of ectopic bone formation. Letournel noted in a study of 195 acetabular fractures treated with the ilio-inguinal approach that no cases of heterotopic ossification occurred [7]. Matta reported a rate of 2% heterotopic ossifications following an ilio-inguinal approach, versus 20% after an ilio-femoral and 8% after a Kocher-Langenbeck approach [12].

4.4.5 Inguinal Hernia

Closure of the inguinal canal must be conducted carefully to avoid hernias. 2–3.5% suffer of an inguinal hernia after the ilio-inguinal approach [5, 7]. Current inguinal or femoral hernias or previous hernia surgery may complicate the surgical approach, particularly in older individuals. In these cases, it may be prudent to limit or omit the second window exposure, and expand visualization through the first and third windows.

Case Report (Figs. 4.8, 4.9, 4.10 and 4.11)

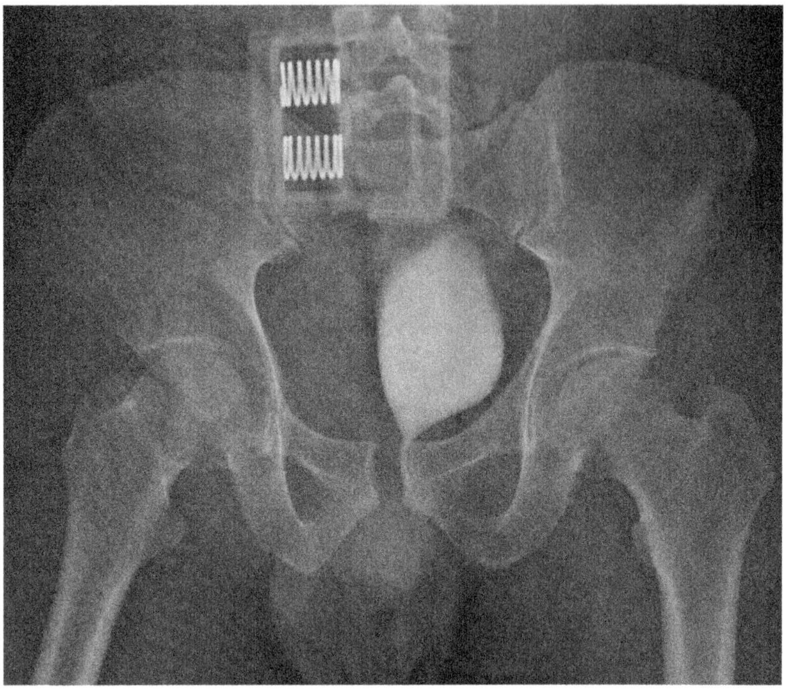

Fig. 4.8 36 year old polytraumatized male patient after a high-energy base-jump accident. The AP-pelvis X-ray shows a dislocated anterior column fracture extending in the ilium, an undislocated hemitransverse fracture, and a pelvic ring fracture type B (open book with rupture of the symphysis and transforaminal fracture of the sacrum left)

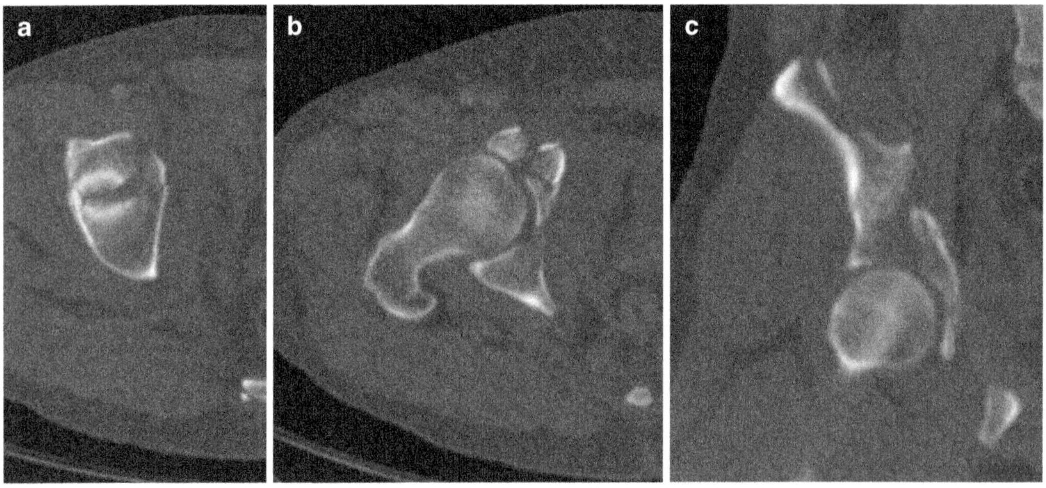

Fig. 4.9 Pre-operative CT scan of the same patient. Axial (**a**, **b**) and coronal (**c**) planes of the fractured acetabulum. Open reduction and internal fixation of the fractures was performed via the ilio-inguinal approach

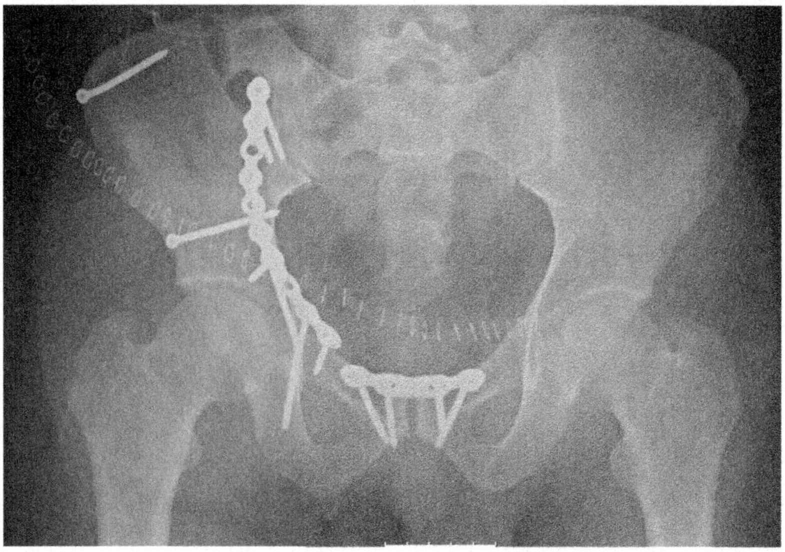

Fig. 4.10 Postoperative AP-pelvis view after fixation of the anterior column with a plate, reduction of the symphysis with a plate and fixation of the ala fracture with two free 3.5 mm cortical screws

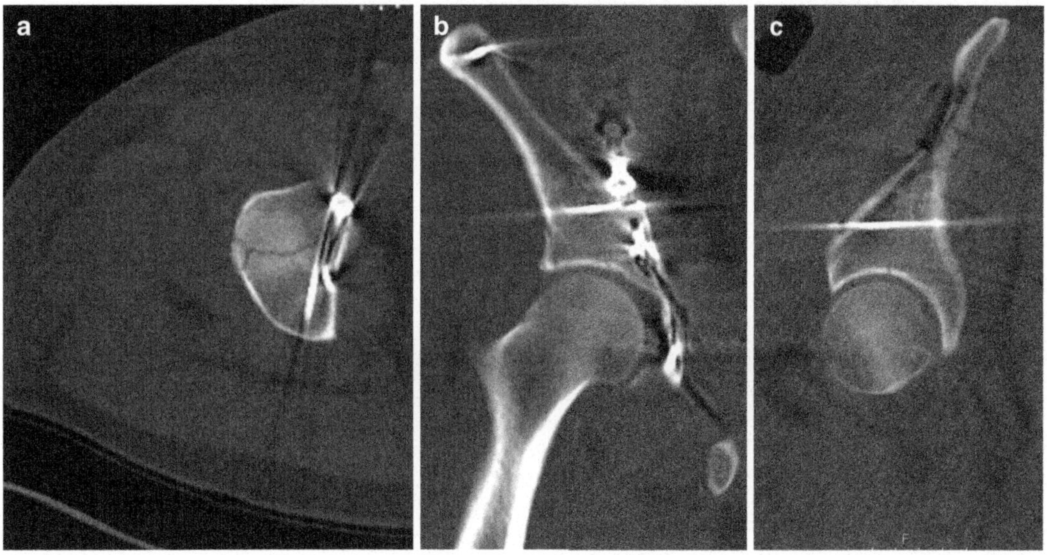

Fig. 4.11 The postoperative CT scan shows anatomical reduction of the fractures in the axial (**a**), coronal (**b**), and sagittal (**c**) planes. Compared to Fig. 4.9, the fracture lines are anatomically reduced

References

1. Judet R, Judet J, Letournel E. Fractures of the acetabulum: classification and surgical approaches for open reduction. Preliminary report. J Bone Joint Surg Am. 1964;46:1615–46.
2. Letournel E. Fractures of the cotyloid cavity, study of a series of 75 cases. J Chir (Paris). 1961;82:47–87.
3. Smith-Petersen MN. A new supra-articular subperiosteal approach to the hip joint. JBJS. 1917;s2–15:592–5.
4. Smith-Petersen MN. Treatment of malum coxae senilis, old slipped upper femoral epiphysis, intrapelvic protrusion of the acetabulum, and coxa plana by means of acetabuloplasty. JBJS. 1936;18:869–80.
5. Letournel E, Judet R. Fractures of the acetabulum. Berlin: Springer; 1993.

6. Letournel E. Acetabulum fractures: classification and management. Clin Orthop Relat Res. 1980;151:81–106.
7. Letournel E. The treatment of acetabular fractures through the ilioinguinal approach. Clin Orthop Relat Res. 1993;292:62–76.
8. Tosounidis TH, Giannoudis VP, Kanakaris NK, et al. The Ilioinguinal approach: state of the art. JBJS Essent Surg Tech. 2018;8:e19.
9. Keel MJ, Bastian JD, Buchler L, et al. Anterior approaches to the acetabulum. Unfallchirurg. 2013;116:213–20.
10. Lehmann W, Hoffmann M, Fensky F, et al. What is the frequency of nerve injuries associated with acetabular fractures? Clin Orthop Relat Res. 2014;472:3395–403.
11. Mardian S, Schaser KD, Hinz P, et al. Fixation of acetabular fractures via the ilioinguinal versus pararectus approach: a direct comparison. Bone Joint J. 2015;97-B:1271–8.
12. Matta JM. Fractures of the acetabulum: accuracy of reduction and clinical results in patients managed operatively within three weeks after the injury. J Bone Joint Surg Am. 1996;78:1632–45.

Anterior Approaches to the Acetabulum

5

Claude H. Sagi

Abstract

A number of surgical approaches exist to allow surgeons the ability to access, reduce, and stabilize acetabular fractures from both the anterior and posterior aspects of the pelvis innominate bone. The anterior approaches in particular have evolved substantially since their inception to the extent that modern acetabular fracture surgery will frequently employ one or more approaches in isolation or in combination. Importantly, while separate camps may exist that favor one "philosophy" or "style," surgeons should recognize the importance and value of each approach such that maximal access can be obtained to optimally expose reduce and stabilize the acetabulum. For example, many surgeons that would consider themselves "purists" in their use of the ilioinguinal approach have come to utilize some form of the "Modified Stoppa" or Anterior Intrapelvic Approach as a more functional medial window for access to the quadrilateral surface and posterior column. This does not represent any form of heresy or deviation; rather, the normal and necessary evolution of surgical techniques that continue to drive the progress and improve the outcomes of fracture surgery and the art of medicine. This chapter will focus on the historical and technical aspects of the "modern" and commonly used anterior surgical exposures for acetabular fracture surgery.

Keywords

Anterior · Surgical exposure · Acetabulum · Ilioinguinal · Iliofemoral · Stoppa · Anterior intrapelvic

5.1 Iliofemoral Approach to the Acetabulum

5.1.1 Introduction and Historical Perspective

As time passes, colloquial usage of various terms tends to overcome the recollection of historical facts; the Iliofemoral and Smith-Petersen approaches are no exception. The anterior approach to the hip joint as originally described by Marius Nygard Smith-Petersen [1] was an inter-nervous surgical exposure for "mold arthroplasty of the hip," not an approach for reduction and fixation of acetabular fractures. While the distal extent of this approach (between the Sartorius and tensor fascia) is similar to other

C. H. Sagi (✉)
Division of Trauma, Department of Orthopaedics and Sports Medicine, University of Cincinnati College of Medicine, Cincinnati, OH, USA
e-mail: sagihc@ucmail.uc.edu

L. Büchler, M. J.B. Keel (eds.), *Fractures of the Hip*, Fracture Management Joint by Joint,
https://doi.org/10.1007/978-3-030-18838-2_5

"versions" of the iliofemoral approach, the proximal portion of the exposure involved elevation of the tensor fascia lata (TFL) and gluteal mass from the outer table of the ilium. The iliofemoral approach for the surgical treatment of acetabular fractures, however, elevates the iliacus muscle (instead of the gluteals and TFL from the outer table) to expose the inner table of the ilium, thus being ideally suited for treatment of fractures involving the anterior column.

The following chapter describes the surgical techniques used to optimize visualization and access using the Iliofemoral approach for reduction and fixation acetabular fractures requiring an anterior surgical approach.

5.1.2 Indications

The iliofemoral approach is useful for accessing the ilium form the iliac crest to the pelvic brim. When combined with either an osteotomy of the anterior superior iliac spine (ASIS) or soft-tissue "sleeve" release of the external oblique, sartorius and inguinal ligament, the anterior column, anterior wall and lateral half of the superior pubic ramus can be visualized. In isolation, the iliofemoral approach can be used to treat high anterior column fractures with or without an associated anterior wall component. In combination with the Anterior Intra-Pelvic approach (see Sect. 5.2) it can be used to successfully treat the Associated Both Column or Anterior plus Posterior Hemitransverse fractures where the cranial extent of the anterior column fracture exits the iliac crest or near the ASIS. This surgical exposure is also very helpful in combined injuries of the acetabulum and pelvic ring when open reduction of the sacro-iliac (SI) joint is required with the patient in the supine position.

5.1.3 Surgical Technique

The patient is positioned flat in the supine position with the lower extremity ipsilateral to the fractured acetabulum draped free. The hip is flexed to approximately 30–45° with a sterile padded triangle or stack of towels under the knee. Ensure that access to the greater trochanter is possible following draping to allow for lateral traction during the course of reduction should it be required. The skin incision is placed along the iliac crest curving distally at the ASIS to proceed longitudinally to the lateral aspect of the patella along the interval between Tensor Fascia Lata (TFL) and Sartorius for a distance of approximately 10 cm. Should proximal extension be required, the incision is turned longitudinally at approximately the mid-axillary line to accommodate the iliac crest which starts to turn back towards the midline posteriorly (Fig. 5.1).

Proximally, the internervous interval between the external oblique (segmental intercostal nerves) and the TFL/Gluteal mass (superficial gluteal nerve) is identified. Recall that from the iliac tubercle posteriorly, the external oblique usually drapes over the crest to varying degrees. The external oblique should be pulled proximally to reveal the interval so that the dissection proceeds straight to bone and does not cut through any muscle fibers of the TFL or external oblique. Adhering to this principle minimizes postoperative pain and facilitates a more reliable fascial closure at the conclusion of the case (Fig. 5.2). The external oblique is then released from its insertion on the iliac crest to expose the fibers of the iliacus muscle on the inner table of the ilium, which is then elevated with a Cobb or other periosteal elevator down to the SI joint pos-

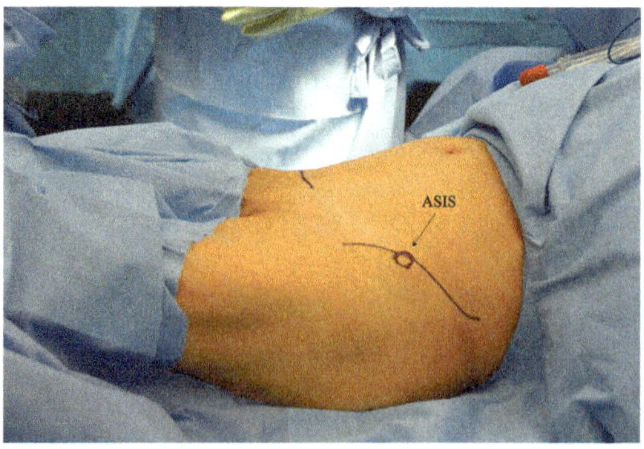

Fig. 5.1 Intraoperative positioning and incision used for iliofemoral approach. Circle delineates the anterior superior iliac spine (ASIS)

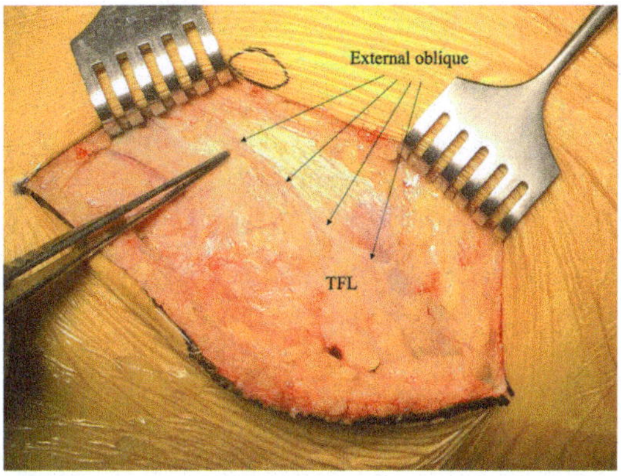

Fig. 5.2 Intraoperative demonstration of the interval between external oblique and tensor fascia (TFL). The forceps are pointing to the ASIS. Note the overhanging nature of the external oblique more posteriorly with the arrows pointing to the inferior margin

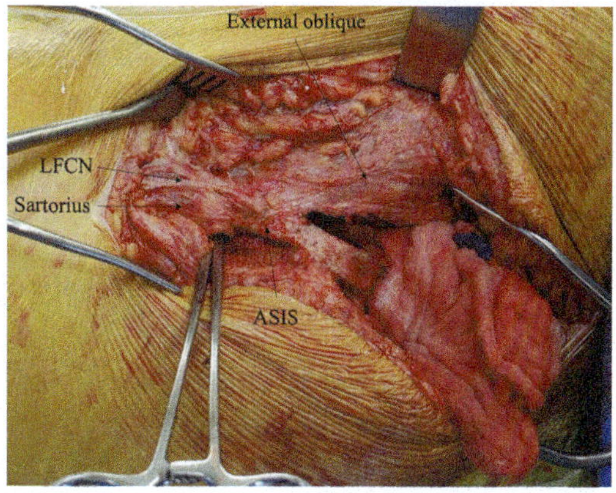

Fig. 5.3 Demonstration of the lateral femoral cutaneous nerve at the level of the ASIS. An incision has been made in the fascia over the lateral border of the sartorius so that the interval between it and the tensor fascia can be developed allowing the nerve to move medially with the sartorius without tension. Sartorius and External Oblique are attached to the ASIS as a digastric ostetomy

teriorly, and to the pelvic brim anteriorly. A small portion (2 cm) of the external oblique insertion just proximal to the ASIS is left attached to the iliac crest so that a "digastric" osteotomy can be performed with the opposing Sartorius if needed (see later).

From the ASIS, an incision is made in the Fascia Lata overlying the TFL and Sartorius muscles taking care to avoid injury to the Lateral Femoral Cutaneous Nerve (LFCN), which has variable anatomic relations to the ASIS and insertion of the Inguinal Ligament. The LFCN should be dissected distally allowing it to be mobilized from the TFL as the Sartorius is retracted medially (Fig. 5.3).

The TFL is then elevated from the external surface of the ilium just enough that the interspinous notch between the ASIS and Anterior Inferior Iliac Spine (AIIS) can be palpated and localized. A small clamp is placed in the interspinous notch to serve as a "target" for the osteotomy, and a curved osteotome is used to osteotomize the ASIS taking care to avoid propagating a crack or fracture line down toward the acetabulum (Fig. 5.4). When the osteotomy is completed both the External Oblique and Sartorius muscles should still be attached to the ASIS to provide opposing muscle tension in digastric fashion after the repair (Fig. 5.5). The osteotomy may take the form of a 90° "step" or

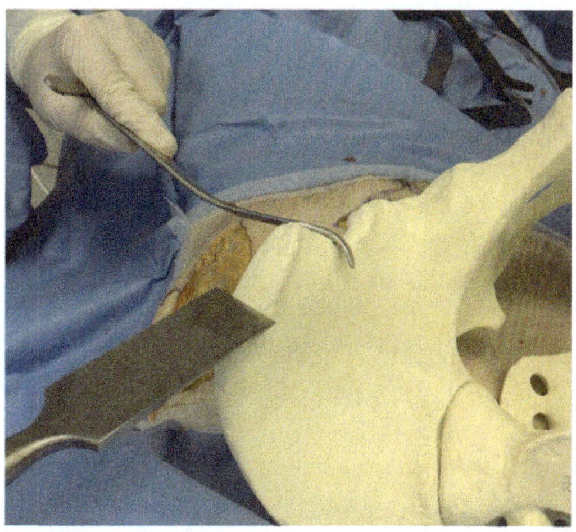

Fig. 5.4 Sawbones model demonstrating a retractor in the interspinous notch serving as a target for the osteotomy which begins on the crest approximately two centimeters posterior to the ASIS

curvilinear path. Alternatively, the external oblique and sartorius can be mobilized as a single sleeve of tissue without an osteotomy if the inguinal ligament is released from its insertion on the ASIS and the LFCN is dissected as described above [2].

With the osteotomy complete, the abdominal wall and iliacus can be retracted medially to a

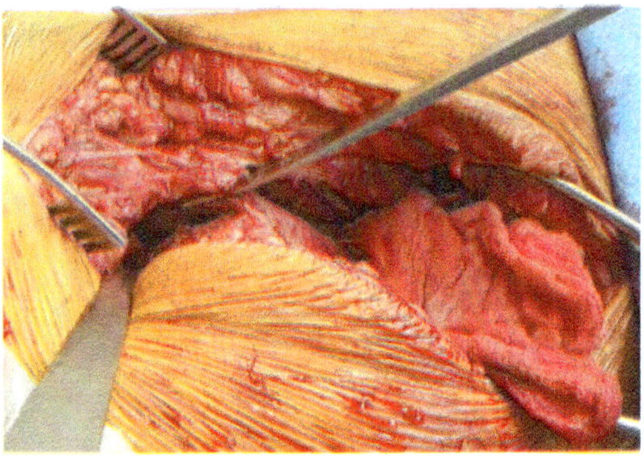

Fig. 5.5 Osteotomy has been performed with sartorius and external oblique remaining attached to the ASIS. The LFCN can be seen moving medially with sartorius and the ASIS, thus protecting it

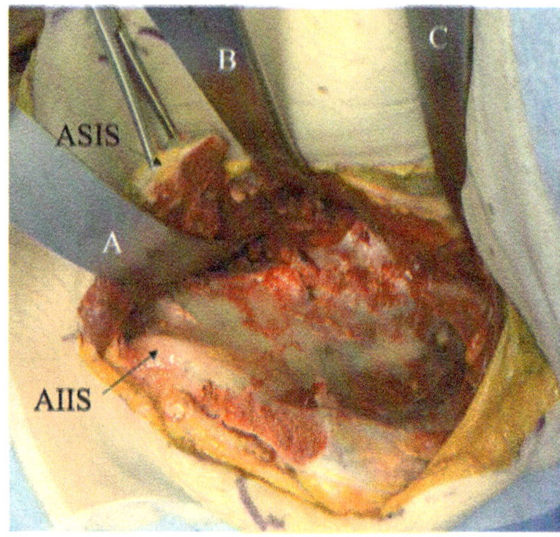

Fig. 5.6 Retractors are positioned over the pelvic brim (A), into the sacral ala lateral to the SI joint (B), and over the iliac crest under the ilio-lumbar ligament (C)

greater extent, giving improved visualization and access to the inner table of the ilium. The LFCN moves with the ASIS and abdominal wall medially and injury is prevented by releasing the fascia over the TFL distally so that the nerve is not tethered and can move freely.

Within the pelvis, the iliacus and iliopsoas tendon are elevated from the psoas gutter/pubic root and retracted medially to expose the lower aspect of the anterior column and pelvic brim down to the lateral aspect of the superior pubic ramus and the base of the anterior wall. If desired, the origin of the direct head of the Rectus Femoris can be detached from the AIIS (leaving a stump of rectus tendon attached to the AIIS for later repair) to provide complete exposure of the anterior wall of the acetabulum. Key retractors and their respective positions are as follows: a sharp Hohmann underneath the iliolumbar ligament at the posterior iliac crest, a sharp Hohmann into the sacral ala just medial to the SI joint, a narrow malleable over the pelvic brim, or a sharp Hohmann at the base of the anterior wall or medial to the pubic root (Fig. 5.6).

5.1.4 Reduction Clamp Opportunities Through the Iliofemoral Approach

5.1.4.1 Sacroiliac Joint

A two-screw technique utilizing a Jungbluth or Farabeuf reduction clamp generally best serves the purpose for reducing the SI joint from an anterior approach. A 3.5 mm screw is placed into the ilium just lateral to the SI joint, directed from the brim posteriorly into the posterior inferior iliac spine (PIIS). A second screw is placed into the sacral ala just medial to the SI joint and directed distally along the length of the sacrum paralleling the SI joint lateral to the sacral foramina (Fig. 5.7).

5.1.4.2 Anterior Column (Cranial Extent to Iliac Crest)

A small window is created by detaching a small portion of the TFL from the iliac crest and a Farabeuf clamp is placed around the iliac crest to manipulate the ilium (Fig. 5.8).

5.1.4.3 Anterior Column (Distal Extent to Pelvic Brim)

Blunt dissection over the brim, down the quadrilateral surface to the lesser sciatic notch lateral to the obturator nerve is undertaken with a periosteal elevator. The distal tine of an angled jaw clamp (quad clamp) is then guided down the quadrilateral surface into the lesser sciatic notch while the proximal tine of the clamp is placed onto the pelvic brim lateral to the anterior column fracture line or onto the outer table of the ilium under the abductors and TFL depending on the vector required (Fig. 5.9). Similarly, the angled

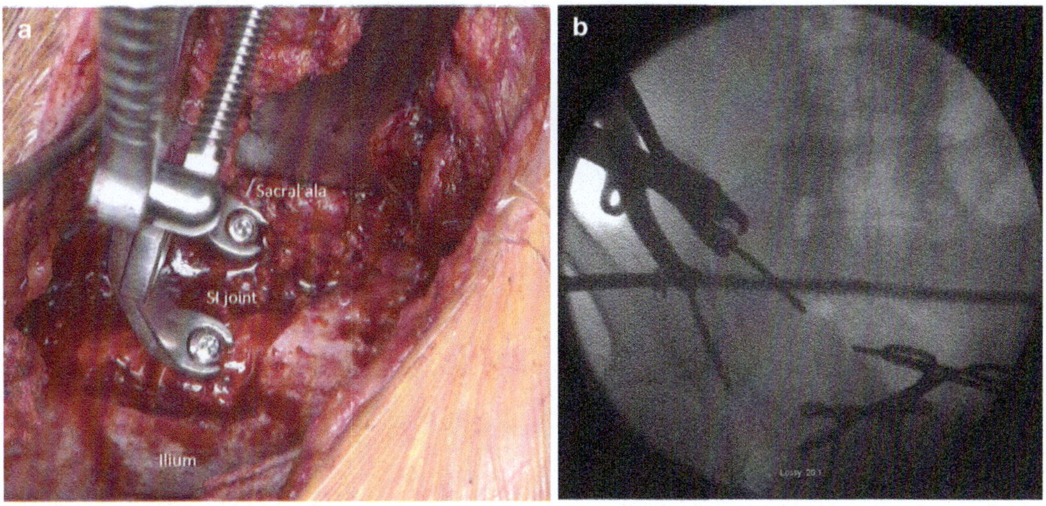

Fig. 5.7 (**a**) Jungbluth retractor reducing the SI joint with screw fixation into the sacral ala and iliac wing. (**b**) Intraoperative fluoroscopic image demonstrating Jungbluth reduction of the SI joint from anterior through the iliofemoral approach

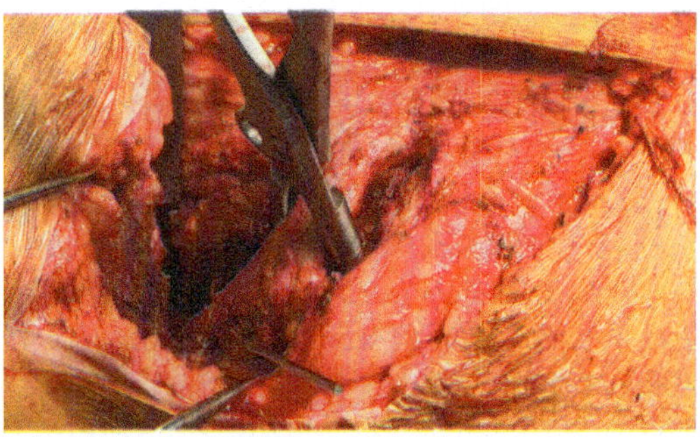

Fig. 5.8 Farabeuf clamp placed through a small window in the tensor fascia to manipulate and facilitate reduction of the iliac wing and cranial portion of the anterior column

jaw clamp can be placed under the abductors onto a posterior and superior wall fragment that is frequently encountered with an associated both column type fracture pattern (Fig. 5.9).

5.1.5 Closure

The direct head of the Rectus femoris is repaired back to the AIIS using a heavy braided non-absorbable suture to re-attach the tendon back to the residual stump of its insertion left behind at the time of tenotomy. The ASIS osteotomy is repaired with a single 3.5 mm lag screw directed from the tip of the ASIS posteriorly into the iliac tubercle after reduction and compression with pointed reduction forceps keeping the opposing external oblique and Sartorius muscles attached (Fig. 5.10). A single drain is placed into the internal iliac fossa. The External Oblique muscle is reattached to the crest by suturing it to the fascial attachment of the TFL/Gluteal mass onto the iliac crest. The superficial and deep fascial layers of the thigh can be closed in a single layer with absorbable suture then subcutaneous tissue and skin in layers. Hip precautions are not necessary for the ASIS osteotomy.

5.2 Anterior Intra-Pelvic Approach to the Acetabulum

5.2.1 Introduction and Historical Perspective

The Anterior Intra-Pelvic (AIP) surgical approach for reduction and fixation of acetabular fractures as we know it today evolved from a technique described by Rives and Stoppa for applying Dacron mesh in the repair of inguinal herniae [3]. The approach utilized a midline ver-

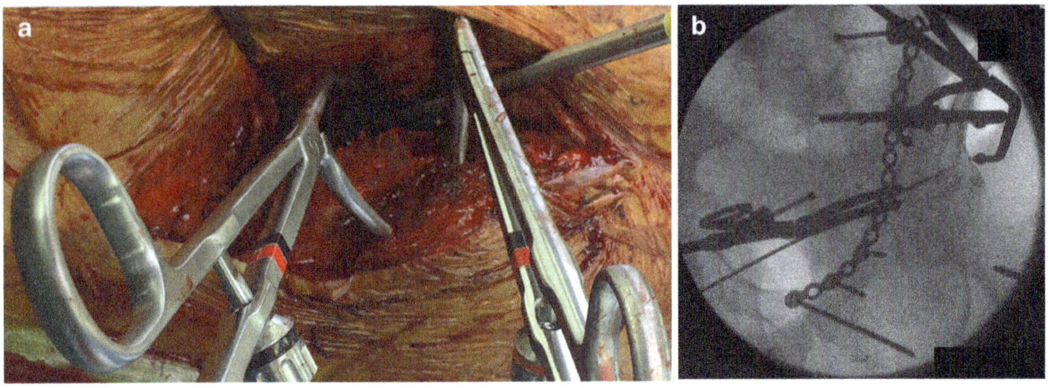

Fig. 5.9 (**a**) Reduction clamp placed around interspinous notch onto the outer table of the ilium to reduce the anterior column, or similarly placed to reduce a high superior posterior wall fragment with an associated both column fracture. (**b**) Intra-operative fluoroscopic image demonstrating clamp reduction described in (**a**)

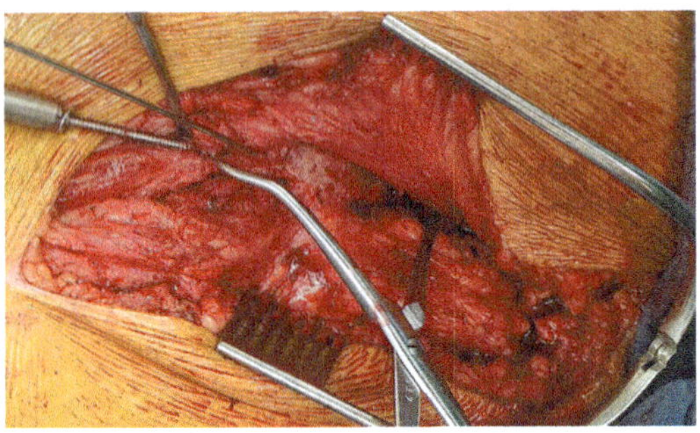

Fig. 5.10 Repair of the ASIS osteotomy with clamp reduction and single lag screw placement into the iliac tubercle. A 2 mm Kirschner wire is placed to help stabilize the fragment while clamping and compressing

tical split in the rectus abdominis followed by dissection along the superior pubic ramus and anterior pelvic brim to expose the inner surface of the anterior abdominal wall. Separate reports by Hirvensalo [4] and Cole/Bolhofner [5], in 1993 and 1994 respectively, reported on the results of acetabular reduction and fixation utilizing an extension of the surgical dissection described by Rives and Stoppa to include exposure along the entire course of the pelvic brim posteriorly to the sacro-iliac joint. These early descriptions of the "Modified Stoppa" described access to the lower portion of the anterior column and pelvic brim from the symphysis to the SI joint. This allowed for reduction and stabilization of the caudal portion of the anterior column as well as the quadrilateral surface with buttress and infra-pectineal plating, respectively. While some attention was paid to the more distal aspects of the quadrilateral surface and posterior column, the initial descriptions of this technique did not focus on manipulation and instrumentation of these areas as such.

Over the last two decades there have been a number of refinements to the surgical technique which have led to improved visualization and access for the placement of reduction clamps and fixation [6]. Recent publications reporting results and complications of acetabular fracture reduction using the AIP approach are similar to those reported using the more traditional ilio-inguinal approach, with 70–80% anatomic reductions and complication rates between 8% and 13% [7–9].

The potential benefits of the AIP approach are:

1. Improved access to comminuted fractures of the quadrilateral surface.
2. Improved access to the posterior column from the sciatic notch to the ischial spine.
3. Avoiding dissection of the inguinal canal, femoral nerve, and external iliac vessels.
4. Avoiding dissection through scarred tissue and mesh from previous herniorraphy.

The following chapter describes the surgical techniques used to optimize visualization and access using the AIP approach for reduction and fixation of acetabular fractures requiring an anterior surgical approach.

5.2.2 Indications

The AIP surgical approach can be used for acetabular fractures that require (either in isolation or in combination with other staged approaches) anterior exposure and access to the pelvis and acetabulum. This would include the following fracture patterns: anterior column, anterior column/anterior wall, anterior plus poster hemitransverse, associated both column, T-shaped fractures (staged and combined with posterior approach), transtectal transverse +/− posterior wall (staged and combined with posterior approach), and acetabular fractures associated with symphyseal and/or sacro-iliac joint disruption. Finally, geriatric acetabular fractures or insufficiency fractures associated with osteopenia/osteoporosis where quadrilateral surface comminution and dome impaction are present are well suited to this surgical approach for reduction and fixation.

5.2.3 Surgical Technique

The patient is positioned supine on the operative table. A urinary catheter is placed to deflate the bladder helping to avoid injury, improve visualization, and monitor urine output/fluid balance during the course of the procedure. The leg ipsilateral to the fractured acetabulum is placed over a padded triangle to flex the hip approximately 35–45°, relaxing the iliacus/psoas muscles, the femoral vein, and the external iliac vessels (Fig. 5.11). The surgeon is positioned on the side of the patient contralateral to the injury. Contrary to popular belief, the patient should NOT be tilted on to the affected side to improve visualization through the AIP window as this places pressure on the greater trochanter, which pushes the femoral head medially into the pelvis and displaces the fracture. Lateral traction via the greater trochanter is applied to extract the femoral head from the pelvis and provide some provisional reduction of the anterior and posterior columns (Fig. 5.12). Longitudinal traction is NOT recommended because this tensions the iliacus and femoral/external iliac neurovascular structures making the dissection more difficult and placing the neurovascular structures at greater risk.

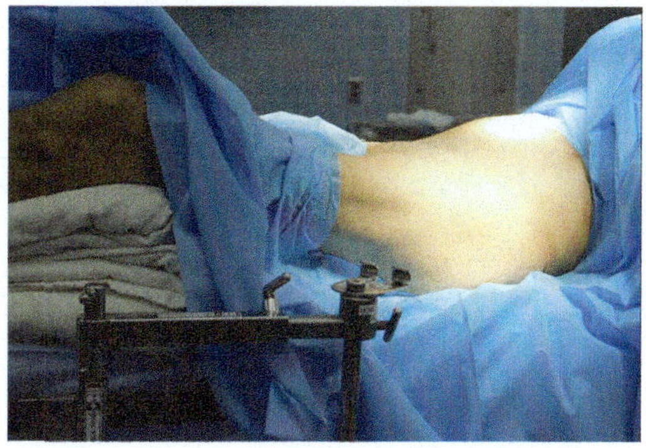

Fig. 5.11 Supine positioning of the patient with ipsilateral leg draped free and hip flexed to ~40°

Depending on various patient factors such as previous incisional scars, exploratory laparotomy or the presence of herniae, the skin incision can be either midline vertical or horizontal in the style of a Pfannenstiel incision. The anterior rectus fascia is exposed to visualize the midline linea alba and decussation of the recuts fascial fibers, but care is taken to avoid excessive undermining of the subcutaneous fatty layer and excessive lateral dissection which can place the spermatic cord and round ligament at risk. Optimal exposure is NOT contingent upon a wide lateral dissection in the superficial layers, it is dependent upon mobilization of the rectus abdominis muscle which requires a high proximal split along the linea alba and a low distal release of the rectus insertion off of the anterior aspect of the pubic body. Reluctance to adhere to this principle will significantly diminish the operating surgeon's field of view and access for reduction clamps/maneuvers. If the midline split of the linea alba proceeds too proximal and the peritoneal cavity is entered, simply take 3-0 chromic suture to repair the peritoneum and place a single figure eight suture in the anterior rectus fascia to prevent further proximal splitting. The rectus abdominis has a broad insertion along the entire superior and anterior aspect of the ipsilateral pubic body and should be released (but not completely detached) anteriorly and lateral to the pubic tubercle (Fig. 5.13).

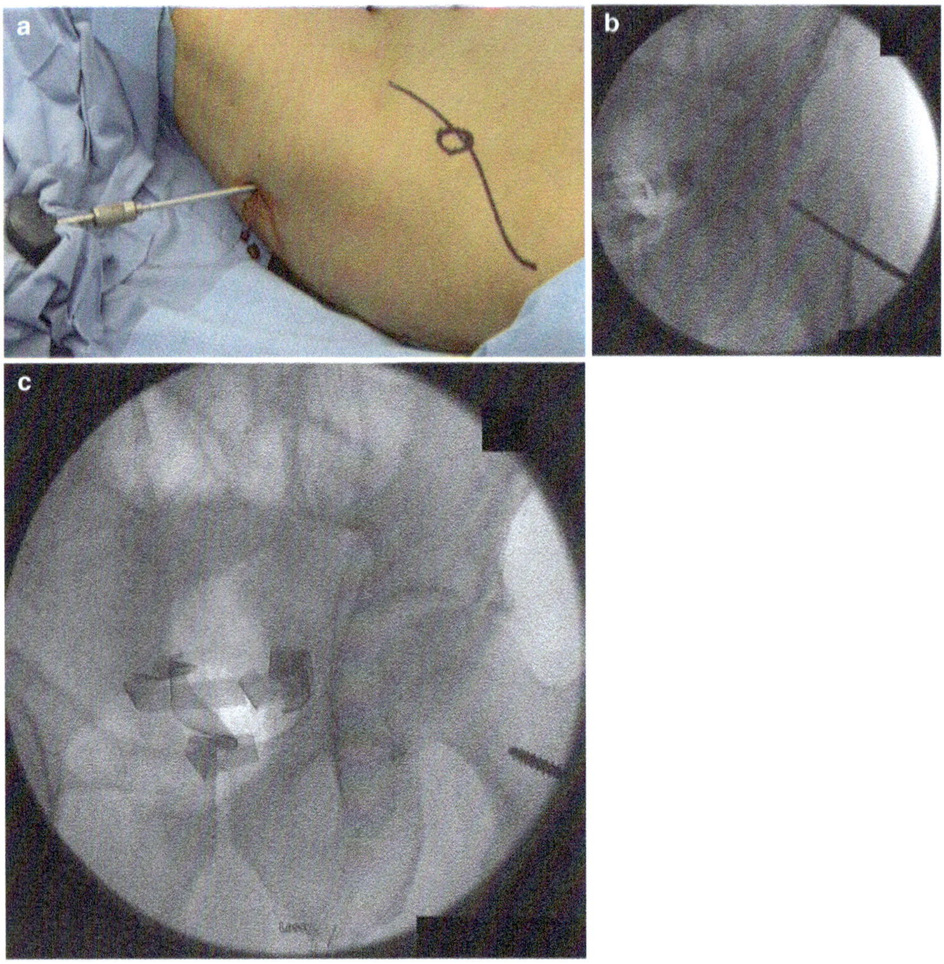

Fig. 5.12 (**a**) Lateral traction applied with Schanz pin through the greater trochanter. (**b**) Intra-operative fluoroscopic view of the acetabulum prior to lateral traction showing intra-pelvic position of the femoral head and displacement of the anterior and posterior columns. (**c**) Intra-operative fluoroscopic view of the acetabulum following lateral traction showing lateralization of the femoral head and improved positioning of the anterior and posterior columns via capsulotaxis

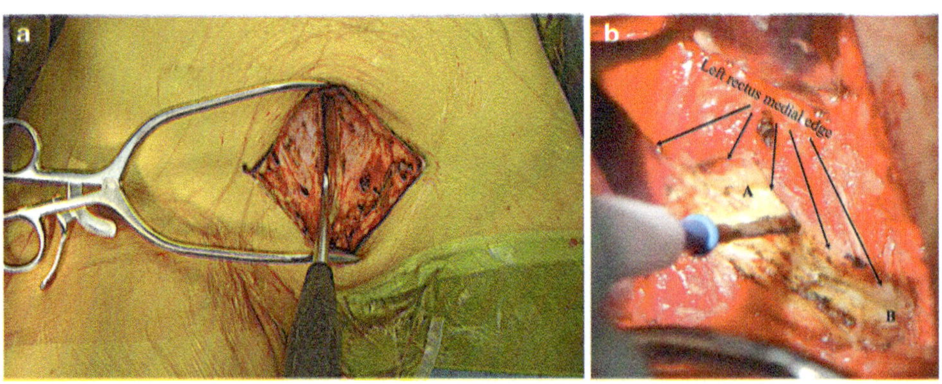

Fig. 5.13 (**a**) Intra-operative clinical photograph showing proximal release of the rectus abdominis. (**b**) Intra-operative clinical photograph showing distal release of the rectus abdominis down the anterior aspect of the pubic body from the pubic tubercle (A) to the lower symphysis (B)

Apart from a single thin layer of transversalis fascia, there is no posterior rectus fascia below the umbilicus and arcuate line. The simplest way to enter the true pelvis and stay out of the peritoneal cavity is to make a small incision in the transversalis fascia just behind the pubic symphysis to enter the potential space of Retzius. With blunt dissection, sweep the index finger between the bladder and posterior surface of the pubic body, then distal to proximal between the superior/anterior surface of the bladder and under surface of the rectus to break down any adhesions. This is important because as the exposure is developed, the rectus will be turned and retracted toward the ipsilateral injured side. The pelvic contents and bladder need to be retracted away from the injured side to allow visualization of the quadrilateral surface and posterior column, if the adhesions to the undersurface of the rectus are not cleared then the pelvic viscera will be pulled into the visual field, hampering the exposure and access to the acetabulum. If during the course of exposure or reduction/fixation the surgeon finds that the bladder is injured, a simple repair with absorbable suture is undertaken. If, however, an injury to the base of the bladder in the region of the trigone, urinary sphincter or urethra is identified then urological consultation is recommended.

A narrow Deaver retractor is placed under the rectus to retract it laterally and a sharp Hohmann retractor is placed lateral to the pubic tubercle anterior to the superior pubic ramus while a lap sponge is placed into the space of Retzius with a malleable retractor to protect the bladder. Care should be taken to avoid excessive downward pressure on the malleable as it can cause damage to the bladder neck and urethra. Similar to the ilioinguinal approach, the ilio-pectineal fascia needs to be released from the superior pubic ramus to allow communication between the true and false pelvis. With the AIP approach this communication is simply developed in the reverse direction: from the true pelvis into the false pelvis. After the iliopectineal fascia is released the underlying muscle fibers of the pectineus muscle come into view and these can be elevated from the superior ramus with a Cobb or other periosteal elevator.

Further dissection along the superior ramus and pelvic brim lateral to the iliopectineal fascia requires releasing the fascia of the iliacus muscle from the pelvic brim so that a retractor can be placed under the iliacus. The external iliac vein and artery are located on the medial edge of the iliacus muscle. In order to prevent injury to the external iliac vein, it should be retracted superiorly and laterally along with the rectus and iliacus muscles to expose the internal iliac fossa. In order to accomplish this safely, the surgeon must address two issues:

Firstly, the surgeon needs to determine if there is a distal branching of the internal iliac vessels. The AIP approach takes place essentially within the axilla created by the branching of the internal and external iliac vessels from the common iliac. Occasionally, the internal iliac has a very distal branching with an "axilla" at the level of the pelvic brim. When this situation occurs, it limits the posterior and distal exposures along the brim and quadrilateral surface respectively, necessitating an alternate exposure such as the ilioinguinal (Fig. 5.14).

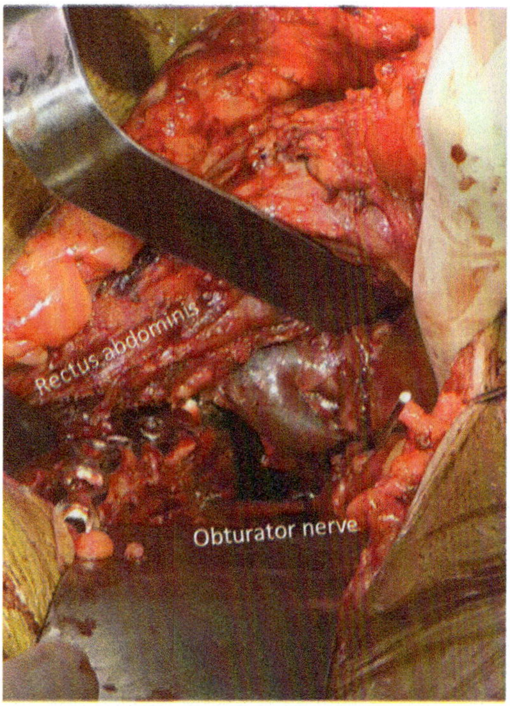

Fig. 5.14 Intraoperative photograph of a low-branching iliac system occurring sitally along the brim (with permission Marcus Sciadini, MD)

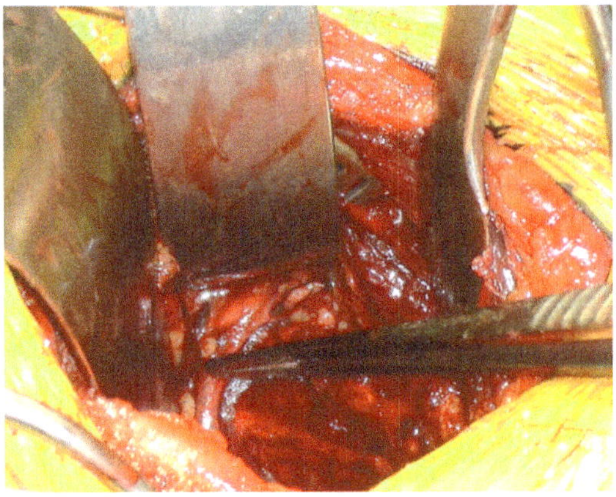

Fig. 5.15 Intra-operative clinical photograph showing the anastomotic vessels, noting the improved access to these vessels with this approach

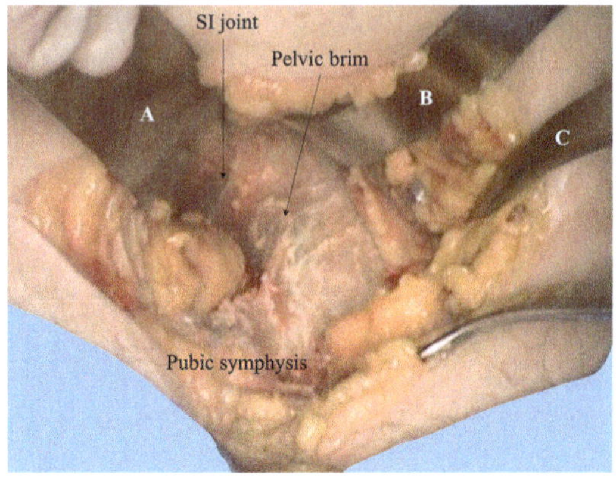

Fig. 5.16 Intra-operative photograph showing retractor placed anterior to SI joint on the pelvic brim (A), underneath the iliacus muscle to expose the internal iliac fossa and protect the external iliac vessels (B) and into the psoas gutter (C) to give a surgeon's view of the pelvic brim from symphysis to SI joint and lower third of internal iliac fossa

Secondly, the surgeon needs to determine if an anastomosis between the external iliac and obturator vessels (the so-called corona mortise) exists. Exposure of the internal iliac fossa by elevation of the external iliac vessels along with the iliacus muscle will not be possible if the external iliac vessels are tethered to the obturator vessels since retraction and elevation will tear the anastomotic or obturator vessels. If these vessels are identified during the course of the dissection, they must be ligated prior to proceeding farther posteriorly along the brim and underneath the iliacus (Fig. 5.15).

With the anastomotic vessels ligated, the external iliac vessels can be retracted farther laterally to expose the underlying iliacus muscle and fascia. A malleable retractor is then gently pushed along the pelvic brim back to the lateral aspect of the SI joint to retract the pelvic viscera away from the acetabulum. While gently retracting the external iliac vein way from the medial edge of the iliacus muscle and pelvic brim, the fascia along the brim is incised from just lateral to the SI joint forward to the pubic root to allow elevation of the iliacus muscle away from the internal iliac fossa. Once this plane is developed, a malleable or other flat retractor is placed underneath the iliacus to protect the external iliac vessels for the duration of the case.

With the iliacus being retracted laterally, sharp dissection is required to continue to release the iliopsoas tendon fibers away from the pubic root and into the psoas gutter. A second sharp Hohmann retractor is then placed into the psoas gutter lateral to the pubic root to retract the iliopsoas tendon, thus completing the more cranial portion of the AIP exposure which allows visualization of the entire lower half of the internal iliac fossa back to the SI joint and lower aspect of the anterior column from anterior inferior iliac spine distally (Fig. 5.16).

The lower portion of the AIP approach involves exposure of the quadrilateral surface and medial surface of the posterior column. At this point, the next order of business is to identify, mobilize, and protect the obturator nerve, which can be found in the fatty tissue immediately below the pelvic brim along the upper portion of the quadrilateral surface laying on the origin of the obturator internus muscle fascia. Acetabular fractures that require anterior approaches often have central dislocation of the femoral head with intra-pelvic intrusion of the quadrilateral surface and posterior column, which places the obturator neurovascular bundle under tension. The surgeon will frequently find that unless the femoral head has been retracted laterally, it can be difficult to isolate and safely mobilize the obturator nerve, making another good case for lateral femoral traction at the beginning of the case. The nerve is traced from the obturator foramen posteriorly to its exit from the lumbosacral plexus so that it can be manipulated easily and the surgeon can work both medial and lateral to the nerve as needed without tension and iatrogenic neuropraxia (Fig. 5.17). Carefully release the upper lateral portion of the obturator membrane to un-tether and further mobilize the obturator nerve.

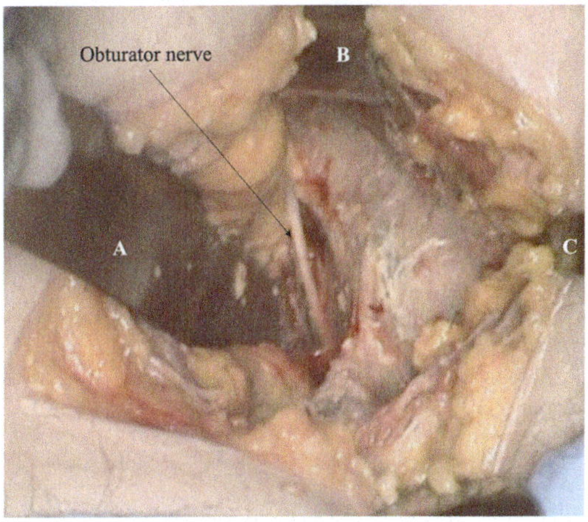

Fig. 5.17 Intra-operative clinical photograph showing mobilization of the obturator nerve so that the surgeon can work both medial and lateral to the nerve. In this photograph the malleable (A) is in the greater sciatic foramen resting on the posterior medial aspect of the posterior column, medial to the obturator nerve to expose the quadrilateral surface without any tension on the nerve. Retractors (B) and (C) are under the iliacus and in the psoas gutter, respectively

Releasing the obturator membrane and mobilizing the obturator nerve from its tunnel also exposes and excellent location for reduction clamp placement (see below).

An important point should be made about the obturator artery and vein at this stage. These vessels are located immediately inferior to the nerve that they accompany and are often traumatically disrupted with fracture patterns that are addressed via an anterior approach. If, however, they are not, they should be isolated and ligated to avoid injury and bleeding during difficult reduction maneuvers involving the quadrilateral surface and distal posterior column. Unlike the obturator nerve, the vessels send many branches into the floor of the pelvis and cannot be mobilized and manipulated as easily as the nerve.

Once the nerve has been mobilized and protected, exposure of the quadrilateral surface and medial aspect of the posterior column is accomplished by elevating the obturator internus muscle from the brim distally to the ischial spine and posteriorly to the greater sciatic foramen (Fig. 5.18). Recall that the hip is flexed during anterior exposures, so the sciatic nerve is under some tension. Careless plunging into the greater sciatic foramen can injure the sciatic nerve in addition to the superior gluteal neurovascular bundle. A malleable retractor can be placed medial to the obturator nerve but lateral to the obturator internus muscle to safely expose the

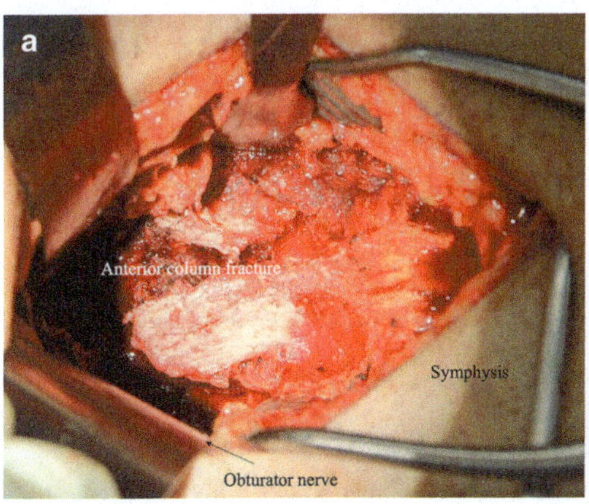

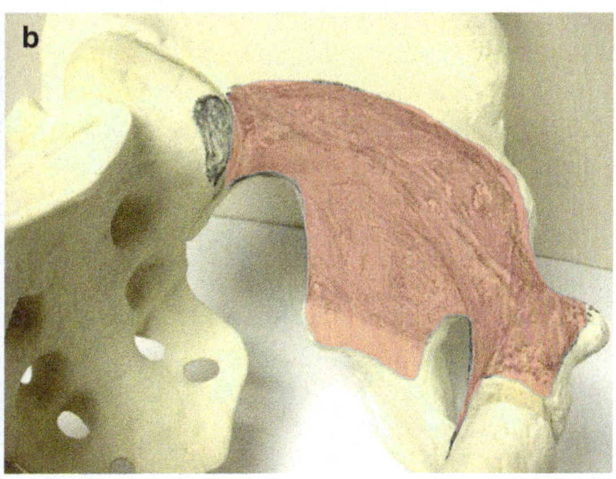

Fig. 5.18 (**a**) Intra-operative clinical photograph showing retraction of the obturator internus muscle medial exposing the quadrilateral surface and posterior column, with no tension on the obturator nerve. (**b**) Schematic demonstrating the visible and accessible territory following complete AIP exposure

entire quadrilateral surface and posterior column form the brim and sciatic notch down to the ischial spine. To keep the pelvic viscera retracted to the contralateral pelvis, retractors can be placed gently into the greater or lesser sciatic foramina.

Should exposure of the upper portion of the anterior column be required to address the full extent of the fracture, a separate lateral surgical window (Ilio-inguinal window #1, or ilio-femoral) along the iliac crest will need to be utilized as discussed above in Sect. 5.1.

5.2.4 Reduction Clamp Opportunities Through the AIP

5.2.4.1 Anterior Column

Reduction of the anterior column generally proceeds from cranial to caudal and from posterior to anterior. If the cranial extent exits the iliac crest or in the region of the interspinous notch, then a separate lateral will be required (see Sect. 5.1). Reduction of the posterior (brim portion) and caudal/anterior (ramus or pubic root) aspects of the anterior column can be accomplished through the AIP window with various pointed reduction forceps (such as a Weber clamp) or an angled-jaw clamp as follows: For the posterior aspect of the anterior column reduction along the brim, one tine of the reduction clamp can be placed over the brim posteriorly into the internal iliac fossa while the other tine can be placed into a drill hole in the quadrilateral surface or the posterior column. For reduction of the caudal or anterior aspect of the anterior column fracture that frequently exits in the region of the pubic root or lateral ramus, one tine can be placed into the psoas gutter while the other tine is placed into the obturator foramen just lateral to the obturator nerve, taking care to visualize the nerve the entire time. Release of the obturator membrane as mentioned above is helpful in mobilizing the nerve to allow clamp placement in this fashion (Figs. 5.19 and 5.20).

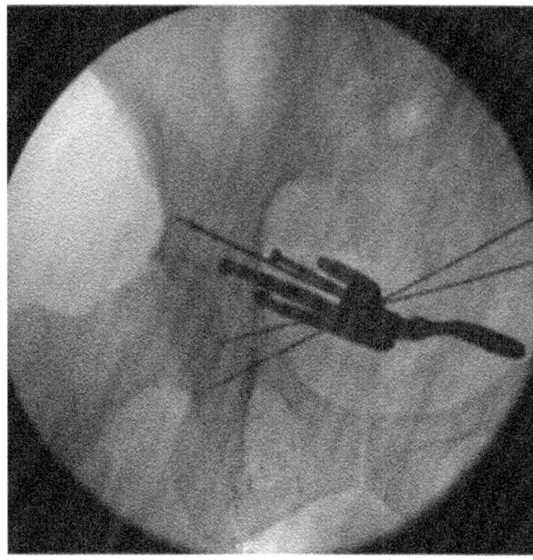

Fig. 5.19 Intra-operative fluoroscopic image demonstrating clamp placement for reduction of the lower more caudal portion of an anterior column fracture through the AIP window

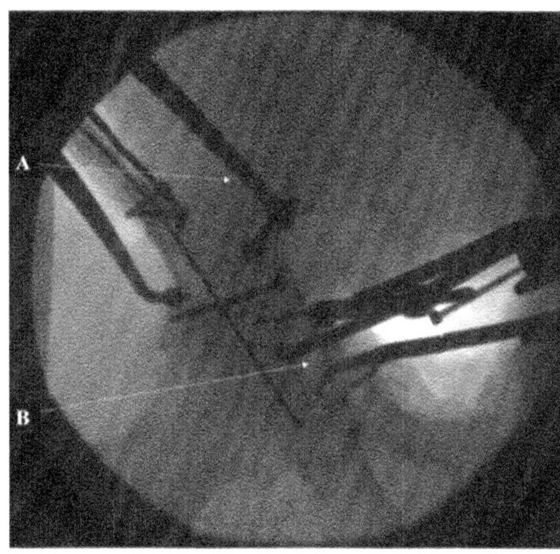

Fig. 5.20 Intra-operative fluoroscopic image demonstrating clamp placement for reduction of a high anterior column fracture (A) requiring use of lateral window for cranial portion of the fracture and "queen tong" placement, and reduction of the lower more caudal portion of the anterior column with a pointed reduction clamp through the AIP window (B)

5.2.4.2 Posterior Column

Reduction maneuvers and clamp placement for the posterior column will depend upon various characteristics of the fracture pattern [10]. If the fracture into the posterior column is high (above or into the greater sciatic notch), then the purchase into the posterior column can be the greater

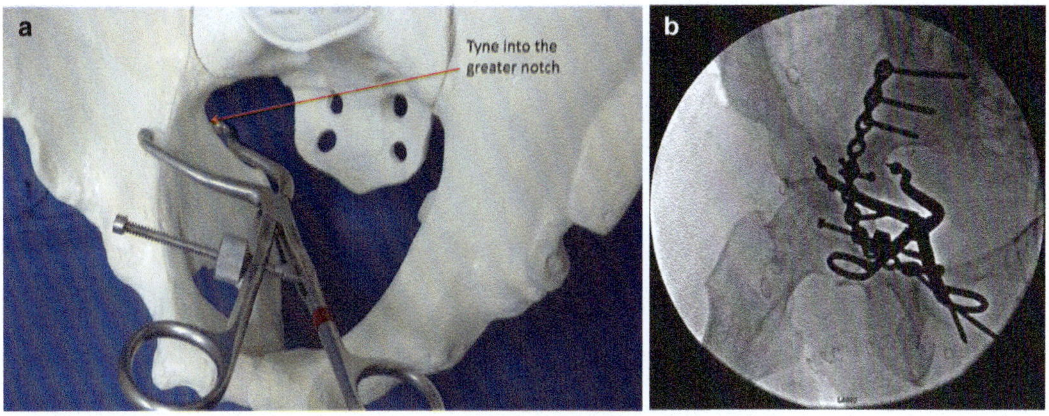

Fig. 5.21 (**a**) Model demonstrating clamp placement for reduction of a high posterior column fracture with the clamp tine in the greater sciatic notch. (A) Tyne into the greater notch. (**b**) Intra-operative fluoroscopic image demonstrating clamp placement for reduction of a high posterior column fracture with lower tine in greater sciatic notch

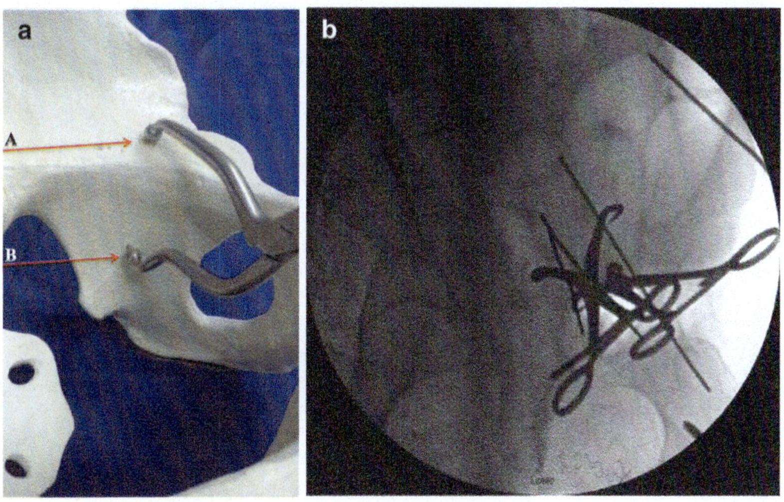

Fig. 5.22 (**a**) Model demonstrating clamp placement for reduction of an intermediate posterior column fracture with the lower clamp tine on the quadrilateral surface. Tine (A) over brim, and tine (B) in drill hole in quadrilateral surface. (**b**) Intra-operative fluoroscopic image demonstrating clamp placement for reduction of an intermediate posterior column fracture with lower clamp tine on the quadrilateral surface

notch itself (Fig. 5.21). If the fracture line exits the posterior column between the sciatic notch and the ischial spine (intermediate), then a drill hole in the posterior column or quadrilateral surface can be used as a point of purchase for the clamp's tine with the other tine up over the brim in the internal iliac fossa (Fig. 5.22). For fractures that exit low in the posterior column around the level of the ischial spine, reduction clamps (such as an angled jaw clamp through the AIP or collinear reduction clamp through the lateral window) will need to be placed into the lesser sciatic foramen with the other tine on the brim of the pelvis (Fig. 5.23). Finally, fractures of the posterior column can have a more atypical orientation running along the length of the column. In this scenario, a clamp can be placed perpendicular to this fracture line with one tine in the obturator foramen and the other tine in the greater sciatic foramen (Fig. 5.24).

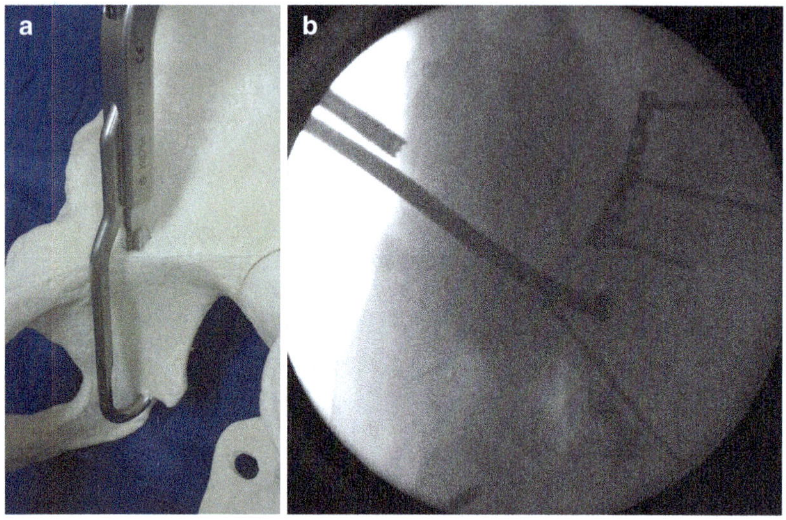

Fig. 5.23 (**a**) Model demonstrating clamp placement for reduction of a low posterior column fracture with the collinear reduction clamp in the lesser sciatic notch (applied through lateral window). (**b**) Intra-operative fluoroscopic image demonstrating clamp placement for reduction of a low posterior column fracture with collinear reduction clamp in the lesser sciatic notch

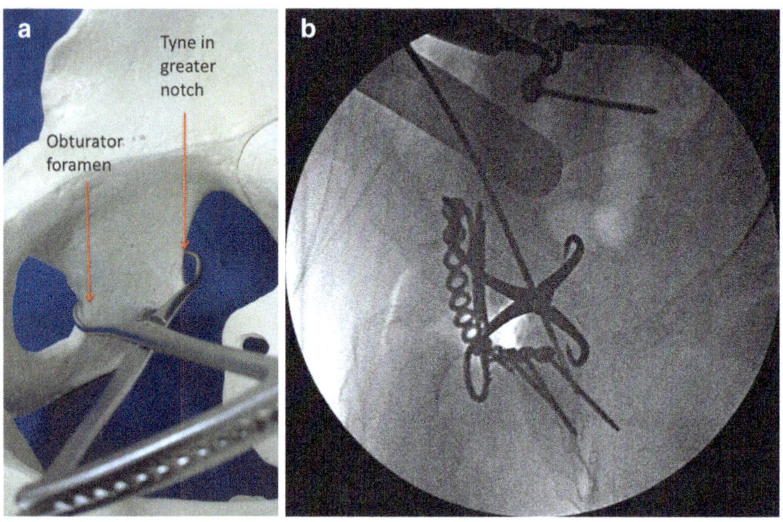

Fig. 5.24 (**a**) Model demonstrating clamp placement for reduction of a vertical oblique posterior column fracture with the clamp tines in the obturator foramen and greater sciatic foramen. (**b**) Intra-operative fluoroscopic image demonstrating clamp placement for reduction of a vertical oblique posterior column fracture with clamp tines in the obturator foramen and greater sciatic foramen

5.2.5 Closure

A single drain is placed into the retropubic space anterior to the bladder. Either a running or interrupted #1 suture is used to re-approximate the anterior rectus fascia. Closure of the single layer of transversalis fascia posterior to the rectus is not necessary. Subcutaneous tissues are closed to assure no dead space remains where a hematoma or seroma may form post-operatively.

References

1. Smith-Petersen MN. Approach to and exposure of the hip joint for mold arthroplasty. J Bone Joint Surg Am. 1949;31A(1):40–6.
2. Sagi HC, Bolhofner B. Osteotomy of the anterior superior iliac spine as an adjunct to improve access and visualization through the lateral window. J Orthop Trauma. 2015;29(8):e266–9.
3. Stoppa RE, Rives JL, Warlaumont CR, Palot JP, Verhaeghe PJ, Delattre JF. The use of Dacron in the repair of hernias of the groin. Surg Clin North Am. 1984;64(2):269–85.

4. Hirvensalo E, Lindahl J, Böstman O. A new approach to the internal fixation of unstable pelvic fractures. Clin Orthop Relat Res. 1993;297:28–32.
5. Cole JD, Bolhofner BR. Acetabular fracture fixation via a modified Stoppa limited intrapelvic approach. Description of operative technique and preliminary treatment results. Clin Orthop Relat Res. 1994;305:112–23.
6. Sagi HC, Afsari A, Dziadosz D. The anterior intrapelvic (modified stoppa) approach for acetabular fracture fixation. J Orthop Trauma. 2010;24(5):263–70.
7. Shazar N, Eshed I, Ackshota N, Hershkovich O, Khazanov A, Herman A. Comparison of acetabular fracture reduction quality by the ilioinguinal or the anterior intrapelvic (modified Rives-Stoppa) surgical approaches. J Orthop Trauma. 2014;28(6):313–9.
8. Elmadağ M, Güzel Y, Acar MA, Uzer G, Arazi M. The Stoppa approach versus the ilioinguinal approach for anterior acetabular fractures: a case control study assessing blood loss complications and function outcomes. Orthop Traumatol Surg Res. 2014;100(6):675–80.
9. Ma K, Luan F, Wang X, Ao Y, Liang Y, Fang Y, Tu C, Yang T, Min J. Randomized, controlled trial of the modified Stoppa versus the ilioinguinal approach for acetabular fractures. Orthopedics. 2013;36(10):e1307–15.
10. Kistler BJ, Sagi HC. Reduction of the posterior column in displaced acetabulum fractures through the anterior intrapelvic approach. J Orthop Trauma. 2015;29:S14–9.

The Pararectus Approach to the Acetabulum

6

Johannes D. Bastian,
and Marius J. B. Keel

Abstract

The appearance of acetabular fractures involving predominantly the anterior column has changed following an increase in elderly trauma. In elderly, a greater prevalence of quadrilateral plate fractures and acetabular dome impaction due to medial protrusion of the femoral head is noticed. The Pararectus approach provides distinct and safe surgical, intrapelvic, extraperitoneal access from anterior directly above the hip joint. The Pararectus approach combines the advantages of the ilioinguinal approach and Stoppa approach with access through the second window, however, without the need to dissect the inguinal canal (ilioinguinal approach) and without losing any direct access to the hip joint (Stoppa approach).

Keywords

Acetabulum · Fracture · Anterior column · Dome impaction · Quadrilateral plate · Exposure · Anterior · Intrapelvic · Extraperitoneal

J. D. Bastian (✉)
Department of Orthopaedic and Trauma Surgery, Inselspital, University Hospital, Bern, Switzerland
e-mail: johannes.bastian@insel.ch

M. J. B. Keel
Trauma Center Hirslanden, Clinic Hirslanden, Zürich, Switzerland

6.1 Introduction and History

The gold standard for anterior surgical treatment of acetabular fractures is the ilioinguinal approach, providing extrapelvic access as described more than 50 years ago [1]. In the 1990s, the modified Stoppa approach was introduced, for the first time providing intrapelvic access to the anterior acetabulum [2, 3]. Subsequently, the modified Stoppa approach was established as a valuable alternative with comparable results to the ilioinguinal approach [2–13]. The modified Stoppa approach avoids dissection within the inguinal canal, which requires time-consuming wound closure with risk of postoperative hernia. Additionally, the modified Stoppa approach reduces operative time, blood loss, and the amount of blood transfusion compared to the ilioinguinal approach.

However, the modified Stoppa approach has some limitations. The second ilioinguinal window is not dissected but only retracted cephalad. Due to this limited access, the first window of the ilioinguinal approach is dissected frequently. Therefore, the surgeon has to switch between the first, third, and fourth windows during fracture reduction and fixation at the level of the hip joint. Traction injuries, especially of the obturator nerve, and postoperative hernia are possible complications. In addition, the appearance of acetabular fractures involving the anterior column has changed within the last decades. Due to demographic changes

L. Büchler, M. J.B. Keel (eds.), *Fractures of the Hip*, Fracture Management Joint by Joint,
https://doi.org/10.1007/978-3-030-18838-2_6

with a significant increase of geriatric patients, new and demanding fracture patterns such as acetabular dome impaction, disruption of the quadrilateral plate and intrapelvic protrusion of the femoral head in elderly patients are current and future challenges [12, 14–17]. These specific fracture patterns are all located within the second window of the ilioinguinal approach.

Accordingly, an ideal surgical approach allows for reduction and fixation of these complex fracture patterns by sufficient visualization of fracture lines through an access directly above the hip joint, comparable to that obtained by the second window of the ilioinguinal approach but without dissection of the inguinal canal. These needs based the concept of the Pararectus approach as initially reported in 2012 [18]. Following the initial published description, further scientific articles confirmed the safety and efficiency of the Pararectus approach [19–21, 22] or describe the technique in detail using a video publication [23].

The potential benefits of the Pararectus approach are:

- Sufficient access to the inner hemipelvis, the acetabular dome, the quadrilateral plate, the posterior column, and the sacroiliac joint.
- Screw placement less limited by soft-tissue tension resulting in a twofold increase in length of the posterior column screws.
- Single approach without the need to change windows.
- No dissection of the inguinal canal.
- Short incision length.
- Simple wound closure.
- Vascular control (iliolumbar vessels, external and internal iliac vessels).
- Safe to use in cases with inguinal hernia or previous hernia repair.
- Safe to use after suprapubic catheter.

6.2 Indications

The Pararectus approach is used for acetabular fractures involving the anterior column (anterior wall, anterior column, transverse and T-shaped fractures with displacement predominantly in the anterior column, associated anterior column-posterior hemitransverse, associated both-column) as a single approach. The Pararectus approach is further used in combination with posterior approaches (digastric trochanteric flip osteotomy, surgical hip dislocation) in complex acetabular fractures (T-shaped fracture, associated anterior column-posterior hemitransverse fracture, or both-column fracture) with an additional severe displacement in the posterior column and/or in the dome, which is not reducible through the anterior approach alone.

6.3 Description of Surgical Technique

6.3.1 Surgical Access

The patient is placed in supine position on a radiolucent operating room table with a Foley catheter in situ. Intravenous antibiotics should be administered preoperatively. The patient is draped with the ipsilateral leg draped freely to allow for reduction maneuvers. The surgeon and scrub nurse are positioned on the contralateral side of the acetabular fracture. The image intensifier is positioned over the injured hip joint, as are the surgical assistants. The landmarks for incision are identified as presented in Fig. 6.1. The skin incision runs along the lateral border of the rectus abdominis muscle and is curved from the lateral to the medial third of the triangle that is built by lines connecting the navel, the anterior superior iliac spine (ASIS) and the pubic symphysis. Superficial dissection develops the rectus sheath, which is incised at the lateral border of the rectus abdominis muscle (Fig. 6.2). Deep dissection is located within the “false” and “true” pelvis (Fig. 6.3) to develop the intrapelvic exposure (Figs. 6.4 and 6.5) with the five surgical windows of the Pararectus approach. Deep dissection starts anteriorly and proceeds posteriorly. The first key structures are the inferior epigastric vessels that are identified easily and circumvented. The next structure is the vas deferens in males or the round ligament in females. Lateral retraction of these structures and posterior retraction of the bladder using a malleable retractor facilitates access to the retroperitoneal space in the fourth

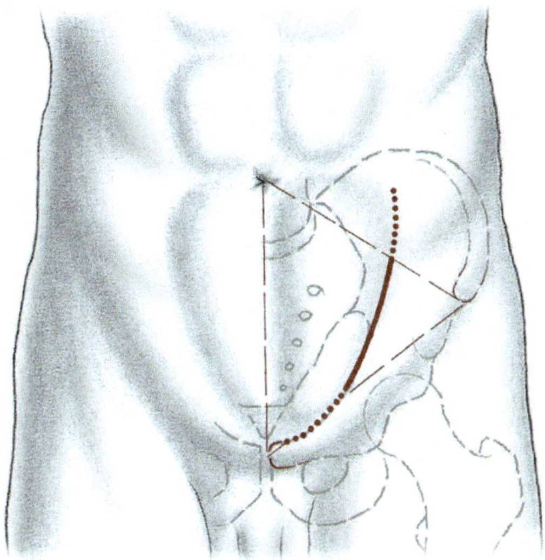

Fig. 6.1 Landmarks for skin incision: The navel, the anterior superior iliac spine (ASIS), and the symphysis are connected (dashed red line). The skin incision (red line) starts cranial at the border between the lateral and middle third of the line connecting the navel with the ASIS. The incision is curved and directed towards the border between the middle and medial third of the line connecting the ASIS with the symphysis. An extension of the incision is possible as presented (dotted lines). Reproduced with permission and copyright © of the British Editorial Society of Bone and Joint Surgery [18]

window. This window visualizes the symphysis and the superior pubic ramus. The periosteum is incised and a Hohmann-retractor placed on the superior pubic ramus. Before visualization of the fractured anterior column and further dissections posteriorly, the third and second windows are developed. The third and fifth windows are located between the inferior epigastric vessels and the external iliac vessels. Accordingly, the next key structures are the external iliac vessels that are digitally identified and mobilized. Before further incision of the periosteum, the Corona Mortis (anastomosis of the obturator and external iliac systems) has to be ligated or clamped in the third window at the level of the superior pubic branch. In the fifth window, the key structure is the obturator neurovascular bundle. Tension to the obturator nerve should be avoided. The periosteum at the quadrilateral plate is incised and the obturator internus muscle is mobilized until the lesser sciatic notch is visible. The second window is located between the iliopsoas muscle and the external iliac vessels. Before deep dissection proceeds with incision of the periosteum in the second window, the iliolumbar vessels

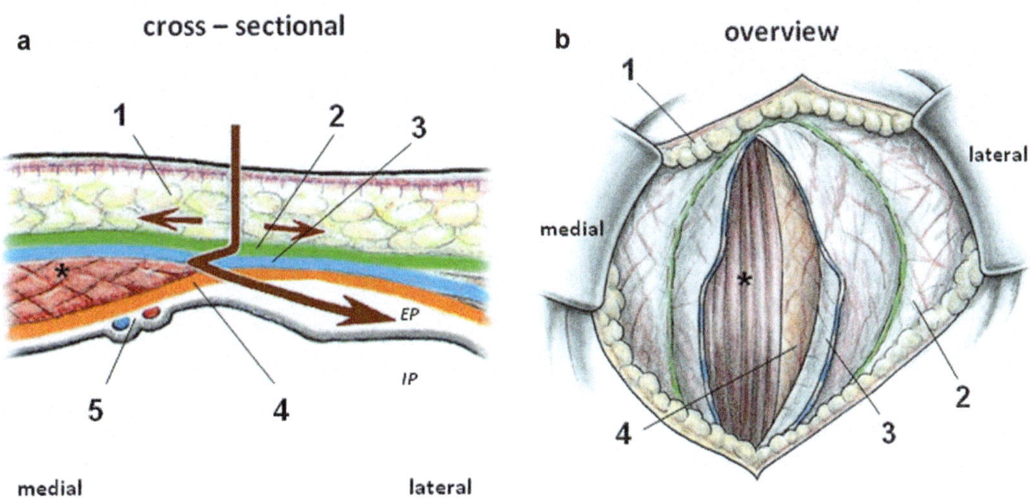

Fig. 6.2 (**a**) Schematic cross-sectional anatomy of the operative field with direction of dissection (red arrows): (1) Subcutaneous tissue, fascia of Camper, (2) deep layer of the anterior abdominal wall (green line), fascia of Scarpa, (3) rectus sheath (blue line), rectus abdominis muscle (star) (4) transversalis fascia (orange line), (5) inferior epigastric vessels. *EP* extraperitoneal space, parietal peritoneum (black line), *IP* intraperitoneal space. (**b**) Schematic overview of the operative field: (1) Subcutaneous tissue, fascia of Camper, (2) deep layer of the anterior abdominal wall, fascia of Scarpa, (3) rectus sheath, rectus abdominis muscle (star), (4) transversalis fascia. Reproduced with permission and copyright © of the British Editorial Society of Bone and Joint Surgery [18]

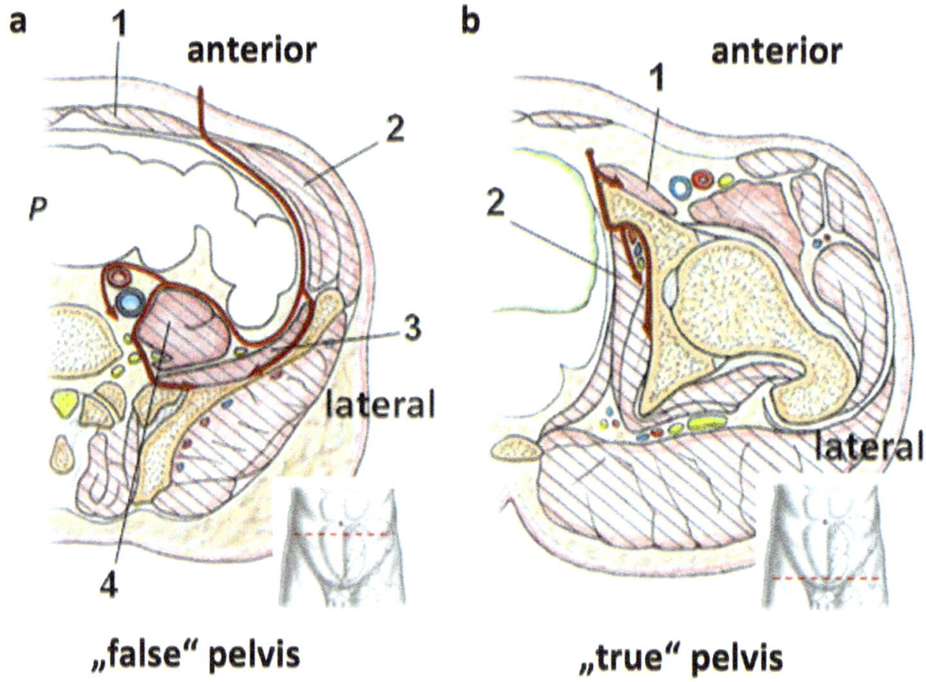

Fig. 6.3 (a) Schematic drawings showing the cross-section at the level of the sacroiliac joint as illustrated by the pictogram. Red arrows indicating the dissection planes within the "false" pelvis: (1) Rectus abdominis muscle, (2) external and internal oblique and transverse abdominis muscles, (3) iliacus muscle, (4) psoas major muscle, *P* peritoneal sac. (b) Schematic drawings showing the cross-section at the level of the hip joint as illustrated by the pictogram. Red arrows indicating the dissection planes within the "true" pelvis: (1) Pectineus and (2) obturator internus muscles. Reproduced with permission and copyright © of the British Editorial Society of Bone and Joint Surgery [18]

Fig. 6.4 Exposure: (1) Ilioinguinal nerve, (2) lateral femoral cutaneous nerve, (3) genitofemoral nerve with femoral and genital branches, (4) external iliac artery/vein, (5) anterior superior iliac spine (ASIS), (6) iliopsoas muscle, (7) roof of the acetabulum, (8) inferior epigastric vessels, (9) anastomosis between obturator and inferior epigastric or external iliac vessels, (10) obturator nerve and vessels (obturator canal), (11) obturator internus muscle, (12) vas deferens, (13) obturator nerve. Reproduced with permission and copyright © of the British Editorial Society of Bone and Joint Surgery [18]

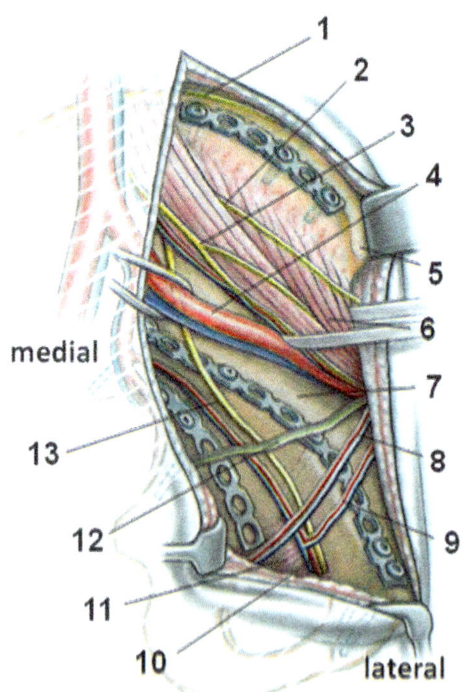

(vascular connection between the internal iliac vessels with the deep circumflex iliac vessels originating from the external iliac vessels) need to be controlled and ligated. The next key structures at the border to the first window are the genitofemoral nerve, the lateral cutaneous femoral nerve, and the iliacus muscle.

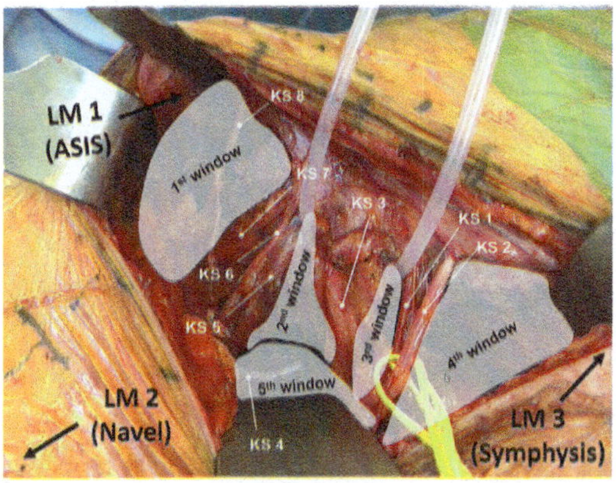

Fig. 6.5 Intraoperative photograph presenting an intrapelvic view from medial to lateral after surgical exposure by the Pararectus approach with the five "surgical windows," essential landmarks (LM) and key structures: (KS 1) inferior epigastric vessels, (KS 2) vas deferens, (KS 3) external iliac vessels, (KS 4) obturator nerve, (KS 5) iliopsoas muscle, (KS 6) genitofemoral nerve, (KS 7) iliacus muscle, (KS 8) lateral cutaneous femoral nerve

6.3.2 Fracture Reduction and Fixation

Once all windows are developed safely, the fracture lines are visualized and cleaned. Lateral traction of the femur supports fracture reduction. Fracture reduction begins at the level of the joint, proceeds with reduction of the anterior column followed by the quadrilateral plate. In presence of an impacted acetabular dome fragment, this can be disimpacted directly through the fracture using a raspatorium, which is a crucial step to obtain anatomic reduction in these articular fractures (Fig. 6.6). The void generated by the disimpaction has to be filled with bone graft to avoid secondary displacement of the reduced dome fragment. An anatomical, preshaped, suprapectineal plate can be used for direct reduction (Fig. 6.7). This plate is inserted from anterior to posterior, fixed preliminary using 2.5 mm threaded K-wires and correct positioning of the plate is confirmed using the image intensifier. A ball-spiked pusher placed on the plate assists in reduction of the anterior column. The plate is fixed posteriorly using 3.5 mm cortical screws. A Verbrugge clamp is used for fixation of the plate to the superior pubic ramus. A curved ball-spiked pusher placed

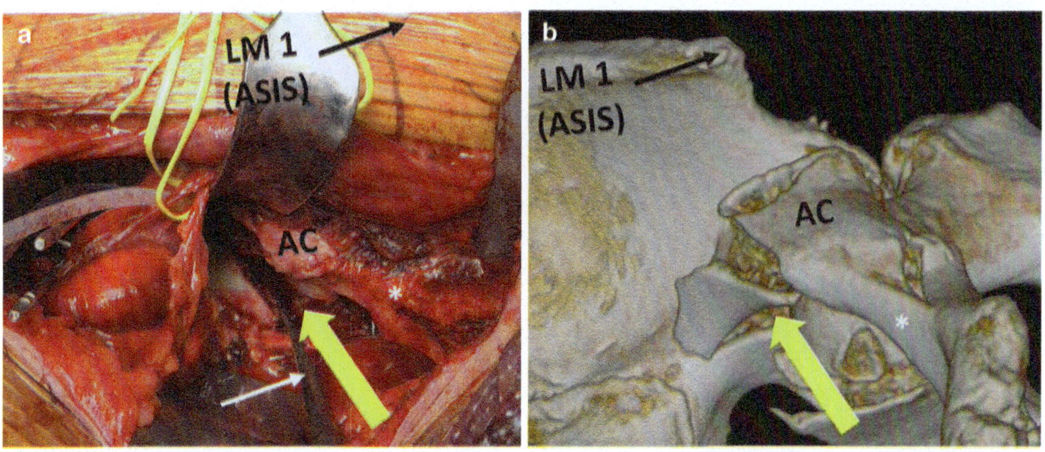

Fig. 6.6 (**a**) Intraoperative photographic showing the medial to lateral intrapelvic view in the third and fifth window obtained by the Pararectus approach in the left hemipelvis in a 79-year-old male patient who sustained an acetabular fracture (compare Fig. 6.8); *LM 1* landmark 1 = ASIS, *AC* anterior column, ∗ superior pubic ramus, *yellow arrow* fracture gap with access to acetabular dome, *white arrow* raspatorium inserted for disimpaction of the acetabular dome. (**b**) Three-dimensional reconstruction of the left-hemipelvis showing the bony structures in correspondence to (**a**)

on the quadrilateral portion of the suprapectineal plate reduces the breakout of the quadrilateral plate. The plate is then fixed anteriorly. A Collinear clamp is used (Fig. 6.7) for compression of the posterior column to the anterior column. The clamp must be hooked into the lesser sciatic notch and compressed against the plate. In fractures with involvement of the posterior column (especially in anterior column posterior hemitransverse fractures), an infra-acetabular screw, a posterior column screw or both should be placed for fixation of the posterior column depending on fracture lines and comminution. Case example presented in Fig. 6.8.

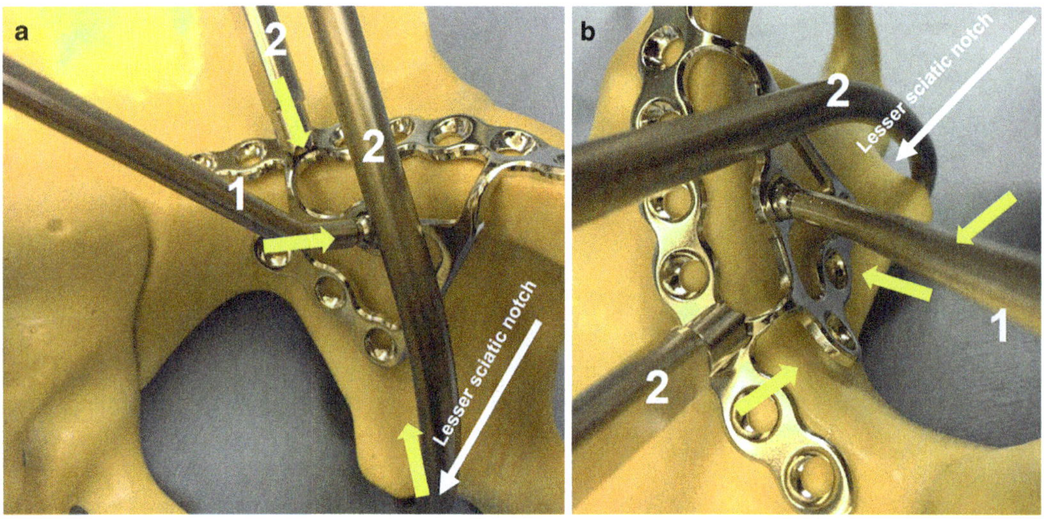

Fig. 6.7 Model showing an intrapelvic view of the quadrilateral plate and the posterior pelvic brim (**a**). A curved ball spiked pusher (1) on the quadrilateral portion on the anatomical, preshaped, suprapectineal plate for direct reduction of the quadrilateral plate and a Collinear clamp (2) for direct reduction of the posterior column (hocked into the lesser sciatic notch and compression against the plate). (**b**) Same model, view from proximal-lateral

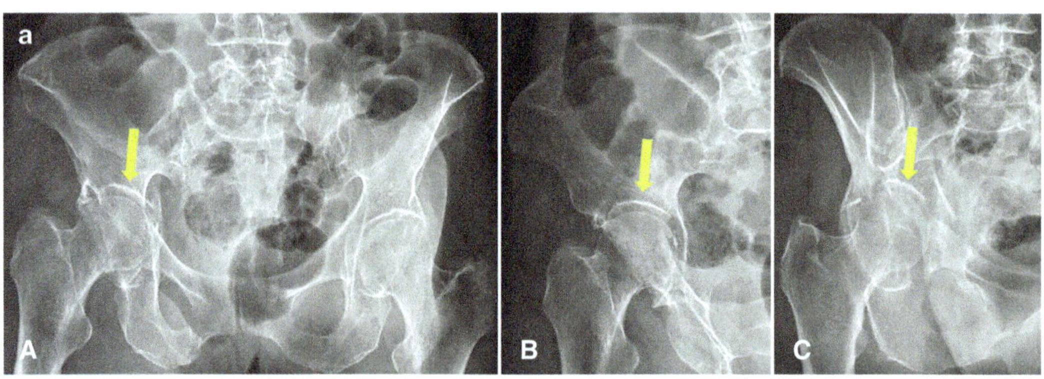

Fig. 6.8 (**a**) Preoperative radiographs with (A) anteroposterior, (B) iliac oblique, and (C) obturator oblique views showing an acetabular fracture (anterior column/ posterior hemitransverse) in a 74-year-old female patient with dome impaction (yellow arrow), breakout of the quadrilateral plate and intrapelvic protrusion of the femoral head. (**b**) Preoperative CT scans with (A) axial (dome level), (B) coronal, and (C) sagittal reconstruction planes showing the acetabular fracture (anterior column/posterior hemitransverse) of the same patient. (**c**) Postoperative radiographs with (A) anteroposterior, (B) iliac oblique, and (C) obturator oblique views showing an anatomic reduction with disimpaction of the dome fragment. A supra-acetabular screw (unfilled yellow arrow) was placed in horizontal direction to buttress the disimpacted dome fragment (unfilled yellow arrow). A posterior column screw was used for compression of the posterior column to the anterior column (filled yellow arrow). (**d**) Postoperative CT scans with (A) axial (dome level), (B) coronal, and (C) sagittal reconstruction planes show an anatomic reduction with disimpaction of the dome fragment (B, yellow arrow). (C): supra-acetabular screw (unfilled yellow arrow), posterior column screw (filled yellow arrow)

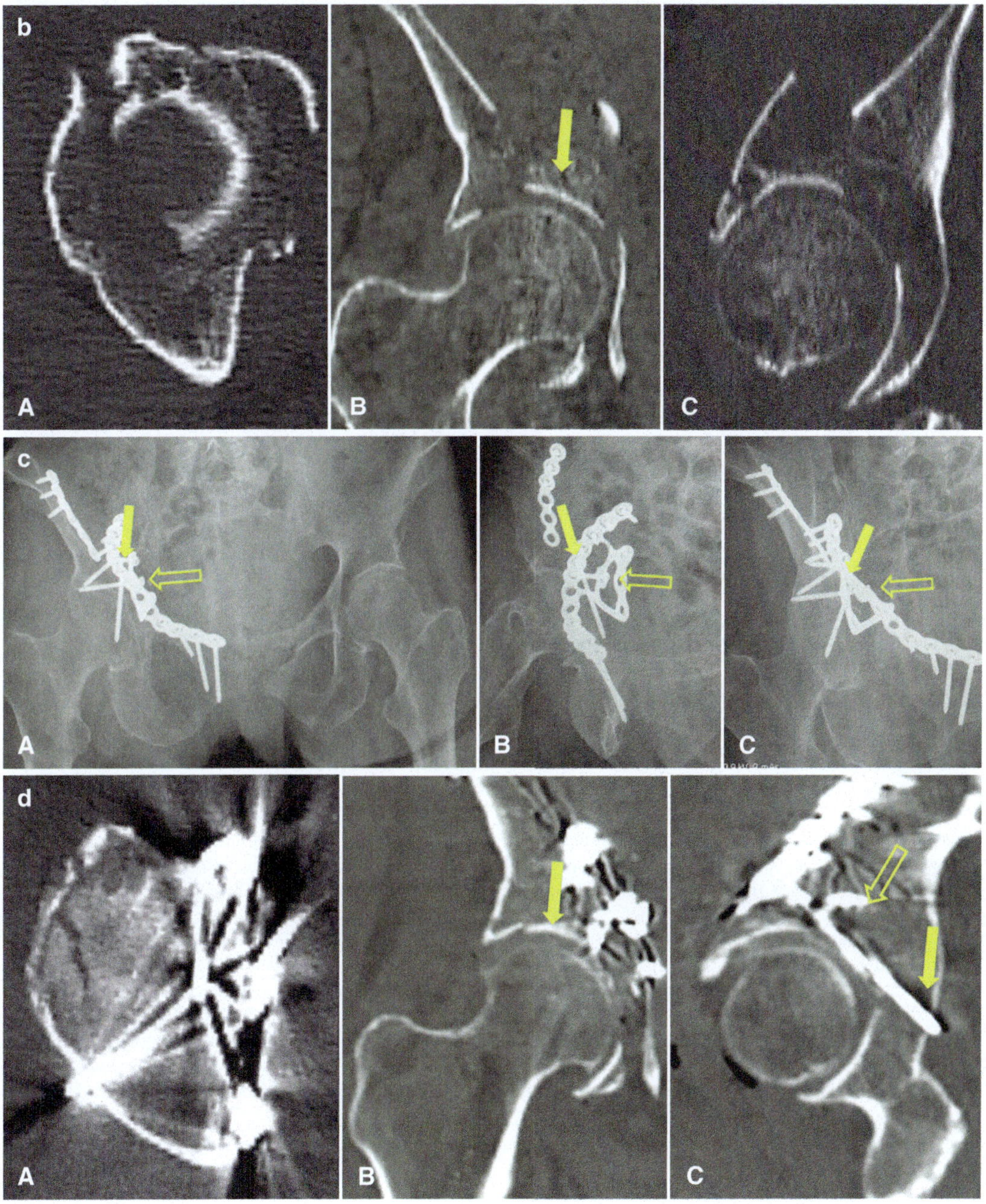

Fig. 6.8 (continued)

6.3.3 Closure

A suction drain is placed in the Retzius space routinely. After wound irrigation, hemostasis and clear urine output, the anterior lamina of the rectus sheath is sutured using absorbable sutures. A layered closure of the subcutaneous tissues follows, and the skin is closed using staples or an intracutaneous suture.

References

1. Judet R, Judet J, Letournel E. Fractures of the acetabulum: classification and surgical approaches for open reduction. Preliminary report. J Bone Joint Surg Am. 1964;46:1615–46.
2. Hirvensalo E, Lindahl J, Bostman O. A new approach to the internal fixation of unstable pelvic fractures. Clin Orthop Relat Res. 1993;297:28–32.

3. Cole JD, Bolhofner BR. Acetabular fracture fixation via a modified Stoppa limited intrapelvic approach. Description of operative technique and preliminary treatment results. Clin Orthop Relat Res. 1994;305:112–23.
4. Ponsen KJ, Joosse P, Schigt A, Goslings JC, Luitse JS. Internal fracture fixation using the Stoppa approach in pelvic ring and acetabular fractures: technical aspects and operative results. J Trauma. 2006;61(3):662–7.
5. Jakob M, Droeser R, Zobrist R, Messmer P, Regazzoni P. A less invasive anterior intrapelvic approach for the treatment of acetabular fractures and pelvic ring injuries. J Trauma. 2006;60(6):1364–70.
6. Sagi HC, Afsari A, Dziadosz D. The anterior intrapelvic (modified Rives-Stoppa) approach for fixation of acetabular fractures. J Orthop Trauma. 2010;24(5):263–70.
7. Andersen RC, O'Toole RV, Nascone JW, Sciadini MF, Frisch HM, Turen CW. Modified Stoppa approach for acetabular fractures with anterior and posterior column displacement: quantification of radiographic reduction and analysis of interobserver variability. J Orthop Trauma. 2010;24(5):271–8.
8. Laflamme GY, Hebert-Davies J, Rouleau D, Benoit B, Leduc S. Internal fixation of osteopenic acetabular fractures involving the quadrilateral plate. Injury. 2011;42(10):1130–4.
9. Khoury A, Weill Y, Mosheiff R. The Stoppa approach for acetabular fracture. Oper Orthop Traumatol. 2012;24(4–5):439–48.
10. Shazar N, Eshed I, Ackshota N, Hershkovich O, Khazanov A, Herman A. Comparison of acetabular fracture reduction quality by the ilioinguinal or the anterior intrapelvic (modified Rives-Stoppa) surgical approaches. J Orthop Trauma. 2014;28(6):313–9.
11. Isaacson MJ, Taylor BC, French BG, Poka A. Treatment of acetabulum fractures through the modified Stoppa approach: strategies and outcomes. Clin Orthop Relat Res. 2014;472:3345–52.
12. Bastian JD, Tannast M, Siebenrock KA, Keel MJ. Mid-term results in relation to age and analysis of predictive factors after fixation of acetabular fractures using the modified Stoppa approach. Injury. 2013;44(12):1793–8.
13. Ma K, Luan F, Wang X, et al. Randomized, controlled trial of the modified Stoppa versus the ilioinguinal approach for acetabular fractures. Orthopedics. 2013;36(10):e1307–e15.
14. Ferguson TA, Patel R, Bhandari M, Matta JM. Fractures of the acetabulum in patients aged 60 years and older: an epidemiological and radiological study. J Bone Joint Surg Br. 2010;92(2):250–7.
15. Anglen JO, Burd TA, Hendricks KJ, Harrison P. The "Gull sign": a harbinger of failure for internal fixation of geriatric acetabular fractures. J Orthop Trauma. 2003;17(9):625–34.
16. Bastian JD, Giannoudis PV. Central acetabular fracture dislocations: are existing classifications comprehensive? Injury. 2014;45(12):1807–15.
17. Prasartritha T, Chaivanichsiri P. The study of broken quadrilateral surface in fractures of the acetabulum. Int Orthop. 2013;37(6):1127–34.
18. Keel MJ, Ecker TM, Cullmann JL, et al. The Pararectus approach for anterior intrapelvic management of acetabular fractures: an anatomical study and clinical evaluation. J Bone Joint Surg Br. 2012;94(3):405–11.
19. Bastian JD, Savic M, Cullmann JL, Zech WD, Djonov V, Keel MJ. Surgical exposures and options for instrumentation in acetabular fracture fixation: Pararectus approach versus the modified Stoppa. Injury. 2016;47:695.
20. Keel MJ, Tomagra S, Bonel HM, Siebenrock KA, Bastian JD. Clinical results of acetabular fracture management with the Pararectus approach. Injury. 2014;45(12):1900–7.
21. Mardian S, Schaser KD, Hinz P, Wittenberg S, Haas NP, Schwabe P. Fixation of acetabular fractures via the ilioinguinal versus Pararectus approach: a direct comparison. Bone Joint J. 2015;97-B(9):1271–8.
22. von Rüden C, Wenzel L, Becker J, Thannheier A, Augat P, Woltmann A, Bühren V, Perl M. The pararectus approach for internal fixation of acetabular fractures involving the anterior column: evaluating the functional outcome. International orthopaedics. 2018. https://doi.org/10.1007/s00264-018-4148-8
23. Keel MJB, Siebenrock KA, Tannast M, Bastian JD. The Pararectus approach: a new concept. JBJS Essent Surg Tech. 2018;8(3):e21.

7 Lateral Approach to the Pelvis and Hip

Joseph M. Schwab, Chad Beck, and Klaus A. Siebenrock

Abstract

Lateral-based surgical approaches to the hip and pelvis are critical to treatment of both traumatic and developmental conditions of the adult hip. This chapter focuses on two lateral-based approaches that can treat a wide array of conditions: The Kocher-Langenbeck approach popularized by Judet and Letournel, and the safe surgical hip dislocation popularized by Ganz. The Kocher-Langenbeck approach has been described over 70 years ago but remains a workhorse approach for certain types of acetabular trauma. Ganz' safe surgical hip dislocation has been described within the past 20 years but has been shown to be safe and effective in the treatment of both traumatic and developmental pathologies. Both approaches are technically challenging and require attention to detail, but with adequate study and practice can be mastered.

J. M. Schwab (✉) · C. Beck
Department of Orthopaedic Surgery, Medical College of Wisconsin, Milwaukee, WI, USA
e-mail: jmschwab@mcw.edu

K. A. Siebenrock
Department of Orthopaedic and Trauma Surgery, Inselspital, Bern University Hospital, Bern, Switzerland

Keywords

Kocher-Langenbeck · Surgical hip dislocation · Acetabular fracture · Femoroacetabular impingement · Trochanteric flip osteotomy

7.1 Kocher-Langenbeck Approach

7.1.1 Introduction

Classically described as a posterior approach, the Kocher-Langenbeck approach is a workhorse approach to the hip and acetabulum that allows complete visualization of the posterior column, as well as palpation of the quadrilateral surface all the way to the pelvic brim. This approach, in its current form, was described by Judet and Lagrange in 1958 [1]. Judet and Letournel described additional extensions to this approach to gain further access to the anterior column in the superior acetabular region. These techniques include splitting the tendinous insertion of the gluteals or extending the incision similar to a triradiate approach. Siebenrock also described expanding anatomic access through a trochanteric flip osteotomy [2]. Despite these extensions, the Kocher-Langenbeck approach in use today remains very similar to the technique described by Judet.

L. Büchler, M. J.B. Keel (eds.), *Fractures of the Hip*, Fracture Management Joint by Joint,
https://doi.org/10.1007/978-3-030-18838-2_7

7.1.2 Indications

The Kocher-Langenbeck approach is still predominantly used for open reduction and internal fixation of fractures about the acetabulum where the fracture pattern is posterior dominant. Specifically, this approach is indicated for the following fracture patterns [3]:

- Posterior wall acetabular fractures.
- Posterior column acetabular fractures.
- Posterior column and posterior wall acetabular fractures.
- Transverse and posterior wall acetabular fractures.
- Transverse acetabular fractures with the major displacement occurring at the posterior column.
- Posterior element reduction and fixation in T-type acetabular fractures.

While this approach provides excellent visual access to the posterior acetabulum and posterior column, as well as palpation access to the quadrilateral surface, it does not provide any adequate access to the anterior elements of an acetabular fracture. Therefore, the following fracture patterns are considered a *contraindication* to the Kocher-Langenbeck approach:

- Anterior wall acetabular fractures.
- Anterior column acetabular fractures.
- Transverse acetabular fractures with the major displacement occurring at the anterior column.
- Associated both-column acetabular fractures.
- Anterior element reduction and fixation in T-type acetabular fractures.
- Anterior column and posterior hemitransverse acetabular fractures.
- Anterior column and anterior wall acetabular fractures.

Finally, when an acetabular fracture is combined with a femoral head fracture, or when it is anticipated that a trochanteric osteotomy would be helpful in gaining exposure to an isolated posterior-superior acetabular wall fracture, it may be preferable to perform the approach in lateral position (see below), rather than the traditional prone position.

7.1.3 Setup

The setup for the Kocher-Langenbeck approach may occur in the lateral position or in the prone position.

7.1.3.1 Lateral Position [3, 4]

The patient is placed in the lateral decubitus position on a flat, radiolucent table, with the operative extremity up, and draped free. This positioning is similar to the posterior approach used in total hip arthroplasty, with the major difference being that the drapes need to extend proximally above the level of the iliac crest and posteriorly to the midline. This allows for palpation of the posterior superior iliac spine as a landmark. The down extremity needs to be appropriately padded to prevent pressure-related complications.

7.1.3.2 Prone Position [5]

For the prone position, traditionally a pelvic table is used to help maintain proper position. Chest rolls are place so that the patient's breasts and areolas are free. Additional padding is placed on the anterior superior iliac spine to help support the pelvis, and a well-padded perineal post is placed. A distal femoral traction pin is placed preoperatively on the operative extremity and attached to an in-line traction component of the table. The foot is placed into the foot holder to allow for positioning the knee in flexion. The table is then adjusted until there is slight extension at the hip and the knee is flexed. This allows tension to be taken off the sciatic nerve for safe retraction during the exposure (Fig. 7.1).

An alternative to a pelvic specialty table is using a completely radiolucent flat top table. For this variation in positioning chest rolls should be placed similar to the pelvic specialty top. Once the patient is in the prone position the hip needs to be slightly extended and the knee flexed. This can be accomplished prior to prepping the patient with pillows under the knee and a stack of blankets at the level of the patient's anterior tibia to hold this position. This can also be accom-

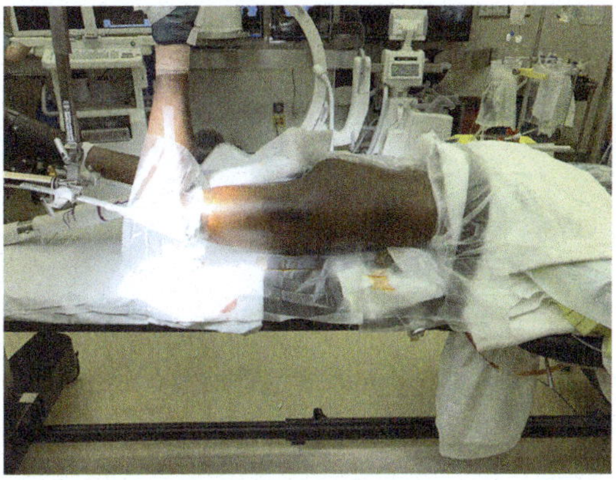

Fig. 7.1 The patient is in the prone position on a fully radiolucent table. A distal femoral traction pin and foot holder are used on the operative side to hold the hip in slight extension and the knee in flexion. The extremity is draped widely to allow access to all necessary bony landmarks. Any catheters, chest tubes, or other drains are positioned under the table to be out of the way of fluoroscopy

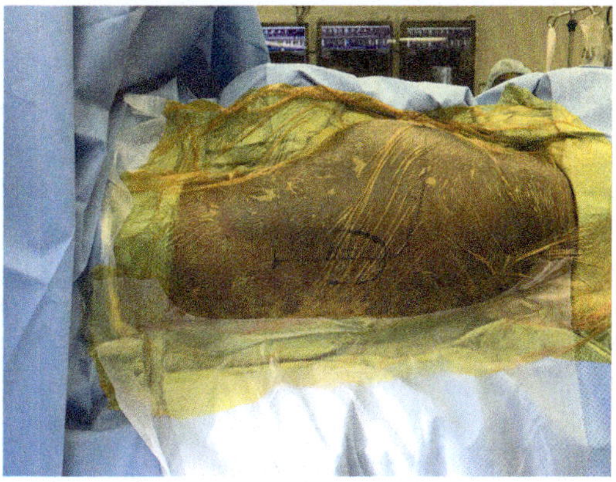

Fig. 7.2 The skin incision is marked. One limb is in line with the femoral diaphysis to the top of the greater trochanter. The second limb then curves towards the posterior superior iliac spine after passing the level of the greater trochanter

plished intra-operatively with an assistant holding the knee flexed while a stack of surgical towels is placed under the anterior thigh allowing for hip extension.

7.1.4 Instruments/Equipment/Implants Required

7.1.4.1 Surgical Table

- A specialty pelvic top traction table is required for the prone position.
- A flat-top Jackson-type table, or imaging table that allows for C-arm fluoroscopy is required for the lateral position.

7.1.4.2 Instruments

- Pelvic retractor set including long curved sciatic nerve retractor.
- For fracture reduction, there are specialized reduction tools, including pelvic reduction clamps and forceps, ball-spike pushers, and bone hooks.

7.1.4.3 Implants

- 3.5 mm cortical screws, 3.5 mm locking screws, and 3.5 mm pelvic reconstruction plates

7.1.4.4 Optional

- Intraoperative autologous blood transfusion (cell-saver).
- Intraoperative imaging with fluoroscopy, O-arm, or CT.
- Additional implants, as needed, such as spring plates, mini-screws, or percutaneous screw sets.

7.1.5 Procedure

7.1.5.1 Exposure

Bony landmarks first need to be located. These include the femoral diaphysis, the posterior superior iliac spine, and the greater trochanter. The skin incision is made in line with the femoral diaphysis, then from distal to proximal, curves towards the posterior superior iliac spine after passing the level of the greater trochanter (Fig. 7.2). In general, the surgeon's palm can be used as a guide for the length of the limbs of this incision. One palm length for the part of the incision along the femoral shaft to the tip of the greater trochanter and two palm widths from the tip of the greater trochanter curving towards the posterior superior iliac spine. This makes the distal limb of the incision from the gluteus maximus tendon to the greater trochanter and the proximal portion double that length. In obese patients or more muscular patients the portion towards the posterior superior iliac spine may have to be increased for easier visualization.

The deeper dissection carries through the subcutaneous fat until you reach the iliotibial band. Be careful to only clear off enough fat from the iliotibial band to allow visualization. Too much cleared off the iliotibial band can cause a large deep space for fluid collection after closure. From here incise the iliotibial band in line with the fibers and in line with your incision. Carry this proximal to the tip of the greater trochanter. From here curve towards the posterior superior iliac spine with incising the gluteus maximus fascia. By following this direction for incising the gluteus fascia you should be in line with the muscle fibers deep to the fascia (Fig. 7.3). The gluteus maximus is now split in-line with its fibers. This should start at the greater trochanter and end once you reach the first neurovascular bundle. This will allow access to the short external rotators. Clear the fat and bursa overlying the tendon insertions of the short external rotators. A blunt retractor placed underneath the gluteus medius muscle belly helps with visualization (Fig. 7.4). Once the two tendons are identified tag both using a strong suture for control. This should be performed 1 cm off the femoral insertions to avoid damage to the femoral head blood supply running up the posterior femur (Fig. 7.5). The confluent tendon from the obturator internus and the gemelli is found deep to the muscle bellies. With these tagged you can now use them as a guide to clear off the retro acetabular surface back to the level of the greater and lesser sciatic notches. The gemelli/obturators can be used to protect the sciatic nerve by

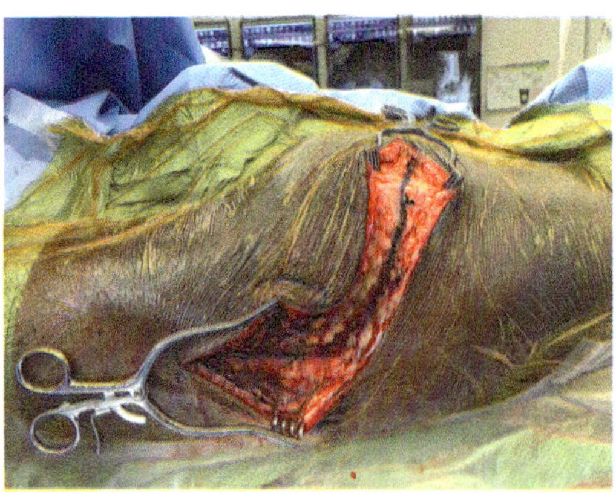

Fig. 7.3 Once the skin and subcutaneous tissues have been incised, the fascial incision follows a similar path as the skin incision

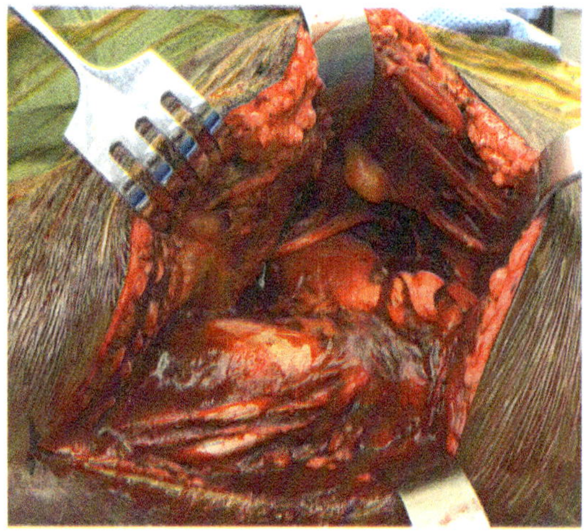

Fig. 7.4 The iliotibial band and gluteus maximus fascia and muscle have been split revealing the posterior structures of the acetabulum and proximal femur. The vastus lateralis tendon and muscle are clearly visible coming off of the greater trochanter. The sciatic nerve can be seen coursing from proximal to distal (right to left) deep in the wound. At this point in the operation, the short external rotators are still intact

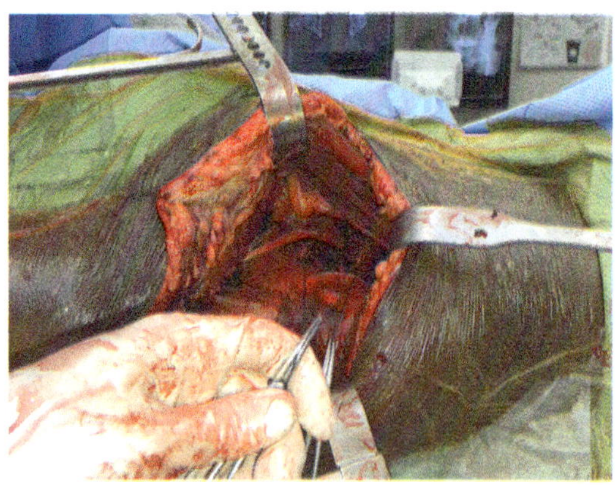

Fig. 7.5 The short external rotators are tagged and reflected off their insertions on the femur. The piriformis tendon (proximal) and confluent tendon of the obturator internus/gemelli (distal) should be transected 1 cm from their insertion on the femur in order to protect proximal femoral blood supply

placing a retractor in the lesser sciatic notch under the muscle bellies (Figs. 7.6 and 7.7). The superior aspect of the dissection will require clearing off the gluteus minimus muscle belly. In the setting of a fracture this should be debrided as well as the short external rotator bellies that look damaged/necrotic. They will be a source of heterotopic ossification if left in the wound. If further visualization is needed in the inferior aspect of the exposure, the quadratus femoris muscle can be elevated off the ischial tuberosity. This muscle belly should never be elevated off the femur during this approach as the blood supply to the femoral head travels along the femur deep to this muscle attachment.

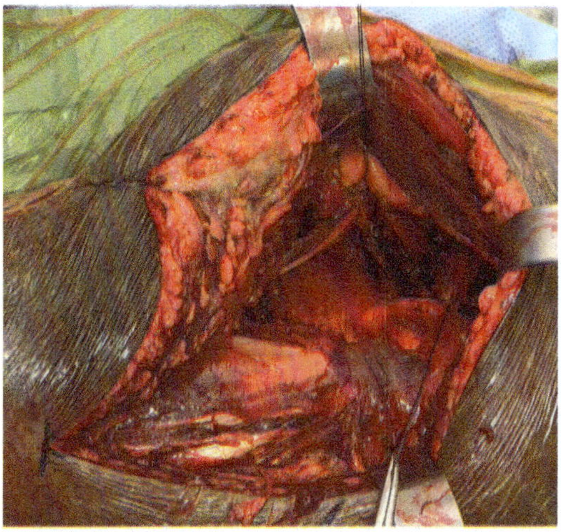

Fig. 7.6 The sciatic nerve typically runs posterior to the confluent tendon. By reflecting this tendon posteriorly, the sciatic nerve can be protected from direct contact with retractors placed in the lesser sciatic notch

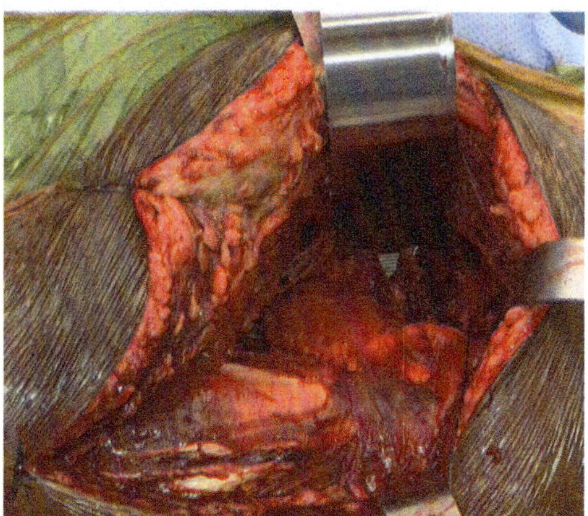

Fig. 7.7 Once the tip of the sciatic nerve retractor is in the lesser sciatic notch, the sciatic nerve can safely be retracted, allowing excellent visualization of the retroacetabular space

7.1.5.2 Wound Closure

A thorough debridement of necrotic muscle, with special attention paid to the gluteus minimus, must occur prior to closure. This is followed by a thorough irrigation of the surgical wound. The short external rotators are repaired to their attachments. Be careful not to suture close to the femur as this repair could accidentally ligate the blood supply to the femoral head. One drain is placed deep to the iliotibial band closure and one deep to the skin closure.

7.1.6 Postoperative Regimen

For most fractures about the hip the patient can be made toe touch weight bearing. This will help reduce the forces across the post-surgical hip. If the patient had a hip dislocation associated with their injury, posterior hip precautions are used for the first 6 weeks post operatively. These precautions include limiting hip flexion to less than 90°, not allowing combined adduction with hip flexion (such as crossing the legs in a seated position), and not allowing the patient to sleep on their side. In addition, a knee immobilizer can sometimes be helpful to prevent the patient from excessively flexing their hip. Heterotopic ossification (HO) prophylaxis is a topic of debate but currently is not used if an adequate debridement of damaged or necrotic musculature, particularly the gluteus minimus muscle, was performed. Increased nonunion rates have been seen with the use of high dose Nonsteroidal anti-inflammatory drugs (NSAID) [6]. Radiation therapy has been shown to reduce rates of clinically relevant (Brooker III-IV) HO when combined with adequate muscle debridement, but it has not clearly been shown to be superior to other forms of prophylaxis [7, 8]. In addition, radiation therapy carries the risk of radiation-induced sarcoma [9, 10].

7.2 Trochanteric Flip and Surgical Hip Dislocation

7.2.1 Introduction

Ganz et al. began using a technique for safe surgical dislocation of the hip in 1992, and subsequently published the technique, along with results on 213 cases, in 2001 [11]. This technique was based on careful anatomic study of the blood supply to the femoral head, with particular focus on the medial femoral circumflex artery being the dominant blood supply to the adult femoral head [12]. This technique uses a trochanteric osteotomy to gain access to the hip capsule, preserving the course of the medial femoral circumflex artery to the retinacular vessels of the femoral head in the process. This technique has led to a greater understanding of hip pathologies such as femoroacetabular impingement, slipped capital femoral epiphysis, Legg-Calve-Perthes disease, and other potential causes of "idiopathic" degenerative changes to the hip [13–21].

7.2.2 Indications

Surgical hip dislocation provides wide access to the proximal femoral and acetabular articular surfaces. This makes it a very powerful approach for a wide variety of intraarticular hip pathology. The following is a list of conditions that can be treated through a surgical hip dislocation:

- Femoroacetabular impingement [14, 15]
- Trauma including femoral head and/or acetabular wall fractures [22]
- Slipped capital femoral epiphysis (acute and chronic) [19, 21]
- Legg-Calve-Perthes disease, and Perthes-like deformities [18, 23]
- Synoproliferative disorders such as synovial chondromatosis and pigmented villonodular synovitis [24]

7.2.3 Setup

The setup for a surgical hip dislocation is similar to that for a traditional posterior-approach total hip arthroplasty [11, 25]. The patient is placed in the lateral decubitus position with the entire operative extremity draped free. The patient should be stabilized in the lateral position to allow intraoperative hip flexion beyond 90°. A tunnel cushion placed over the non-operative extremity protects it from injury and provides a supportive surface for the operative extremity during the procedure (Fig. 7.8). A sterile bag, or pocket, on the anterior side of the patient is used while the hip joint is dislocated.

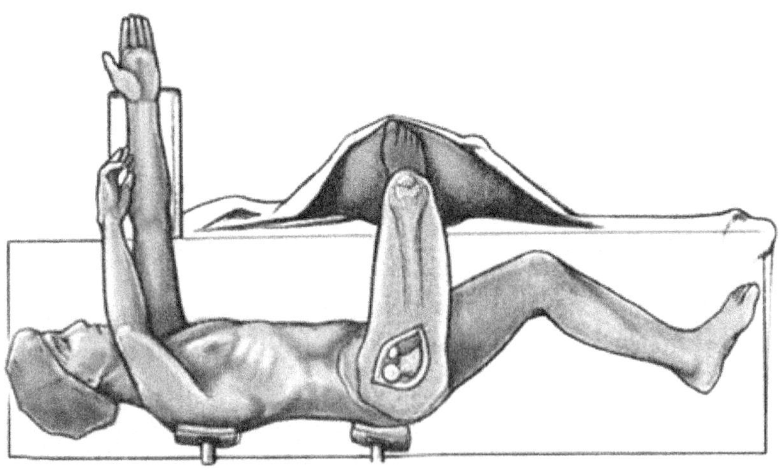

Fig. 7.8 The patient is secured in the lateral decubitus position and a tunnel cushion is placed over the down extremity to provide protection to the extremity and act as a stable surface for the surgical limb. Reproduced with permission and copyright © of Springer [26]

7.2.4 Instruments/Equipment/ Implants Required

7.2.4.1 Surgical Table

- A flat-top Jackson-type table, or imaging table with padded positioners to hold the patient in the lateral decubitus position.

Instruments

- Langenbeck-style, curved spoon-style, and double bent Hohmann retractors are helpful for atraumatic soft-tissue retraction.
- A long, curved scissors is helpful to transect the ligamentum teres during hip dislocation.
- Curved osteotomes and/or a high-speed burr can be used for femoral head and acetabular rim trimming.
- An arthroscope can be used to provide close-up inspection of the joint during dislocation, without the need for a fluid pump.
- Plastic hemispherical femoral head templates of multiple sizes are helpful for determining when adequate femoral head resection has been performed in cases of cam-type femoro-acetabular impingement.

Implants

- 3.5 mm cortical screws for trochanteric fragment fixation
- Suture anchors for labral repair, refixation, or reconstruction.
- Mini-screws or headless screws for articular surface fixation (i.e., femoral head fracture, head reduction osteotomy, etc.)
- Proximal femoral fixations plates for fixation of femoral derotational osteotomies.

Optional

- Arthroscopic shaver for synovial debridement (e.g. PVNS, synovial chondromatosis).

7.2.5 Procedure

7.2.5.1 Exposure

The skin incision is typically 20–25 cm long and is centered over the tip of the greater trochanter in line with the anterior third of the femur. The hip is approached through a Gibson interval [11, 25, 27], just anterior to gluteus maximus muscle. Branches of the inferior gluteal artery run within the fascia between the gluteus medius and the gluteus maximus and perforate the fascia lata at the anterior border of the gluteus maximus [25] (Fig. 7.9). These vessels continue into the subcutaneous fat after perforating the fascia lata. This is most easily identified by starting the dissection distally, identifying the fascia lata, and proceeding proximally until the perforating vessels are encountered. The fascia overlying the gluteus medius muscle is incised at the anterior border of the gluteus maximus muscle. The gluteus maximus muscle is retracted posteriorly keeping the overlying fascia of the gluteus medius with it. This helps to protect the superior cluneal nerves, as well as branches of the superior gluteal artery, which can run in that fascia.

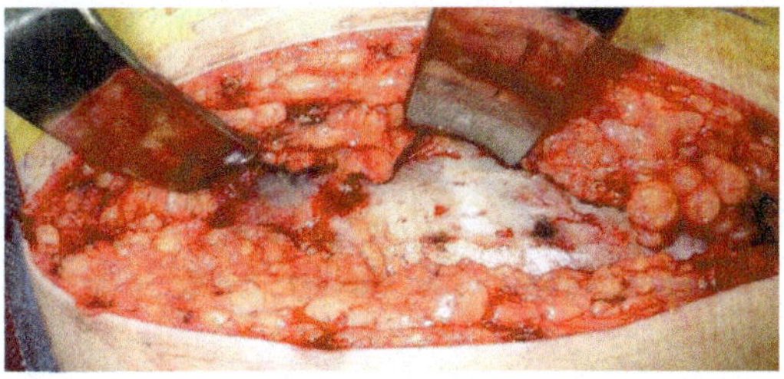

Fig. 7.9 Perforating vessels are a relatively constant anatomic indicator of the anterior border of the gluteus maximus. After identifying these vessels, the fascia can be incised, anterior to the vessels, in line with femur

The leg is then internally rotated to expose the gluteus minimus, piriformis, and short external rotators. Care must be taken at this point to avoid disrupting these posterior structures as they protect the medial femoral circumflex artery (MFCA), the major blood supply to the femoral head [12].

7.2.5.2 Trochanteric Osteotomy

An osteotomy of the greater trochanter is then performed. This can either be a flat-cut or step-cut osteotomy depending on the goals of surgery specific to that patient. For instance, if a trochanteric advancement or relative neck lengthening is indicated, a flat-cut osteotomy is recommended. Step-cut osteotomy provides greater resistance to superior migration secondary to pull from the gluteus medius and may allow for more accelerated rehabilitation [28, 29]. Whether performing a flat or stepped osteotomy, the femur should be internally rotated approximately 15°–20° to compensate for femoral anteversion. Before performing the osteotomy, mark a line from the tip of the greater trochanter to the posterior border of the vastus lateralis ridge with electrocautery. This also cauterizes the trochanteric branch of the MFCA, which can otherwise cause bleeding during the osteotomy. It is also important to avoid cutting the trochanter too medial proximally, as this can damage the retinacular vessels from the medial femoral circumflex artery as they course into the femoral head. This could lead to iatrogenic avascular necrosis, a devastating complication.

7.2.5.3 Variation: Step-Cut Osteotomy [26, 28, 29] (Fig. 7.10)

Pass a narrow oscillating saw from posterior to anterior starting at the tip of the greater trochanter and extending approximately ½ of the length of the osteotomy. The blade is left in the osteotomy and used as a plane of reference. A broad oscillating saw is then passed starting just distal to the vastus lateralis ridge and extending to the distal end of the first cut, approximately 6 cm more medial. A 6 mm osteotome is then passed to connect the two ends of the step and the trochanteric fragment is mobilized.

7.2.5.4 Variation: Flat-Cut Osteotomy (Fig. 7.11)

Pass an oscillating saw from posterior to anterior along the cauterized line. If anatomic fixation is desired, the anterior, or anterosuperior portion of cortical bone can be left intact and fractured by prying the fragment up. This would provide an area to "key in" when fixing the osteotomy. Otherwise, if mobility of the fragment is desired (as in the case of a trochanteric advancement), the osteotomy should be completed with the saw. Thickness of the mobilized trochanteric fragment is approximately 1.5 cm.

7.2.5.5 Capsular Exposure

Once the trochanteric osteotomy has been performed, the leg is taken out of internal rotation while the trochanteric fragment is mobilized anteriorly. Fibers of the vastus lateralis muscle are released from the femur down to the midpoint of the insertion of the gluteus maximus tendon to achieve mobilization of the fragment. Proximally 1–2 mm of gluteus medius tendon remains on the

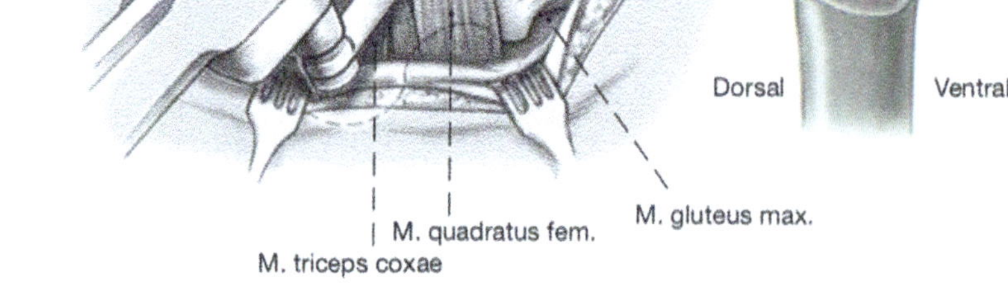

Fig. 7.10 Step cut trochanteric osteotomy is performed by first (A) passing the saw blade from the proximal tip to approximately 3/5 the length of the osteotomy. A second saw blade is used to place a second limb of the osteotomy, more medial, along the distal 2/5 of the osteotomy. The two limbs are connected with the use of a narrow (approximately 6 mm) osteotome to complete the osteotomy. Reproduced with permission and copyright © of Springer [26]

stable portion of the greater trochanter and must be released to mobilize the fragment anteriorly. Often a few fibers of the piriformis tendon remain attached to the mobile fragment and must be carefully released to allow mobilization.

Dissection is then carried out between the gluteus minimus and piriformis muscles, which allows visualization of the joint capsule. To facilitate exposure of the capsule, the hip should now go into slight flexion and external rotation while the gluteus medius and minimus are retracted superiorly.

7.2.5.6 Capsulotomy (Fig. 7.12)

Z-shaped capsulotomy is performed starting with the anterolateral capsule in-line with the femoral neck. After initial capsule penetration with the scalpel, an "inside-out" capsulotomy helps protect the cartilage and labrum from iatrogenic injury. The capsulotomy is extended to the rim of the acetabulum proximally and to the anterolateral tip of the stable trochanter distally. An anteroinferior limb of the capsulotomy is then performed, and care must be taken to stay anterior to the lesser trochanter to protect the MFCA. The supe-

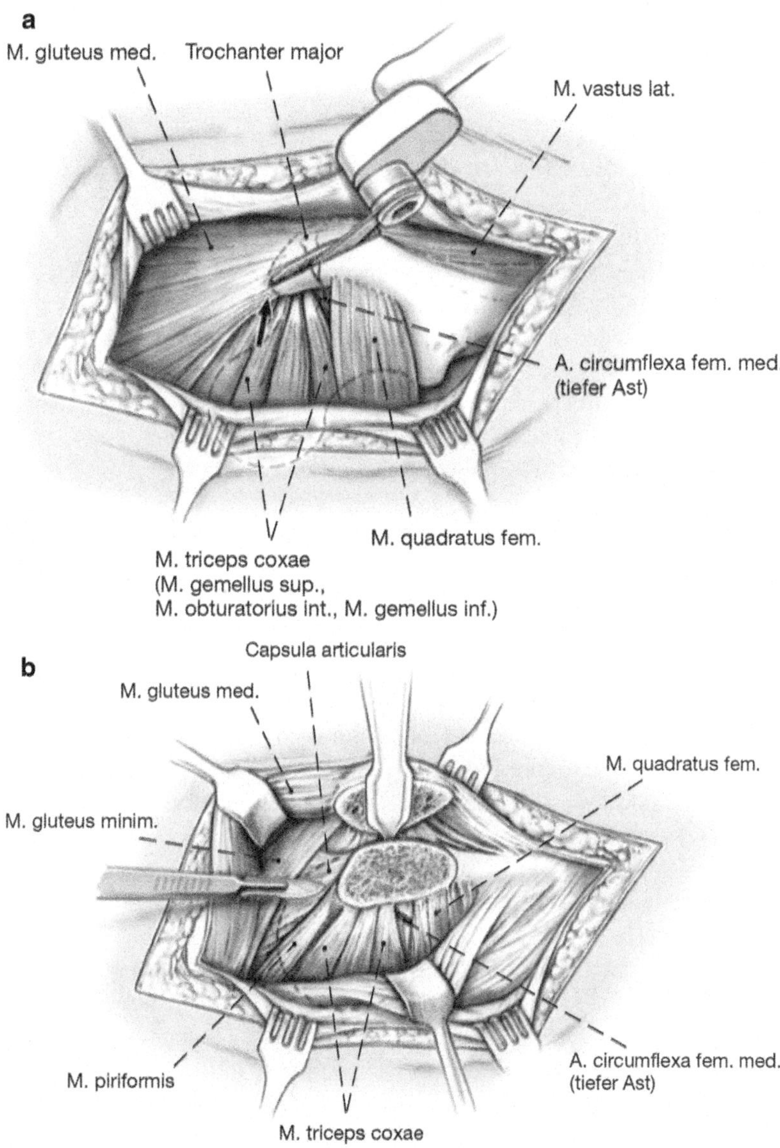

Fig. 7.11 Flat cut trochanteric osteotomy (**a**) is designed to be approximately 15 mm in depth and extend from the medial border of the tip of the greater trochanter to just distal to the vastus lateralis ridge. A saw blade is passed most of the way through the greater trochanter with care not to aim to medial proximally. (**b**) Once the osteotomy is complete the trochanteric fragment can be reflected anteriorly and fibers of the vastus lateralis released from the femur to allow fragment mobilization. Reproduced with permission and copyright © of Springer [26]

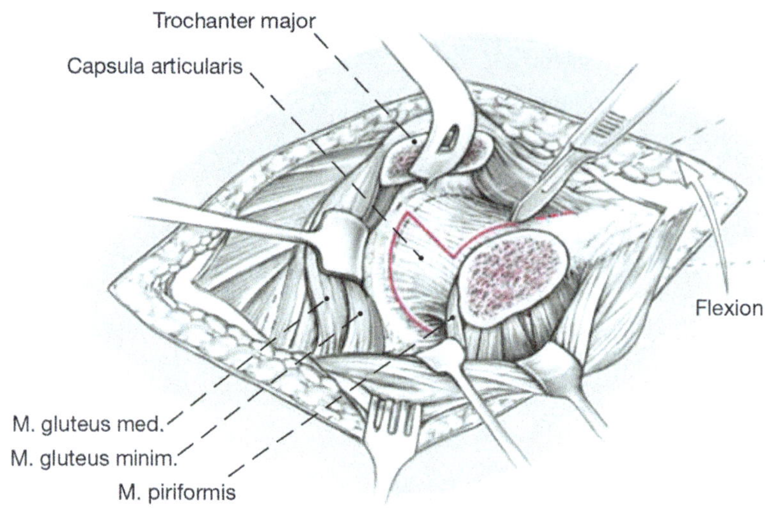

Fig. 7.12 Capsulotomy is performed along the femoral neck starting at the junction where the trochanter meets the femoral neck anteriorly. This capsulotomy is performed in an "inside-out" fashion to protect the cartilage and labrum. The proximal portion of the capsulotomy is extended posteriorly along the acetabular rim, and the distal portion is extended medially towards the lesser trochanter. Reproduced with permission and copyright © of Springer [26]

rior limb of the capsulotomy is then developed along the rim of the acetabulum posteriorly until it reaches the retracted piriformis tendon.

7.2.5.7 Dislocation

Bringing the hip into flexion and external rotation leads to dislocation. We routinely use a bone hook around the inferior neck to gently apply the appropriate force to the proximal femur to aid in dislocation. A curved scissors is used to transect the ligamentum teres, allowing full dislocation. Once dislocated, the operative leg is placed in the sterile bag anterior to the patient. The proximal femur and acetabulum can now be circumferentially inspected. The remaining ligamentum teres is excised from the fovea capitis.

7.2.5.8 Wound Closure

The capsulotomy is closed anatomically with absorbable suture. A watertight closure of the capsule is not necessary as efflux of the hemarthrosis may reduce the risk of iatrogenic osteonecrosis secondary to increased joint pressure. After capsule closure the mobile trochanteric fragment is reduced and fixed with two to three 3.5 or 4.5 mm cortical screws aimed towards the inferior neck and lesser trochanter (Fig. 7.13). The gluteus maximus fascia and proximal iliotibial band are then closed with a running absorbable suture. Subcutaneous tissue and skin are closed in routine fashion.

Both deep and superficial drains can be used to reduce hematoma formation and allow for more comfortable early passive motion.

7.2.6 Postoperative Regimen

Postoperatively patients are placed in a continuous passive motion machine to minimize intraarticular adhesions. Mechanical and pharmacologic DVT prophylaxis are maintained while in the hospital, and pharmacologic prophylaxis is continued for at least 30 days following surgery.

Patients with a flat-cut trochanteric osteotomy are made touchdown weight bearing and advanced to full weight bearing between 6 and 8 weeks postoperatively. Once they are full weight bearing, they may begin abductor strengthening [25].

Patients with a step-cut osteotomy are made 50% body weight bearing and may advance to full weight bearing between 3 and 6 weeks postoperatively depending upon the clinical situation [28, 29]. Abductor strengthening may begin after the patient is full weight bearing.

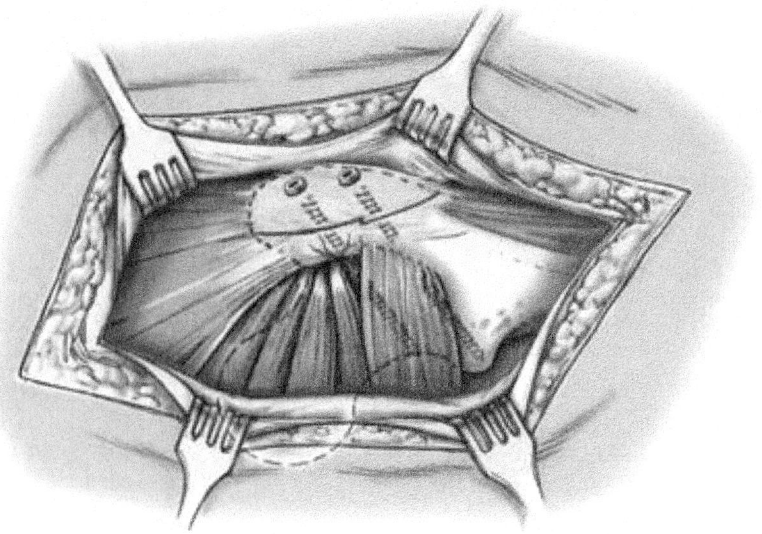

Fig. 7.13 Fixation of the trochanteric osteotomy is performed with two 3.5 mm cortical screws aimed towards the lesser trochanter. While this image depicts the step-cut osteotomy, the same fixation can be used for a flat-cut osteotomy. Reproduced with permission and copyright © of Springer [26]

References

1. Judet R, Judet J, Lagrange J. Gibson's postero-external approach without section of the trochanter in surgery of femur neck fractures and in osteotomies. Presse Med. 1958;66:263–4.
2. Siebenrock KA, Gautier E, Ziran BH, Ganz R. Trochanteric flip osteotomy for cranial extension and muscle protection in acetabular fracture fixation using a Kocher-Langenbeck approach. J Orthop Trauma. 1998;12:387–91.
3. Tosounidis TH, Giannoudis VP, Kanakaris NK, Giannoudis PV. The Kocher-Langenbeck approach: state of the art. JBJS Essent Surg Tech. 2018;8:e18. https://doi.org/10.2106/JBJS.ST.16.00102.
4. Negrin LL, Benson CD, Seligson D. Prone or lateral? Use of the Kocher-Langenbeck approach to treat acetabular fractures. J Trauma. 2010;69:137–41. https://doi.org/10.1097/TA.0b013e3181b28ba6.
5. Letournel E, Judet R. Surgical approaches to the acetabulum. In: Elson RA, editor. Fractures of the acetabulum. Berlin: Springer; 1993. p. S-363–97.
6. Sagi HC, Jordan CJ, Barei DP, et al. Indomethacin prophylaxis for heterotopic ossification after acetabular fracture surgery increases the risk for nonunion of the posterior wall. J Orthop Trauma. 2014;28:377–83. https://doi.org/10.1097/BOT.0000000000000049.
7. Davis JA, Roper B, Munz JW, et al. Does postoperative radiation decrease heterotopic ossification after the Kocher-Langenbeck approach for acetabular fracture? Clin Orthop Relat Res. 2015;474:1430–5. https://doi.org/10.1007/s11999-015-4609-y.
8. Rath EMS, Russell GV, Washington WJ, Routt MLC. Gluteus minimus necrotic muscle debridement diminishes heterotopic ossification after acetabular fracture fixation. Injury. 2002;33:751–6.
9. Farris MK, Chowdhry VK, Lemke S, et al. Osteosarcoma following single fraction radiation prophylaxis for heterotopic ossification. Radiat Oncol. 2012;7:140. https://doi.org/10.1186/1748-717X-7-140.
10. Mourad WF, Packianathan S, Shourbaji RA, et al. Radiation-induced sarcoma following radiation prophylaxis of heterotopic ossification. Pract Radiat Oncol. 2012;2:151–4. https://doi.org/10.1016/j.prro.2011.06.005.
11. Ganz R, Gill TJ, Gautier E, et al. Surgical dislocation of the adult hip a technique with full access to the femoral head and acetabulum without the risk of avascular necrosis. J Bone Joint Surg Br. 2001;83:1119–24.
12. Gautier E, Ganz K, Krügel N, et al. Anatomy of the medial femoral circumflex artery and its surgical implications. J Bone Joint Surg Br. 2000;82:679–83.
13. Beck M, Kalhor M, Leunig M, Ganz R. Hip morphology influences the pattern of damage to the acetabular cartilage: femoroacetabular impingement as a cause of early osteoarthritis of the hip. J Bone Joint Surg Br. 2005;87:1012–8. https://doi.org/10.1302/0301-620X.87B7.15203.
14. Clohisy JC, St John LC, Schutz AL. Surgical treatment of femoroacetabular impingement: a systematic review of the literature. Clin Orthop Relat Res. 2010;468:555–64. https://doi.org/10.1007/s11999-009-1138-6.
15. Espinosa N, Rothenfluh DA, Beck M, et al. Treatment of femoro-acetabular impingement: preliminary results of labral refixation. J Bone Joint Surg Am. 2006;88:925–35. https://doi.org/10.2106/JBJS.E.00290.
16. Ganz R, Parvizi J, Beck M, et al. Femoroacetabular impingement: a cause for osteoarthritis of the hip. Clin Orthop Relat Res. 2003;417:112–20. https://doi.org/10.1097/01.blo.0000096804.78689.c2.

17. Ross JR, Schoenecker PL, Clohisy JC. Surgical dislocation of the hip: evolving indications. HSS J. 2013;9:60–9. https://doi.org/10.1007/s11420-012-9323-7.
18. Siebenrock KA, Anwander H, Zurmühle CA, et al. Head reduction osteotomy with additional containment surgery improves Sphericity and containment and reduces pain in Legg-Calvé-Perthes disease. Clin Orthop Relat Res. 2014;473:1–10. https://doi.org/10.1007/s11999-014-4048-1.
19. Slongo T, Kakaty D, Krause F, Ziebarth K. Treatment of slipped capital femoral epiphysis with a modified Dunn procedure. J Bone Joint Surg Am. 2010;92:2898–908. https://doi.org/10.2106/JBJS.I.01385.
20. Steppacher SD, Huemmer C, Schwab JM, et al. Surgical hip dislocation for treatment of femoroacetabular impingement: factors predicting 5-year survivorship. Clin Orthop Relat Res. 2014;472:337–48. https://doi.org/10.1007/s11999-013-3268-0.
21. Ziebarth K, Zilkens C, Spencer S, et al. Capital realignment for moderate and severe SCFE using a modified Dunn procedure. Clin Orthop Relat Res. 2009;467:704–16. https://doi.org/10.1007/s11999-008-0687-4.
22. Haefeli PC, Marecek GS, Keel MJB, et al. Patients undergoing surgical hip dislocation for the treatment of acetabular fractures show favourable long-term outcome. Bone Joint J. 2017;99-B:508–15. https://doi.org/10.1302/0301-620X.99B4.37681.
23. Albers CE, Steppacher SD, Schwab JM, et al. Relative femoral neck lengthening improves pain and hip function in proximal femoral deformities with a high-riding trochanter. Clin Orthop Relat Res. 2015;473:1378–87. https://doi.org/10.1007/s11999-014-4032-9.
24. Sink EL, Beaulé PE, Sucato D, et al. Multicenter study of complications following surgical dislocation of the hip. J Bone Joint Surg Am. 2011;93:1132–6. https://doi.org/10.2106/JBJS.J.00794.
25. Espinosa N, Beck M, Rothenfluh DA, et al. Treatment of femoro-acetabular impingement: preliminary results of labral refixation. Surgical technique. J Bone Joint Surg Am. 2007;89(Suppl 2 Pt.1):36–53. https://doi.org/10.2106/JBJS.F.01123.
26. Tannast M, Siebenrock KA. Die offene Therapie des femoroazetabulären Impingements. Oper Orthop Traumatol. 2010;22:3–16. https://doi.org/10.1007/s00064-010-3001-7.
27. Gibson A. Posterior exposure of the hip joint. J Bone Joint Surg Br. 1950;32-B:183–6.
28. Bastian JD, Wolf AT, Wyss TF, Nötzli HP. Stepped osteotomy of the trochanter for stable, anatomic refixation. Clin Orthop Relat Res. 2009;467:732–8. https://doi.org/10.1007/s11999-008-0649-x.
29. Schoeniger R, LaFrance AE, Oxland TR, et al. Does trochanteric step osteotomy provide greater stability than classic slide osteotomy? A preliminary study. Clin Orthop Relat Res. 2009;467:775–82. https://doi.org/10.1007/s11999-008-0668-7.

8 Extended Iliofemoral and Combined Approaches

Marius J. B. Keel

Abstract

The indications for the extended iliofemoral (EIF) approach are transverse, T-shaped, or both-column acetabular fracture types with some complicating factors such as the transtectal transverse fracture subtype, associated anterior pelvic ring pathologies, sacroiliac joint injuries, a separate sciatic notch fragment, extended posterior wall fractures, separate dome fracture or impaction or the late reconstruction (>3 weeks after accident) of complex acetabular fractures. Due to the high incidence of complications of the EIF approach such as ectopic ossifications and fair or poor functional outcome combined approaches become more popular. The simultaneous intrapelvic Pararectus approach and trochanteric flip osteotomy with surgical hip dislocation allow anatomic reconstruction of complex acetabular fractures with a lower incidence of complications.

Keywords

Complex acetabular fractures · Extended iliofemoral approach · Combined approaches · Surgical hip dislocation · Intrapelvic approach · Pararectus approach · Floppy lateral position

8.1 Extended Iliofemoral (EIF) Approach

8.1.1 Concept of EIF Approach

The extended iliofemoral (EIF) approach was developed by Letournel [1]. The idea was to achieve both columns simultaneously through one single anatomic approach. It provides direct access to the entire external aspect of the innominate bone from the crest to the ischial tuberosity. In addition the internal iliac fossa can also be exposed to the iliopectineal eminence and psoas tendon as medial border. The dissection follows an interval between the muscles innervated by the femoral nerve, which are retracted medially, and the muscles innervated by the superior and inferior gluteal neural vascular bundles, which are retracted postero-laterally [2].

8.1.2 Surgical Technique of EIF Approach

The patient is placed in the lateral decubitus position with a mobile leg or on a skeletal traction table. The skin incision begins posteriorly at the

M. J. B. Keel (✉)
Trauma Center Hirslanden, Clinic Hirslanden, Zürich, Switzerland
e-mail: mkeel@traumazentrum.ch

L. Büchler, M. J.B. Keel (eds.), *Fractures of the Hip*, Fracture Management Joint by Joint,
https://doi.org/10.1007/978-3-030-18838-2_8

posterior superior iliac spine and courses anteriorly along the iliac crest. At the level of the anterior superior iliac spine, the distal arm of the incision is directed toward the supero-lateral pole of the patella at the medial border of the tensor muscle. The gluteal muscles and the tensor fascia lata are subperiosteally released from the external aspect of the iliac wing. The sheath of the tensor fascia lata is opened and the tensor muscle belly is retracted laterally. The anterior superior spine is dissected from both arms of the exposure. The tensor-gluteal myocutaneous flap is completed by abductor tenotomy or by an osteotomy of the greater trochanter. The greater sciatic notch is visualized under careful control of the superior gluteal neurovascular bundle. After identification of the sciatic nerve the short external rotator tendons are released according to the Kocher-Langenbeck approach. The rectus muscle belly is retracted medially. Distally the ascending branches of the lateral femoral circumflex vessels are ligated. The reflected head of the rectus is dissected off the hip capsule. The external oblique insertion on the crest is released with the attachment of the sartorius and inguinal ligament at the anterior spine. Alternatively an osteotomy of the anterior superior iliac spine (ASIS) can be carried out. Finally the iliac fossa is developed completely. A marginal capsulotomy can be made over the posterior and cranial aspect of the joint (Fig. 8.1). As extension of the approach the femoral insertion of the gluteus maximus can be released. After reduction and fixation, all dissected tendons are reattached in sequence or the greater trochanter and/or the ASIS are attached with screws.

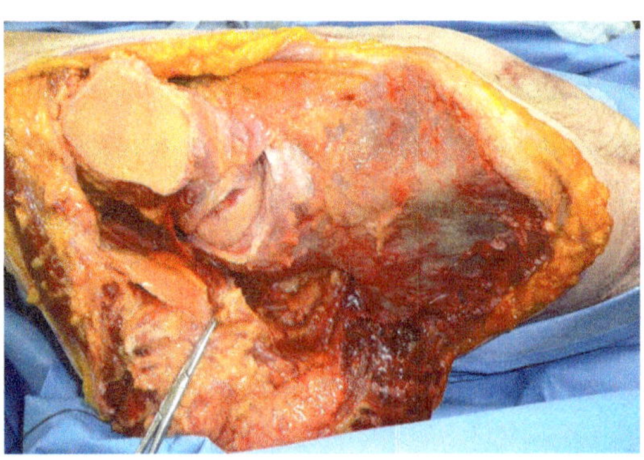

Fig. 8.1 Extended iliofemoral approach in a cadaver dissection. The tensor-gluteal myocutaneous flap is completely mobilized with osteotomy of the greater trochanter and a marginal capsulotomy is done. The internal iliac fossa is not yet exposed

8.1.3 Indication for EIF Approach

The indications for the EIF approach are transverse, T-shaped, or both-column fracture types with some complicating factors [2]. These factors are the transtectal subtype in transverse or T-shaped fractures, associated anterior pelvic ring pathologies, sacroiliac joint injuries (Fig. 8.2), a separate sciatic notch fragment (Fig. 8.3), extended posterior wall fractures or separate

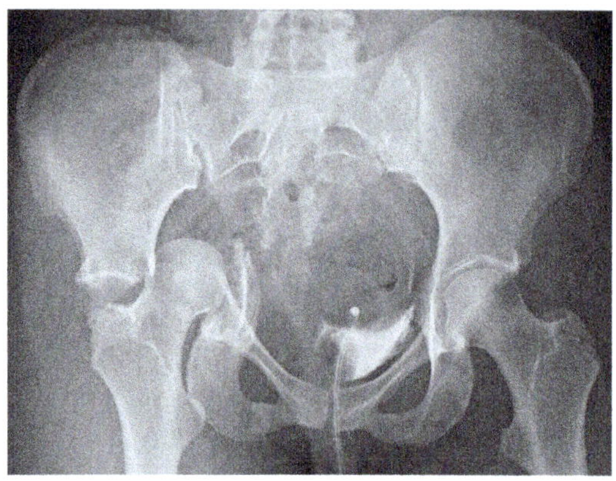

Fig. 8.2 AP pelvis of a transtectal T-shaped acetabular fracture with an associated ipsilateral sacroiliac joint injury

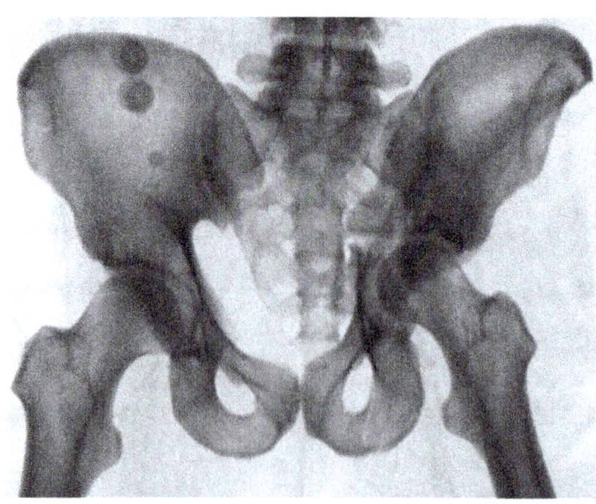

Fig. 8.3 AP 3D computed tomography image of a both-column acetabular fracture with a separate sciatic notch fragment

dome fracture or impaction. In addition late reconstruction (>3 weeks after accident) of complex acetabular fractures is also a classic indication for the EIF approach. The use of the EIF approach was decreased in the series of Matta by the increased experiences for single approaches like the ilioinguinal or the Kocher-Langenbeck approaches [3]. In a retrospective study, increase in single approach surgery resulted in shorter mean surgical time, significant increase in anatomical reduction, and reduction of frequency of intra- and postoperative complications [4].

8.1.4 Complications and Outcome of EIF

The advantage of the EIF for complex acetabular fractures is the concept of one single anatomic approach. However the approach is at risk for infections, heterotopic ossifications, total flap necrosis, and prolonged postoperative morbidity due to the devascularization of the innominate bone and the gluteus medius and minimus muscles [2].

In a series of Matta with 106 patients involving in 60% both-column fractures, 64% good or excellent results could be observed 6.3 years (2–17) postoperatively [5]. 36% developed fair or poor results. Functional outcome correlated significantly with the accuracy of the reduction. The reduction was graded as anatomical (0–1 mm of displacement) in 72%, imperfect (2–3 mm) in 22%, and poor (>3 mm) in 6%. Operation was undertaken in less than 3 weeks after injury in 67% and in 33% the procedure was carried out later. Significant heterotopic ossification developed in 30% and was associated with a worse outcome.

In a series of 50 cases published by Stöckle in 2002 complications included 8% loss of reduction, 13% significant heterotopic ossifications, and 4% avascular femoral head necrosis [6]. At the two-year follow-up there were 74% good or excellent radiographic and clinical results. Four patients had already total hip replacements. In summary, between 30% and 40% of complex acetabular fractures operated through the EIF approach ended in fair or poor results with a high incidence of ectopic ossifications. The use of the EIF approach is finally a risk for poor outcome with implantation of a total hip arthroplasty [3].

8.2 Combined Approaches

8.2.1 Concept and Indications of Combined Approaches

As alternative to the EIF approach anterior and posterior approaches can be combined for complex approaches. This can be carried out sequentially or simultaneously. If the anterior approach is followed by the posterior approach or vice versa in the same operation or in two separate operations the fixation of the anterior or posterior column should not block the opposite column in a malposition. The indications for combined approaches are the similar like for the EIF approach.

8.2.2 Techniques of Combined Approaches

Routt described the open reduction and internal fixation through combined anterior and posterior exposures during the same period of anesthesia in a sequential procedure [7]. The simultaneous use of the ilioinguinal and Kocher-Langenbeck approaches in floppy lateral position was primarily described in 1989 by Goulet [8]. However these simultaneous approaches are technically complicated by the limitations of both approaches in the semi-lateral position. The combination of an intrapelvic approach, the modified Stoppa or especially the Pararectus approach [9], with the trochanteric flip osteotomy and surgical hip dislocation is easier to proceed and allows an absolute anatomic reduction because of the full exposure of the joint and the verification of the anatomic reduction [10]. The success of the combined approaches depends on the experience of the surgeon carrying out each single approach.

8.2.3 Complications and Outcome of Combined Approaches

Goulet showed in his series of 31 cases excellent in 35% and good results in 42% [8]. Routt achieved in 24 cases anatomic reduction in 88%. Significant ossifications developed in 16%. In another series of ten patients with sequential ilioinguinal and Kocher-Langenbeck approaches, only in three patients of seven patients anatomic reduction could be achieved [11]. Moroni published 18 patients affected by both-column fractures operated on by staged combined ilioinguinal and Kocher-Langenbeck approaches with a low rate of anatomical reduction in 28% [12]. Clinical and radiological results of combined intrapelvic and posterior approaches are missing. However, first experiences as shown by the presented cases (Figs. 8.4 and 8.5) demonstrate excellent results with a low incidence of complications.

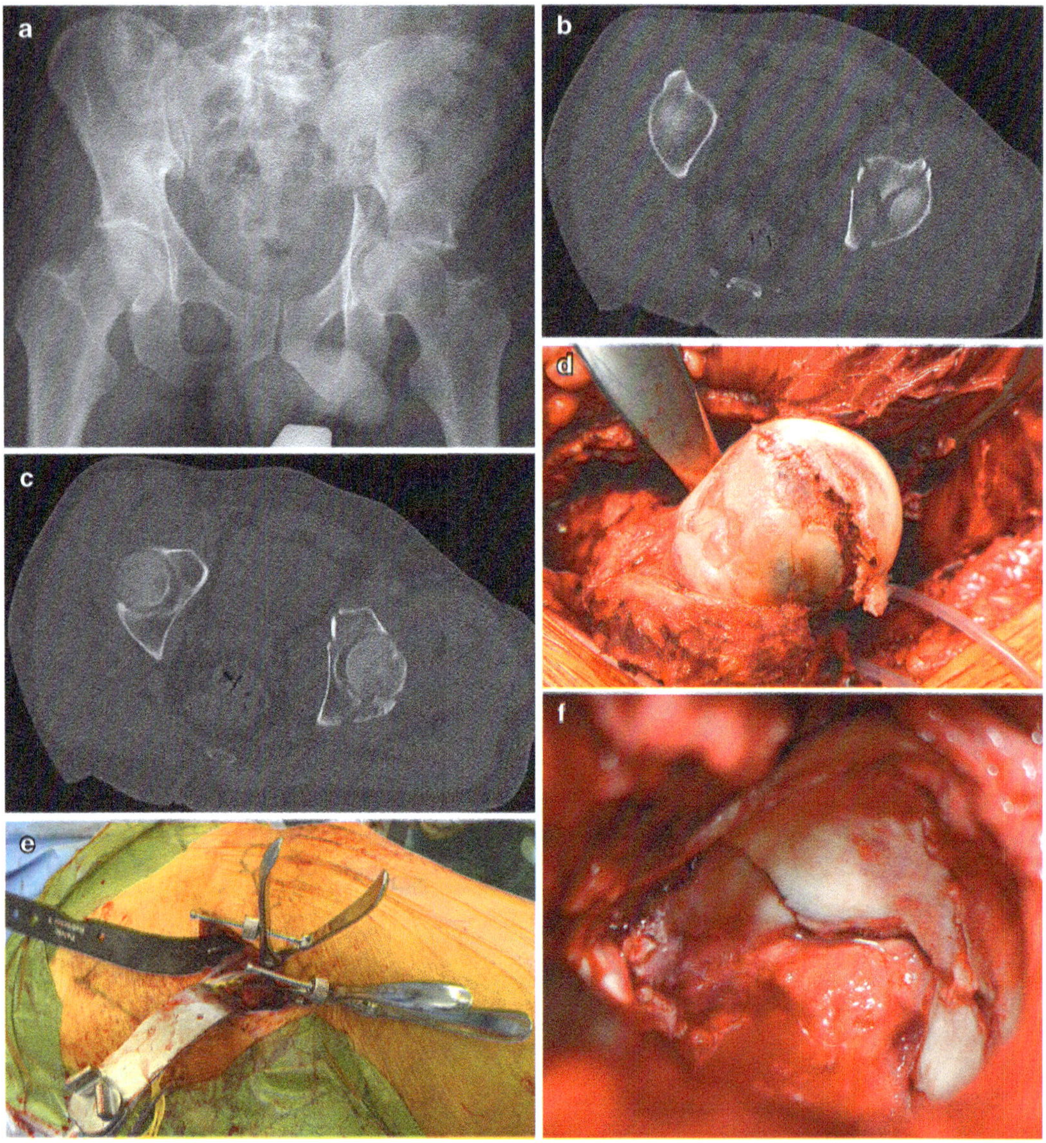

Fig. 8.4 46 year old man with transtectal T-shaped fracture and a femoral head impaction on the left side after ski accident. AP pelvis (**a**) and axial CT cuts on the dome level (**b**) and distally with the displacement in the posterior column and impaction of the femoral head (**c**). Intraoperative views on the femoral head impaction during surgical hip dislocation (**d**), the Pararectus approach with retractors and reduction clamps in situ (**e**) and into the joint after anatomic reduction and fixation (**f**) in the floppy lateral position. Postoperative AP pelvis (**g**) and axial CT cut on the dome level (**h**) with demonstration of the anatomic reconstruction. AP pelvis (**i**) 2 years after surgery of the pain-free patient

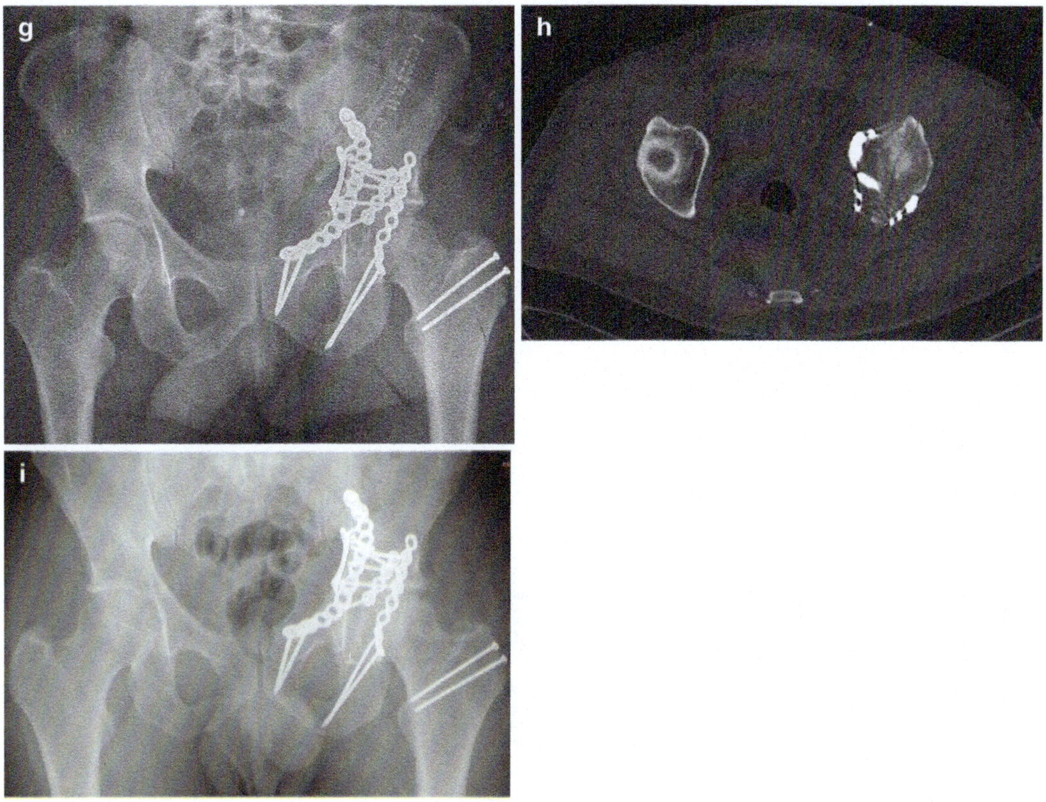

Fig. 8.4 (continued)

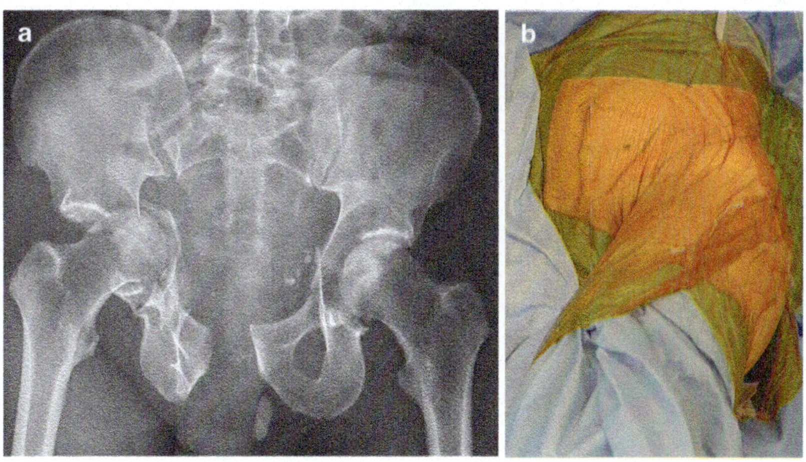

Fig. 8.5 62 year old man with juxtatectal T-shaped fracture on the left side, a posterior hip dislocation on the right side with a transtectal transverse fracture and associated sacroiliac joint dislocation on the right side and symphysis dislocation after a bicycle accident. AP pelvis after closed reduction of the right hip (**a**). Intraoperative view of the floppy lateral position for the reconstruction of the left hip joint (**b**) in the first operation. Intraoperative views of the reduction maneuver of the sacroiliac joint on the right side with a Jungbluth clamp (**c**) and the plates on the anterior column and the symphysis through the Pararectus approach on the right side (**d**) in the second operation in the same anesthesia. AP pelvis postoperatively (**e**) and 8 months after surgery with equal bilateral hip functions however with some ectopic ossifications (**f**)

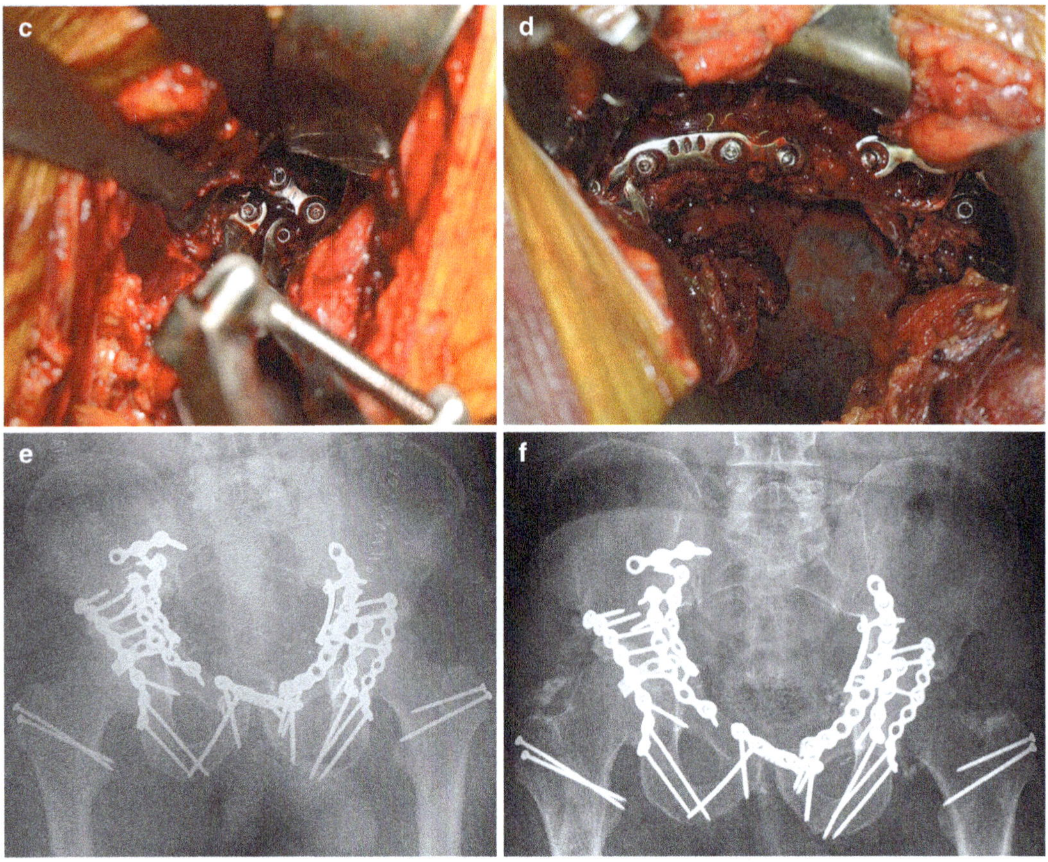

Fig. 8.5 (continued)

References

1. Letournel E. Les fractures du còtyle. Etude d'une serie de 75 cas. J Chir. 1961;87:83–92.
2. Mayo KA. Surgical approaches to the acetabulum. Tech Orthip. 1990;4:24–35.
3. Tannast M, Najibi S, Matta JM. Two to twenty-year survivorship of the hip in 810 patients with operatively treated acetabular fractures. J Bone Joint Surg Am. 2012;94:1559–67.
4. Gusic N, Sabalic S, Pavic A, Ivkovic A, Sotosek-Tokmadzic V, Cicvaric T. Rationale for more consistent choice of surgical approaches for acetabular fractures. Injury. 2015;46S:S78–86.
5. Griffin DB, Beaulé PE, Matta JM. Safety and efficacy of the extended iliofemoral approach in the treatment of complex fractures of the acetabulum. J Bone Joint Surg (Br). 2005;87-B:1391–6.
6. Stöckle U, Hoffmann R, Südkamp NP, Reindl R, Haas NP. Treatment of complex acetabular fractures through a modified extended iliofemoral approach. J Orthop Trauma. 2002;16:220–30.
7. Routt ML Jr, Swiontkowski MF. Operative treatment of complex acetabular fractures. Combined anterior and posterior exposures during the same procedure. J Bone Joint Surg Am. 1990;72:897–904.
8. Goulet JA, Bray TJ. Complex acetabular fractures. Clin Orthop Relat Res. 1989;240:9–20.
9. Keel MJB, Ecker TM, Cullmann JL, Bergmann M, Bonel HM, Büchler L, Siebenrock KA, Bastian JD. The Pararectus approach for anterior intrapelvic management of acetabular fractures. An anatomical study and clinical evaluation. J Bone Joint Surg Br. 2012;94-B:405–11.
10. Keel MJB, Ecker TM, Siebenrock KA, Bastian JD. Rationales for the Bernese approaches in acetabular surgery. Eur J Trauma Emerg Surg. 2012;38:489–98.
11. Guerado E, Cano JR, Cruz E. Simultaneous ilioinguinal and Kocher-Langenbeck approaches for the treatment of complex acetabular fractures. Hip Int. 2010;20(Suppl 7):S2–S10.
12. Moroni A, Caja VL, Sabato C, Zinghi G. Surgical treatment of both-column fractures by staged combined ilioinguinal and Kocher-Langenbeck approaches. Injury. 1995;26:219–24.

Traumatic Hip Dislocations

9

Mark Rickman and Lorenz Büchler

Abstract

Pure hip dislocations are relatively unusual, but represent an injury with significant capacity for resulting in long-term disability. The femoral head most commonly dislocates posteriorly (80–90%), typically caused by axial force on the femur with the hip flexed as seen in dash board injuries. Concomitant pathomorphologies of the hip such as cam-type impingement, or femoral retrotorsion are a risk factor for posterior dislocation. Anterior dislocations are not that unusual, forming approximately 10% of most series. Other forms of pure dislocation are very unusual, i.e. obturator and central dislocation and are mostly a fracture dislocation. Early reduction is essential to improve outcome, and certainly within 12 h of injury, although as early as is safely possible is ideal. CT scanning is the current standard imaging; examination under anesthesia to assess stability aids planning and early post-operative mobility is probably beneficial. Surgery is reserved for irreducible dislocations, associated fractures, incongruence after reduction, or significant instability found at examination under anesthesia (EUA). Long-term hip outcomes are mostly excellent or good, but avascular necrosis (AVN) and post-injury arthritis affect up to 20% of cases. Associated injuries are common in this group, and often determine the overall patient outcome.

Keywords

Hip · Joint dislocation · Traumatic dislocation · Obturator dislocation · Femoral head · Open reduction · Closed reduction · Hip outcome

9.1 Epidemiology, Mechanism of Injury

The hip is an intrinsically stable joint, with the femoral head typically well seated within the acetabulum. Stability is further improved by surrounding musculature, as well as the labrum, capsule and associated thickenings/ligaments (especially iliofemoral ligament and zona orbicularis), and the ligamentum teres. The energy required to dislocate a native hip joint therefore is immense, and as a result concomitant life-threatening injuries and fractures are reported to occur in up to 95% of cases [1]. Apart from ace-

M. Rickman (✉)
Centre for Orthopaedic and Trauma Research, Discipline of Orthopaedics and Trauma, University of Adelaide, Adelaide, SA, Australia

Department of Orthopaedics and Trauma, Royal Adelaide Hospital, Adelaide, SA, Australia
e-mail: mark.rickman@sa.gov.au

L. Büchler
Department of Orthopaedic Surgery, Kantonsspital Aarau, Aarau, Switzerland

L. Büchler, M. J.B. Keel (eds.), *Fractures of the Hip*, Fracture Management Joint by Joint,
https://doi.org/10.1007/978-3-030-18838-2_9

tabular fractures, imaging must therefore be carefully scrutinized to identify femoral head or neck fractures, and patients carefully examined looking for distant injuries. Posterior dislocations commonly occur in conjunction with knee injuries and are most frequently seen in drivers of vehicles, prompting the theory of a dashboard strike as the mechanism; however, other theories have been put forward including a brake-pedal injury [2]. Sciatic nerve injuries are seen in around 10% of posterior dislocations [3], and more likely to occur with delayed reduction [4] . As well as direct injuries, the blood supply to the femoral head can be compromised by this injury, resulting in avascular necrosis.

Epstein et al. postulated that posterior impingement at the extreme of external rotation acts as a lever, to force the femoral head anteriorly [5]. Upadhyay et al. found a decrease in femoral anteversion in a group of patients who had suffered a posterior dislocation, suggesting that the hip would impinge during internal rotation and posterior dislocation would then occur [6]. More recently several authors have linked cam-type femoro-acetabular impingement to posterior dislocation through a similar postulated mechanism [7–10].

No matter what the exact mechanism, there is significant contact between the femoral head and acetabular rim at the time of dislocation, with a combination of compression and shear forces; this frequently results in either an acetabular rim fracture or chondral damage to the femoral head or acetabulum. It is generally believed that an anterior dislocation will fare worse than a posterior one, in view of the femoral head damage typically being posterior in these cases—however there is a paucity of evidence in the literature either to confirm or refute this.

As the femoral head dislocates, the ligamentum teres is necessarily rendered incompetent. True ligament ruptures occur, but frequently there is a bony avulsion from either the femoral head (which can lead to a significant femoral head injury) or from the foveal surface; these bony avulsions often come to lie in the joint after reduction, causing incongruence and further damage if not retrieved.

Post-traumatic arthritis is the commonest long-term complication of hip dislocation, primarily as a result of the joint surface damage sustained, combined with effects from retained loose bodies and subtle post-injury instability.

Avascular necrosis is the second most common and severe complication. The exact incidence of AVN remains unclear in the literature, and AVN rates are reported in the range of 1–15% [11–14]. In the past treatment involved a long period of traction but it is now recognized that there seems to be no correlation between the period of traction and the incidence of either avascular necrosis or recurrent instability following hip dislocation. It remains unknown whether early weight bearing affects outcome [5, 15]. The importance of immediate reduction of the dislocation is also difficult to state with any certainty. The purest series, that is with the longest follow-up, is that published by Upadhyay and Moulton in 1981 [16]. They had 53 posterior dislocations without fracture, in a series of over 80 cases. The follow-up was greater than 10 years in 55 of these cases, and the avascular necrosis rate of the whole series was 6%, which is in the midrange of other authors on the topic. The numbers of avascular necrosis in Upadhyay's paper were too small to give any indication regarding the timing of relocation and avascular necrosis rate although in both dislocations that were missed avascular necrosis developed and subsequently had a poor outcome. However, Reigstad reported no incidences of AVN in hips reduced within 6 h, and Hougard similarly showed poorer results in hips dislocated for longer than this in a series of 127 cases. Kellam and Ostrum [17] published a systematic review of the literature on this issue in 2015, and concluded that AVN was approximately twice as likely to occur after posterior dislocations compared to anterior, and that reduction before 12 h has a significant effect on the likely risk of AVN overall. There is no evidence that anything less than 6 h has a significant effect, thus reduction should be planned as soon as is feasible, but not rushed in an unsafe manner. Any dislocation that is missed for a significant period will result in a poorer outcome with a higher incidence of avascular necrosis, osteoarthritis, and subsequent requirement for arthroplasty.

9.2 Clinical and Radiographic Assessment

Most orthopedic surgeons are familiar with patients presenting with dislocated total hip replacements, and the position of the leg; dislocated native hips are little different from a clinical perspective, with the exception of the higher energy involved. Posterior dislocations (Fig. 9.1) will tend to result in the lower limb becoming fixed in internal rotation with or without flexion and adduction, and anterior dislocations (Fig. 9.2) typically result in external rotation, abduction, and extension. Obturator dislocations have a more variable position, but the main defining factor is typically that the leg rests in a degree of abduction.

It is critical to examine the patient at this stage for signs of neurological or vascular compromise, and to document these findings; the discovery of sciatic nerve palsy after a closed reduction of a dislocated hip is impossible to interpret without sound knowledge of the pre-reduction state, and can lead to unnecessary urgent surgery.

In most hospitals, the initial imaging will involve a simple plain AP pelvic radiograph. The vast majority of dislocations are easily identified on plain films, but both the direction of dislocation and associated injuries can be much more difficult to elucidate. CT scanning allows a more formal assessment of the injury; if one studies pre-operative radiographs and CT scans carefully, it is often possible to identify small posterior wall flake fractures and hence these really

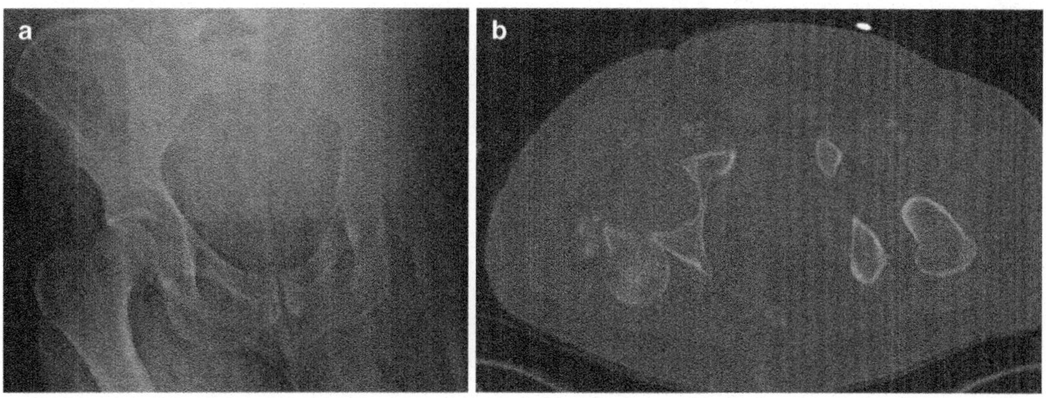

Fig. 9.1 (**a**) AP radiograph of a posterior hip dislocation at presentation. (**b**) CT scan of the same case, showing the femoral head locked behind the posterior acetabulum

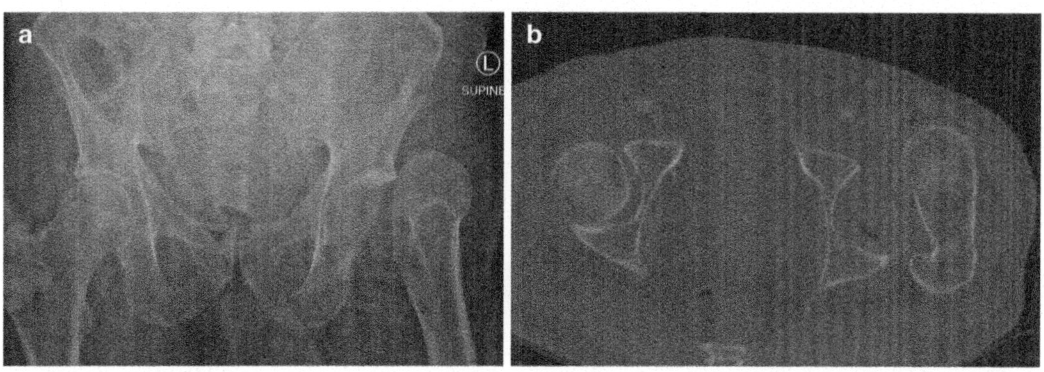

Fig. 9.2 (**a**) AP radiograph of an anterior hip dislocation at presentation. (**b**) CT scan of the same case, showing the direction of dislocation more clearly

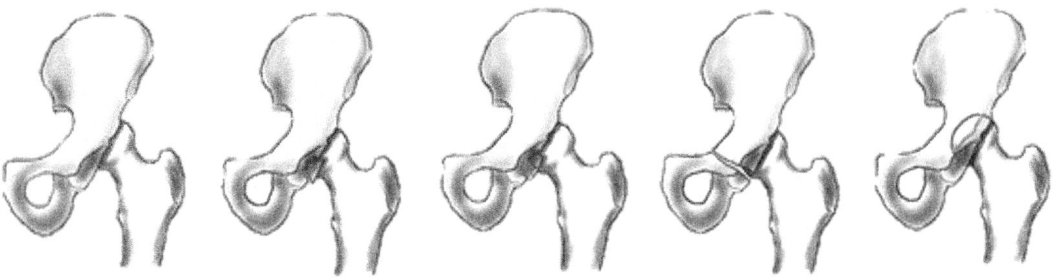

Fig. 9.3 Classification of Traumatic Hip Dislocations from Thompson & Epstein. (1) With or without minor fracture. (2) With large single fracture of posterior acetabular rim. (3) With comminuted fracture of rim of acetabulum, with or without major fragment. (4) With fracture of acetabular rim and floor. (5) With fracture of femoral head. Reproduced with permission and copyright © of Springer [19]

need to be classified as wall fractures rather than pure dislocations.

The role of MRI scanning remains controversial. Whilst it may add useful information regarding the vascularity of the femoral head [18] as well as identify labral or chondral damage, its main role remains as an adjunct to follow-up, or for investigation of the incongruent hip after reduction, especially in skeletally immature patients.

9.2.1 Classification

Classification of hip dislocation can either be done based on direction or associated injuries. In its pure form (i.e., without any associated acetabular or femoral head fractures) the dislocated hip can be classified as being posterior, anterior, or obturator in decreasing order of frequency. Central fracture-dislocations are also often described, but these represent an acetabular fracture with medial displacement of the femoral head, rather than a true dislocation. This descriptive classification helps the treating surgeon when thinking about reduction maneuvers, and has some prognostic information with regard to AVN rates and possibly long-term outcomes.

The most commonly used injury related classification is that of Thompson and Epstein [11], although all five of their categories potentially had associated fractures, types 2–4 had acetabular fractures and type 5 had femoral head fractures (Fig. 9.3). Only Type 1 was said to be "with or without minor fracture." Nevertheless, this is a useful and widely applied classification, and their results show nicely that from 116 cases, the anterior dislocations fared well, and 20 of 30 Type 1 posterior dislocations had good or excellent outcomes compared to only 13 of 68 Types 2–5. It must be noted though that a good result in this report allowed for a 25% decrease in range of motion with minimal X-ray changes (at a mean of 3 years and 9 months), and it is likely that these cases would deteriorate and become arthritic in time.

9.3 Reduction and Assessment/Decision Making

All pure dislocations will require reduction. In the absence of a femoral neck fracture this is generally possible using manual maneuvers, but requires muscle relaxation in the form of either heavy sedation or general anesthesia. In addition, immediate confirmation of reduction using image intensifier is necessary, and some assessment of the level of instability is helpful, and for these reasons it is desirable for reduction to be performed where possible in the operating theater. However, a balance needs to be struck between these desires and the need for rapid reduction. If immediate or very early access to an environment where image intensifier is available is not possible, then reduction in the emergency department is reasonable provided safe sedation is available.

9.3.1 Reduction Methods

In basic terms, reduction of a dislocated joint requires traction with or without rotational maneuvers, and some form of counter-traction. Regardless of the direction of dislocation, manual in line traction will reduce many dislocations. Two more advanced methods for reduction of a dislocated hip have been described.

Allis [20] described his technique over 100 years ago. The patient is supine, and counter-traction applied to the pelvis—in the original report this was done with bandages passed through hooks in the floor, running up and over the pelvis, more commonly an assistant will place each hand on an anterior superior iliac spine and hold the pelvis still. With the hip and knee both flexed to 90° traction is applied in a vertical direction, with the addition after a few seconds of sustained traction of slight adduction/rotation in order to facilitate the femoral head clearing the lip of the acetabulum. In order to gain mechanical advantage the surgeon must be above the patient—this is typically achieved either by the patient being very close to (or on) the floor or by the surgeon standing on the bed; this maneuver is very difficult if not impossible to do with the surgeon standing on the floor and the patient in bed at a routine height.

Stimson [21] described a gravity assisted method even earlier—in 1889. This technique involves having the patient lie prone, with the affected leg hanging off the side of the bed. The hip and knee are again flexed to 90°, and traction applied this time to the back of the calf. This maneuver is in fact the same as the Allis maneuver, but as it is gravity assisted it is mechanically easier to perform. It has the disadvantage however of requiring a prone patient, which in the trauma situation is rarely possible in a safe manner.

Numerous other techniques have been described [22–26], most of which in various forms attempt to increase the mechanical advantage of the surgeon, using either a fulcrum or assistants.

9.3.2 Failed Reduction

If closed reduction is not possible, then open reduction is mandated. This situation requires careful planning around the surgical skills available—not only is the surgical approach more difficult due to displaced structures, but ideally any associated injuries should be dealt with at the same time. This situation confers a poorer prognosis—McKee et al. [27] recorded a series of 25 patients with high-energy dislocations that could not be reduced closed. Not surprisingly there were a high incidence of other injuries including sciatic nerve palsy (28%), femoral head or neck fractures (36%), and only 6 of the 25 patients had a good or excellent outcome. Canale and Manugian [28] also discussed the irreducible hip, and described the causes as being the femoral head button-holed through the capsule, or piriformis being displaced across the acetabulum. In cases with associated fractures, a large intra-articular bone fragment may prevent reduction; in addition, if there is a large posterior wall fracture, then reduction can be unstable enough that it appears impossible to reduce the hip, whereas reduction is in fact achieved but stability is impossible.

If an open reduction is necessary, then a CT is mandated prior to surgery; this will give essential information regarding associated injuries and possible causes for failed reduction which may impact directly on the proposed procedure.

9.3.3 Assessment of Reduction

After closed reduction, careful assessment of the imaging is required to assess congruence. In some cases, a plain film will show a perfect reduction, and it is safe to plan further management; however in a number of cases, although the hip will be relocated, incongruence is seen as a result of either bone, cartilage or labrum typically being interposed between the joint surfaces (Figs. 9.4, 9.5 and 9.6). Any doubt regarding congruence should lead to further imaging. CT scanning will show incongruent reductions and

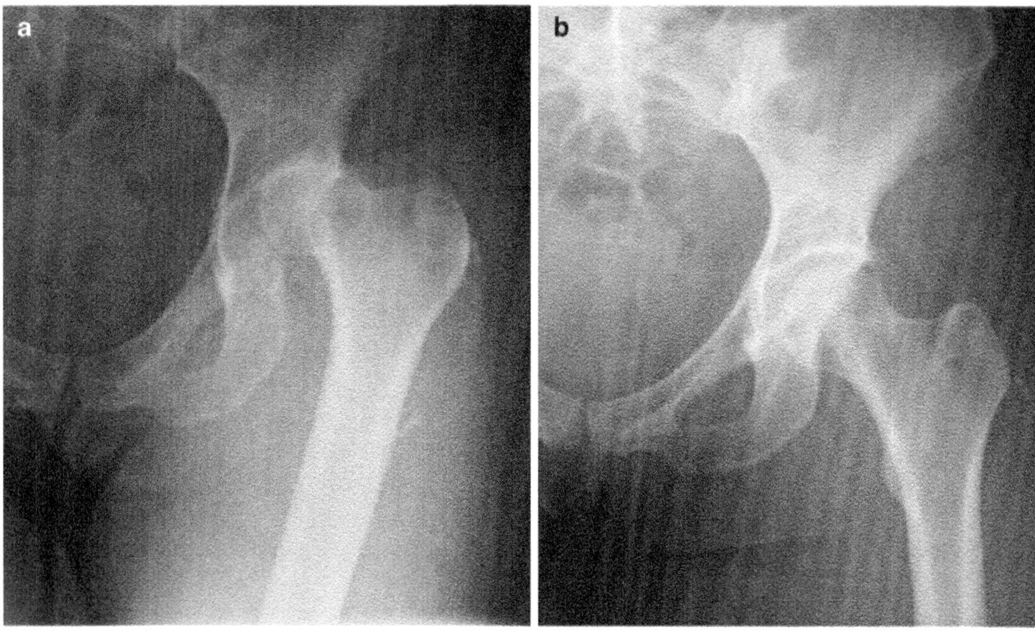

Fig. 9.4 (a) AP radiograph of a hip showing posterior hip dislocation. (b) AP radiograph after reduction showing an incongruent joint with a slightly increased joint space

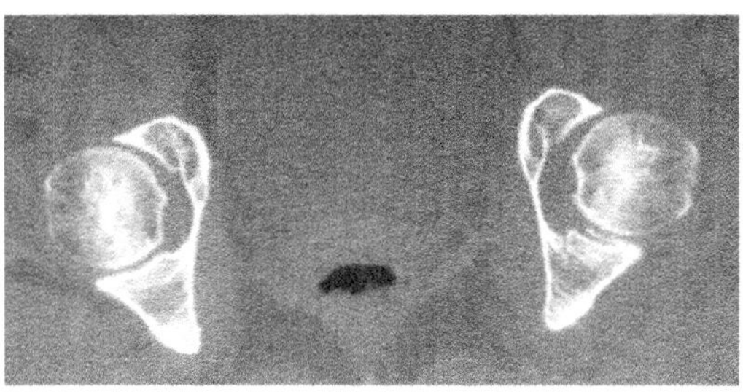

Fig. 9.5 CT scanning revealed a loose fragment in the joint

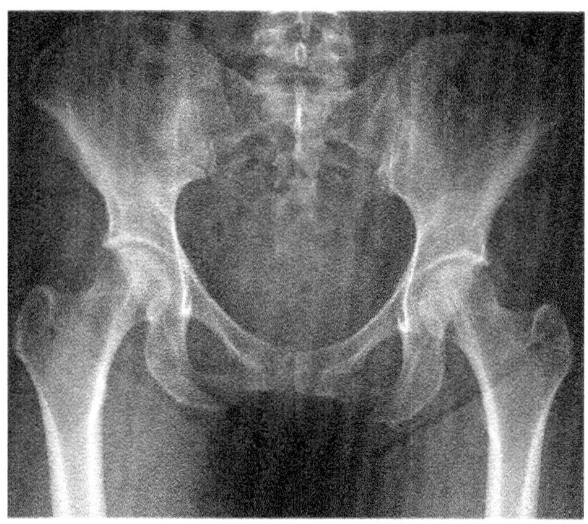

Fig. 9.6 The loose body was retrieved arthroscopically—the AP film subsequently shows a congruent hip joint

bone fragments well, is typically more readily available but involves radiation; MRI scanning whilst being less easy to organize in most institutions will give additional information regarding the labrum, and any other associated soft tissue damage that may be causing incongruence. The accuracy of MRI scanning for assessment of chondral injuries however appears less good, with Tannast et al. [18] reporting observed chondral injuries in only 16–21% of cases, whereas surgery on the same cases revealed damage in 67%. In practice, CT scanning gives more relevant information and is simpler to organize, meaning that the role of MRI scanning remains predominantly in the follow-up phase, or rarely for cases where CT has demonstrated no cause for post-reduction incongruence.

Of note—there are a number of cases where reduction is congruent, but CT scanning shows a small fragment of bone sitting in the acetabular fossa. Provided the fragment is definitely not interposed between the articular surfaces, then it is safe for this small fragment to be left alone; in most cases, it will be seen to be resorbed and disappear over time, after having become locked in place in the fossa by early scar tissue.

9.3.4 Assessment of Stability

After reduction (whether open or closed), an assessment of instability is helpful for further management decisions. Typically the hip is flexed to 90°, then internal rotation/abduction applied until the hip is seen to start to sublux (or external rotation/adduction for anterior dislocations). After a closed reduction, a very unstable hip requires careful consideration of surgical exploration and repair; in most cases, there is a significant tear in the capsule, as well as labral detachment. Again, these are well visualized on MRI scanning, although the decision is aided more by stability testing than imaging. Stable, congruent hips can be managed non-operatively with the expectation of good results, even in the presence of soft tissue damage.

9.4 Conservative Treatment

Until fairly recently these injuries were managed with differing amounts of bed rest and traction, with the presumed benefit of avoiding re-dislocation, allowing the soft tissues to heal, and limiting joint damage by avoiding weight bearing in this potentially unstable phase. However, if the hip is proven to be stable on testing, then careful activity management should avoid re-dislocation; more recent papers have shown no disadvantage to early weight bearing, and in fact the opposite may in fact be true [29].

Patients with pure dislocations that have been reduced anatomically and shown on examination under anesthetic to be stable can therefore be managed simply with full weight bearing as soon as the patient is comfortable. It is prudent to avoid flexion beyond 90° for 6 weeks, and internal rotation beyond 10°. A pair of crutches for 6 weeks may also serve to "remind" patients of their injury, as symptoms subside over the early weeks.

9.5 Operative Treatment

The only absolute indications for operative management of a pure hip dislocation are the irreducible hip and the incongruent reduction. Relative indications are instability demonstrated at EUA, repair of large soft tissue lesions identified on MRI scanning, and surgery to assess chondral impaction identified on CT scanning.

The irreducible hip is an emergency situation, whereas the incongruent hip can be delayed for a day or two if necessary; most surgeons would apply traction in the meantime to avoid further articular damage as a result of the interposed structures. Surgery for instability, soft tissue lesions or femoral head damage can be planned more leisurely, but should still ideally be performed within a few days.

The choice of surgical approach is made based on injury factors as well as the skills of the surgeon; most pure dislocations with or without femoral head damage can be safely approached via lateral or posterior approach, and a trochanteric osteotomy added if necessary. This will give access to the entire posterior capsule and labrum, as well as the entire femoral head if chondral injuries are to be addressed. However, for irreducible anterior dislocations an anterior approach (e.g. Smith-Petersen) is recommended, as the block to reduction is more likely to be out of the field of view of a posterior approach, even after a trochanteric osteotomy. In all approaches performed for irreducible dislocations, extreme care must be taken as structures are displaced from their usual positions, and often under tension.

Femoral head impaction lesions or abrasion of the cartilage are difficult to manage, and undoubtedly have a negative effect on overall long-term outcomes. Management options are the same as discussed in Chap. 11, Pipkin Fractures. As well as achieving anatomic joint reduction, the soft tissues should be repaired as far as possible, in order to achieve stability. This involves repairing the labrum where torn, as well as closing the damaged capsule and reattaching any torn tendons when possible.

9.5.1 Hip Arthroscopy After Dislocation

In recent years, interest has increased in the role of hip arthroscopy after hip dislocations. Use of hip arthroscopy can be divided into early (predominantly removal of loose bodies or labral repair) or late (similar indications, but also allowing assessment of healed chondral surfaces).

Keene and Villar [30] were the first to publish two case reports of arthroscopic loose body removal after hip relocation—they also stressed the importance of careful joint distraction to avoid further damaging the femoral head blood supply.

Mullis and Dahners [31] reported 36 patients undergoing hip arthroscopy after dislocated hips at a mean of 15 days, with no specific clinical indication. They found loose bodies in 92% of cases, but no patient outcomes were provided.

Wylie et al. [32] performed arthroscopies on 12 cases of dislocation (11 within 30 days of injury), performed for ongoing hip symptoms, and found eight patients to have loose bodies and the same number to have labral injuries. Patient outcomes however were again not given in the paper.

A summary of the available literature regarding hip arthroscopy after dislocation would be that it is possible to treat specific lesions identified on imaging, and routine arthroscopy may identify previously unappreciated pathology, but whether this translates into any clinical benefit for the patient is yet to be proven.

One of the concerns regarding early hip arthroscopy after dislocation is the possibility of fluid extravasation and the development of compartment syndrome. Whilst case reports [33] of abdominal compartment syndrome exist, there are none within the literature at the present time related to post-traumatic hip arthroscopies; nevertheless, it remains a theoretical risk, and one which surgeons must bear in mind. Mullis stated that extravasation was commonly seen, but had not resulted in any clinical problems.

9.6 Overall Outcomes

The two largest series of anterior dislocation of the hip were reported by Epstein in 1980 and Brav in 1962. There were 54 cases with a mean follow-up of 17 months in Epstein's series and 34 cases with a mean follow-up of 18 months in Brav's—88 cases in all. Drainhoffer et al. in 1994 have reported a further 12 cases with a mean follow-up of 8 years.

The overall incidence of an excellent or good result (using Thompson/Epsteins method) was 76%, with a quarter being fair or poor. There was a 5% avascular necrosis rate. Post-traumatic arthritis was 17% and myositis ossificans was seen in 4%.

Thompson & Epstein's series and classification of posterior dislocation types I, II, III, IV, and V are difficult to interpret as they are almost combining posterior dislocation with some form of acetabular fracture in three of the five injuries.

Upadhyay described the long-term (mean 14.5 years) outcome of 74 simple posterior dislocations, presumably managed by only closed methods. 56 (76%) hips had good or excellent results, but six hips had developed AVN by 3 years, and a further 16% developed osteoarthritis. Manual laborers fared much worse, with the incidence of osteoarthritis in patients injured in mining accidents as high as 45%.

CT scanning was not widely available at the time of any of these reports, and one of the reasons for the poor results is the fact that although the acetabular rim does not break, the femoral head will be indented and impacted; these injuries would have gone undetected, whereas today they are more likely to be seen and addressed. However, no large series of patients exist using modern imaging and treatment methods.

References

1. Hak DJ, Goulet JA. Severity of injuries associated with traumatic hip dislocation as a result of motor vehicle collisions. J Trauma. 1999;47(1):60–3.
2. Monma H, Sugita T. Is the mechanism of traumatic posterior dislocation of the hip a brake pedal injury rather than a dashboard injury? Injury. 2001;32(3):221–2.

3. Cornwall R, Radomisli TE. Nerve injury in traumatic dislocation of the hip. Clin Orthop Relat Res. 2000;377:84–91.
4. Hillyard RF, Fox J. Sciatic nerve injuries associated with traumatic posterior hip dislocations. Am J Emerg Med. 2003;21(7):545–8.
5. Epstein HC. Traumatic dislocations of the hip. Clin Orthop Relat Res. 1973;92:116–42.
6. Upadhyay SS, Moulton A, Burwell RG. Biological factors predisposing to traumatic posterior dislocation of the hip. A selection process in the mechanism of injury. J Bone Joint Surg. 1985;67(2):232–6.
7. Steppacher SD, Albers CE, Siebenrock KA, Tannast M, Ganz R. Femoroacetabular impingement predisposes to traumatic posterior hip dislocation. Clin Orthop Relat Res. 2013;471(6):1937–43.
8. Berkes MB, Cross MB, Shindle MK, Bedi A, Kelly BT. Traumatic posterior hip instability and femoroacetabular impingement in athletes. Am J Orthop (Belle Mead NJ). 2012;41(4):166–71.
9. Manner HM, Mast NH, Ganz R, Leunig M. Potential contribution of femoroacetabular impingement to recurrent traumatic hip dislocation. J Pediatr Orthop B. 2012;21(6):574–8.
10. Krych AJ, Thompson M, Larson CM, Byrd JW, Kelly BT. Is posterior hip instability associated with cam and pincer deformity? Clin Orthop Relat Res. 2012;470(12):3390–7.
11. Thompson VP, Epstein HC. Traumatic dislocation of the hip; a survey of two hundred and four cases covering a period of twenty-one years. J Bone Joint Surg Am. 1951;33-a(3):746–78.
12. Upadhyay SS, Moulton A, Srikrishnamurthy K. An analysis of the late effects of traumatic posterior dislocation of the hip without fractures. J Bone Joint Surg. 1983;65(2):150–2.
13. Paus B. Traumatic dislocations of the hip; late results in 76 cases. Acta Orthop Scand. 1951;21(2):99–112.
14. Stewart MJ, Milford LW. Fracture-dislocation of the hip; an end-result study. J Bone Joint Surg Am. 1954;36(A:2):315–42.
15. Brav EA. Traumatic dislocation of the hip. JBJS. 1962;44-A:1115–34.
16. Upadhyay SS, Moulton A. The long-term results of traumatic posterior dislocation of the hip. J Bone Joint Surg. 1981;63b(4):548–51.
17. Kellam P, Ostrum RF. Systematic review and meta-analysis of avascular necrosis and posttraumatic arthritis after traumatic hip dislocation. J Orthop Trauma. 2016;30(1):10–6.
18. Tannast M, Pleus F, Bonel H, Galloway H, Siebenrock KA, Anderson SE. Magnetic resonance imaging in traumatic posterior hip dislocation. J Orthop Trauma. 2010;24(12):723–31.
19. Kanakaris NK, Giannoudi MP. Fractures-dislocations of the hip. In: Lasanianos NG, Kanakaris NK, Giannoudis PV, editors. Trauma and orthopaedic classifications. A comprehensive overview. London: Springer; 2014. p. 293–8.
20. Allis OH. XI. Everted dorsal dislocations of the hip. Ann Surg. 1911;54(3):371–80.
21. Stimson LA. Five cases of dislocation of the hip. Clin Orthop Relat Res. 1988;231:3–6.
22. Dahners LE, Hundley JD. Reduction of posterior hip dislocations in the lateral position using traction-countertraction: safer for the surgeon? J Orthop Trauma. 1999;13(5):373–4.
23. Lefkowitz M. A new method for reduction of hip dislocations. Orthop Rev. 1993;22(2):253–6.
24. Marya SK, Samuel AW. Piggy back technique for relocation of posterior dislocation of the hip. Injury. 1994;25(7):483–4.
25. Nordt WE 3rd. Maneuvers for reducing dislocated hips. A new technique and a literature review. Clin Orthop Relat Res. 1999;360:260–4.
26. Schafer SJ, Anglen JO. The East Baltimore lift: a simple and effective method for reduction of posterior hip dislocations. J Orthop Trauma. 1999;13(1):56–7.
27. McKee MD, Garay ME, Schemitsch EH, Kreder HJ, Stephen DJ. Irreducible fracture-dislocation of the hip: a severe injury with a poor prognosis. J Orthop Trauma. 1998;12(4):223–9.
28. Canale ST, Manugian AH. Irreducible traumatic dislocations of the hip. J Bone Joint Surg Am. 1979;61(1):7–14.
29. Schlickewei W, Elsasser B, Mullaji AB, Kuner EH. Hip dislocation without fracture: traction or mobilization after reduction? Injury. 1993;24(1):27–31.
30. Keene GS, Villar RN. Arthroscopic loose body retrieval following traumatic hip dislocation. Injury. 1994;25(8):507–10.
31. Mullis BH, Dahners LE. Hip arthroscopy to remove loose bodies after traumatic dislocation. J Orthop Trauma. 2006;20(1):22–6.
32. Wylie JD, Abtahi AM, Beckmann JT, Maak TG, Aoki SK. Arthroscopic and imaging findings after traumatic hip dislocation in patients younger than 25 years of age. J Hip Preserv Surg. 2015;2(3):303–9.
33. Fowler J, Owens BD. Abdominal compartment syndrome after hip arthroscopy. Arthroscopy. 2010;26(1):128–30.

Acetabular Fractures

10

Ippokratis Pountos and Peter V. Giannoudis

Abstract

Acetabular fractures are the result of high-energy trauma in young individuals or low-energy impacts in elderly. They are rare injuries and can be associated with morbidity and mortality. These injuries constitute a challenging joint-reconstruction problem. The goal of surgery is to restore the congruency of the joint and minimize or prolong the appearance of arthritis. A step or gap of more than 2 mm is regarded an indication for surgery. Our armamentarium includes a variety of approaches and implants for the fixation of these injuries. Primary arthroplasty has a role in the management of acetabular fractures especially in elderly individuals with pre-existing osteoarthritis, and severe impaction with a compromised bone stock.

Keywords

Acetabular fractures · Pelvis · Trauma · Triradiate cartilage · Internal fixation · Total hip arthroplasty

I. Pountos · P. V. Giannoudis (✉)
Academic Department of Trauma & Orthopaedics, School of Medicine, University of Leeds, Leeds, UK
e-mail: p.giannoudis@leeds.ac.uk

10.1 Epidemiology and Mechanism of Injury

Acetabular fractures are rare injuries that are associated with significant morbidity and mortality. Their incidence in the USA and Europe has remained unchanged over the years. The annual incidence of pelvic fractures is approximately 35–40 cases per 100,000 population. Acetabular fractures are only seen in about 10% of these cases [1, 2].

The epidemiology of acetabular fractures shows a bimodal age distribution. The first peak represents young adults sustaining high-energy trauma following motor vehicle collisions or falls from height. The second peak corresponds to older patients with decreased bone density and low-energy injuries. It has been previously estimated that approximately 80% of acetabular fractures are the result of motor vehicle collisions and 11% the outcome of falls [3]. The implementation of strict road safety regulations has decreased the incidence of high-energy acetabular fractures, but on the other hand, low-energy fractures are becoming increasingly common due to the increased life expectancy together with a more active lifestyle [4]. Some studies quantify the incidence of low energy acetabular fracture to 25% of all acetabular fractures [5–7]. It is possible that the observed increase in the incidence of acetabular fractures in elderly is also due to increased diagnosing, as computed tomography

L. Büchler, M. J.B. Keel (eds.), *Fractures of the Hip*, Fracture Management Joint by Joint,
https://doi.org/10.1007/978-3-030-18838-2_10

(CT) scans are readily available in the assessment of hip pain after simple low energy falls.

There is a male preponderance to the acetabular fractures, which is evident in the elderly as well. This later finding contrasts with common fragility fractures like distal radius and hip fractures which have a strong female predominance [2, 5]. Common associated injuries in high-energy acetabular fractures include pelvic and lower limb fractures as well as head, chest, and abdominal life-threatening injuries [3, 8]. Not uncommonly, bone fragments can injure adjacent neurovascular structures or penetrate the bowel or the genitourinary tract.

The fracture configuration depends on the position of the femoral head at the time of impact, magnitude, and vector of the causative force as well as the underlying strength of the bone. In young individuals they occur as a result of high energy trauma and most commonly associated with multiple injuries. Internal rotation of the femoral head at the time of impact is associated with a posterior column fracture while anterior column fractures occur with external rotation. Equally, abduction of the femoral head can lead to fractures of the inferior aspect of the dome, while adduction leads to fracture of the acetabular roof. The fracture-dislocation of the femoral head is closely related to the magnitude of the causative force. Likewise, the degree of comminution and articular impaction are also associated with the amount of the transmitted energy and the strength of the underlying bone.

In elderly, fracture characteristics show a higher degree of variability. Lower energy is transmitted with the force vector applied from the greater trochanter and directed towards the anteromedial aspect of the acetabulum. Fractures with a quadrilateral-plate component or roof impaction as well as those configurations causing medial displacement are more common in elderly patients [5]. Fractures involving the anterior wall of the acetabulum are more prevalent in elderly as well as the anterior column with a posterior hemitransverse extension and the both column patterns [5, 9].

10.2 Clinical and Radiological Evaluation

An acetabular fracture can be the result of significant trauma and can be associated with other life-threatening injuries. Consequently, trauma patients should be initially assessed and managed according to Advanced Trauma Life Support (ATLS) principles. The primary aim is to stabilize the patient, identify, and treat life-threatening conditions and initiate supportive treatment. Only once the patient is stable, further evaluation of the injuries can be commenced together with plans for the operative or non-operative management of the acetabular fractures.

The major cause of mortality within the first 24 h following pelvic and acetabular fractures is acute blood loss. Thereafter, multiorgan failure is the commonest cause of death. The patient's age, early physiologic derangement, and presence of other injuries (head or trunk) are negative predictors for survival [10]. Unstable acetabular fractures are likely to receive blood transfusions. In one study the average transfusion requirement for "both column" acetabular fractures was 8.8 units while anterior column posterior hemitransverse was 6.4 units [10]. The ideal volumes of plasma, platelets, cryoprecipitate, and other coagulation factors in relationship to the red blood cell transfusion volume are currently unknown [9, 11]. Current data incline towards a target ratio of plasma: red blood cell: platelet transfusions of 1:1:1 [11]. Transfusion of blood and blood products should be guided by clotting profiles and an assessment of the degree of coagulopathy. Conventional clotting tests are still used as standard but other markers like thromboelastography and rotational thromboelastometry could allow real time assessment of clotting. At present, the transfusion of fluids, blood, and blood products is guided by local protocols as a joint effort and agreement between trauma physicians.

Clinical evaluation requires a thorough history together with a systematic clinical examination. Establishing the past medical history and current medications is essential. Effective analgesia is always required to reduce patient suffering and facilitate the clinical examination. The primary or secondary surveys can identify the personality of the injury, for example leg position after posterior hip dislocation. The presence of a hip dislocation requires a prompt reduction. Closed reduction should be performed under sedation in the emergency department. In cases where this is unsuccessful, CT scanning is required to establish the obstruction to reduction and the formulation of an operative plan. Occasionally general anesthesia and fluoroscopy are required, however, if the surgeon's experience in open reduction is limited, transfer of the patient to a center capable in dealing with these injuries is recommended. In patients with sciatic nerve injury following posterior hip dislocation, prompt reduction is associated with better outcomes.

The radiographic examination provides the essential information for acetabular fracture classification and CT with or without multiplanar reconstruction is always recommended. X-ray examination should include three main views: anteroposterior, iliac oblique, and obturator oblique (Judet views), (Fig. 10.1). The anteroposterior (AP) view is essential in evaluating a patient following trauma and should be always obtained under the ATLS protocol. During the evaluation of patient with pelvic injuries, the AP view can give information of the congruency of several structures. The six fundamental landmarks visible in this view include the anterior and posterior wall of the acetabulum, the teardrop, the roof, and the iliopectineal (anterior column) and ilioischial (posterior column) lines (Fig. 10.2). The iliac oblique view provides an en face view of the iliac wing and profile of the obturator ring, hence it brings the posterior column and anterior wall into relief. For this view the patient is rolled 45° towards the injured side. The obturator oblique view, on the other hand, is used to assess the obturator ring, posterior wall and anterior column and requires the patient to be rotated 45° towards the uninjured side on the radiographic table.

CT is useful in showing the finer details [12]. The entire pelvis should be included and axial cuts with thin 1.5–3 mm intervals and corresponding slice thicknesses should be acquired (Fig. 10.3) [13]. CT allows the visualization of additional fragments and obscure fracture lines not previously visible with plain films. CT can

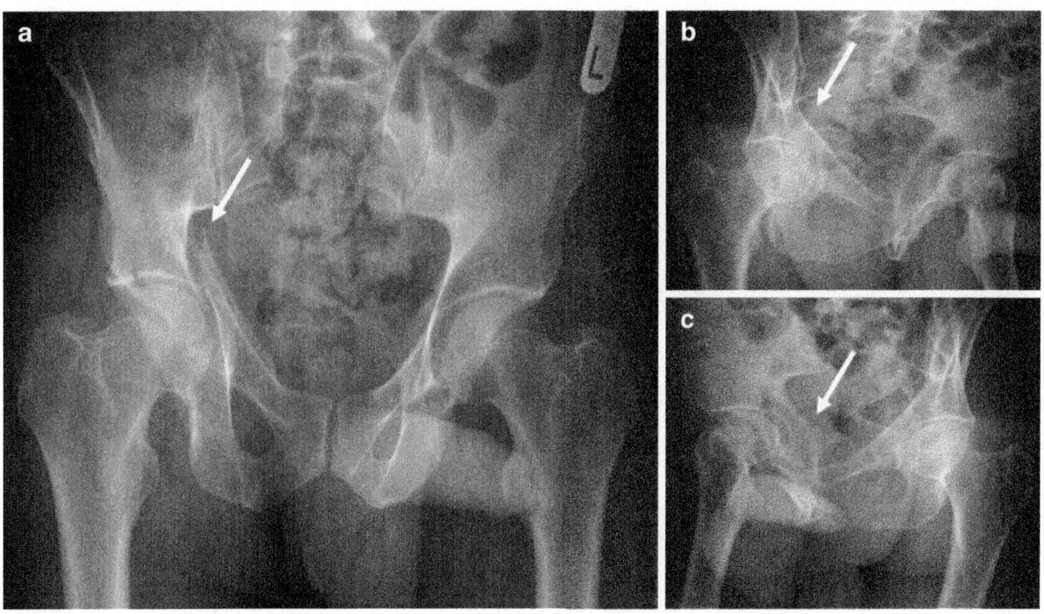

Fig. 10.1 Pelvic radiographs: AP (A) and Judet views: Obturator oblique (B) and iliac oblique view (C). Arrow illustrates fracture location

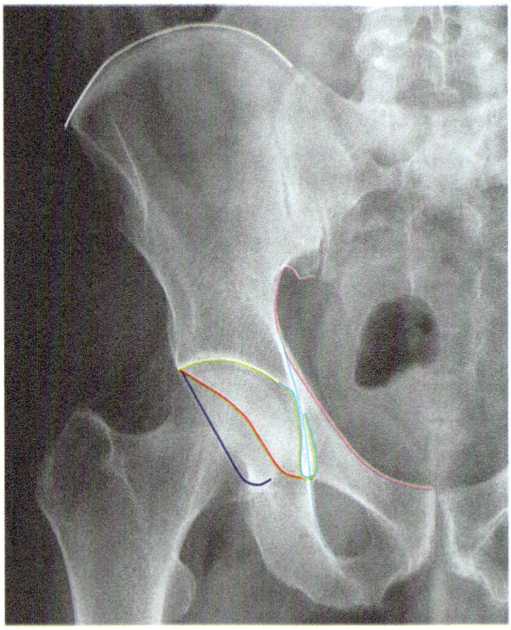

Fig. 10.2 Radiological landmarks of acetabulum: Pink line = Iliopectineal line (anterior column), Light blue line = Ilioischial line (posterior column), Dark blue line = Posterior wall, Red line = Anterior wall, Green line = Teardrop, Yellow line = Roof, White line = Iliac wing

show the number and size of bony fragments, the presence of articular comminution, impaction or incongruency (steps of the articular cartilage), the extent of displacement and the rotation of the columns, and the presence of retained bony fragments inside the joint (Fig. 10.4). It can also identify associated injuries in the pelvis like sacral fractures, injuries of

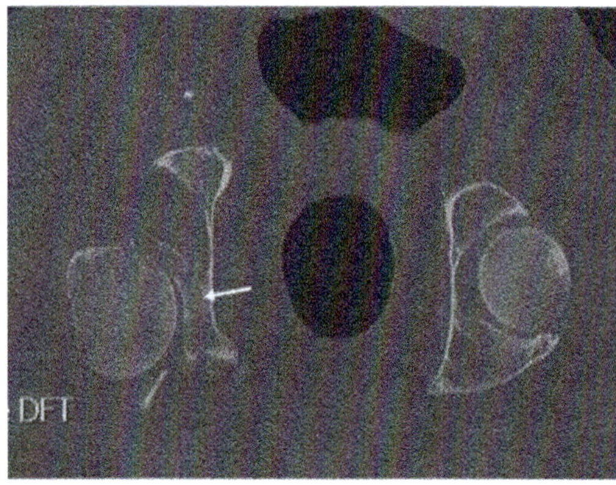

Fig. 10.4 Axial cut demonstrating marginal impaction (white arrow) of right acetabulum

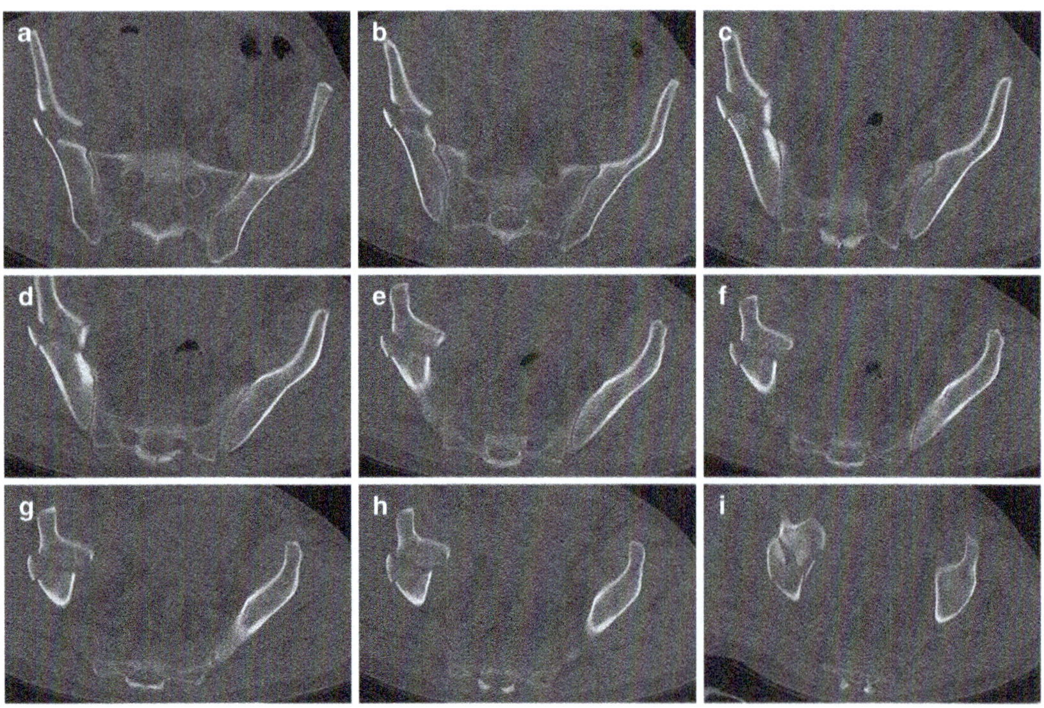

Fig. 10.3 A–I: Axial cuts demonstrating a two-column fracture of the left acetabulum, showing the complete separation of the joint from the proximal pelvic ring

the sacroiliac joint, soft tissues injuries, and the presence of hematoma. An artificial pelvic model is often helpful to draw and understand the fracture patterns and template the fracture fixation. 3D reconstruction or the more recent advance of 3D printing can be of great assistance to the surgeon.

A 3-dimentional CT (3D CT) reconstruction transforms the scanned CT data into standard coordinates to create a 3D-image. Current software may help better visualize the major fracture lines by the disarticulation of the femoral head from the acetabulum and removing rectal or intravenous contrast material [14]. Several studies have shown that 3D reconstructions improve the surgeons understanding for fracture configuration however, caution is required as during the process some vital information could be eliminated by the software, for example minimally displaced fractures [15–17]. An alternative approach which is gaining popularity is the rapid prototyping and 3D printing technology [18, 19]. This technology can allow the fabrication of complex real models based on CT scans. The surgeon could be assisted not only by the model but also by the fabrication of guiding templates but also pre-bended or custom metalwork [18, 19]. This aims to improve the placement accuracy and safety of the metalwork [18, 19].

10.3 Classification

The accurate classification of acetabular fractures is crucial to guide the appropriate management. Early classification systems initially described the direction of hip dislocation, followed by the "clock face" classification of Knight and Smith and the "triradiate" of Rowe and Lowell [20, 21]. In 1961, the Letournel and Judet classification was developed which represents the most comprehensive and widely adopted system to date [22].

Letournel and Judet divided acetabular fractures into simple and associated types (Fig. 10.5) [22]. The simple fractures are isolated fractures of one wall or one column along with transverse fractures; the five subtypes of simple fractures include fractures of the posterior wall, posterior column, anterior wall, anterior column, and transverse fractures. The associated fracture types are of more complex configuration and include T-type fractures, combined fracture of the posterior column and posterior wall, combination of transverse and posterior wall fracture, anterior column fracture with hemitransverse posterior fracture and both column fractures.

The classification of Letournel and Judet is based on the morphological characteristics of the innominate bone. The authors realized that the acetabulum was located centrally between two columns, an anterior and a posterior, which acted as struts to provide stability. The iliac crest, iliac spines, pubis, and the anterior aspect of the acetabulum compose the anterior column while the posterior column consists of the ischium, posterior half of the acetabulum till the bone of the sciatic notch. As result, anterior column fractures disrupt the iliopectineal line while posterior ones disrupt the ilioischial lines. In addition to the columns, the acetabular walls or rims represent only the anterior or posterior articular surface of the acetabulum. The transverse acetabular fractures are limited to the acetabulum with the fracture line involving both the anterior and posterior aspects of the acetabulum. The fracture line is on a transverse plane relative to the acetabulum, with the fracture components coursing medially and superiorly from the acetabulum. On X-rays, both the iliopectineal and ilioischial lines are disrupted and the obturator ring is intact. Both column fractures represent fractures that divide the ilium so that the sacroiliac joint is not connected by any articular segment (see Fig. 10.3). Characteristic of both column fractures is the spur sign seen on the obturator oblique view, which represents the posterior displacement of the sciatic buttress, in essence disconnecting the roof of the acetabulum from the axial skeleton. Finally, T-type acetabular fractures represent a combination of a transverse fracture that extends inferiorly into the obturator ring. Similarly, to both column fractures, these fractures disrupt the obturator ring causing discontinuity of both the iliopectineal and ilioischial lines during roentgenographic evaluation. These fractures do not

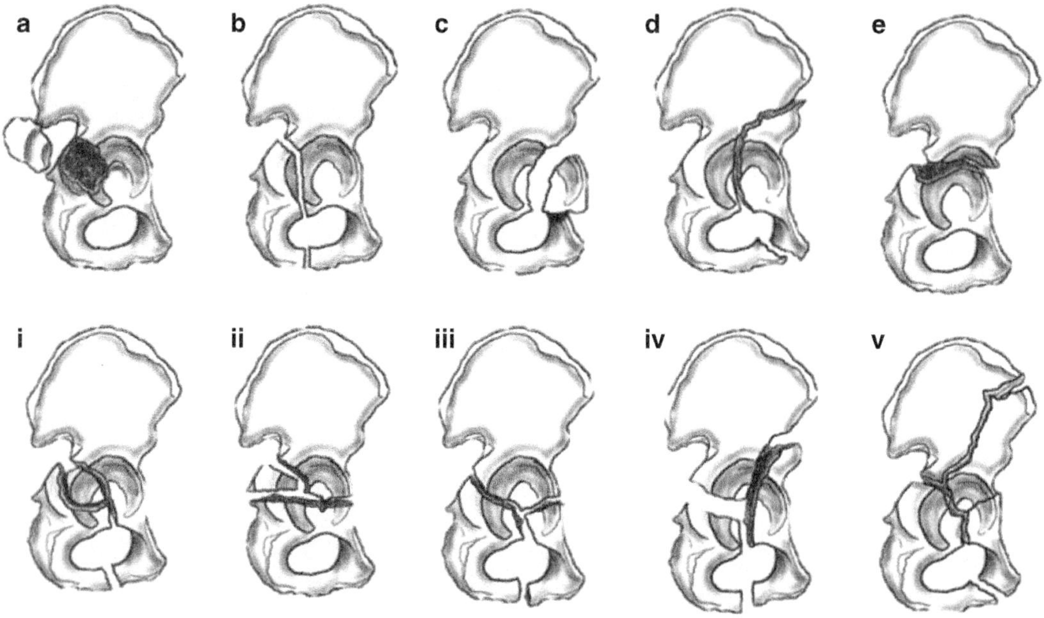

Fig. 10.5 Judet-Letournel fracture classification of acetabular fractures. Elementary fractures include the (A) posterior wall, (B) posterior column, (C) anterior wall, (D) anterior column, and (E) transverse fractures. Associated fractures include the (I) posterior wall with posterior column, (II) transverse with posterior wall, (III) T-shaped fracture, (IV) anterior wall/column hemitransverse, and (V) both column fractures. Reproduced with permission and copyright © of Springer [23]

involve the iliac wing, hence can be differentiated from the both column fractures.

Attempts to expand and improve the classification of Letournel and Judet have been reported. Among them, Harris classification utilized a CT based scheme able to classify more fracture subtypes and introduce more symmetry between the walls and columns [24, 25]. The two main differences of this classification is firstly the way of definition of walls and columns (lips of the acetabulum referred to as walls while medial aspect referred to as columns) and secondly the shortening of anterior column that reaches only to the top of the iliopectineal line. Harris et al. categorized the fractures according to the involved columns with subcategories for the fracture line extension.

The AO group has also developed an alphanumeric classification system adopting and expanding the Letournel and Judet classification. The AO classification aims to describe the severity and predict the final outcome. Type A fractures include partial articular of a single wall or column. Type B fractures are partially articular transverse oriented fractures including the transverse and posterior wall (B1), T-type (B2) and anterior and posterior hemitransverse fracture types (B3). Finally, type C injuries include fractures of both columns with all articular segments, including the roof, detached from the ilium. This is also referred to as "floating acetabulum." Qualifiers aiming to add information and document the condition of the articular surfaces were added in an attempt to improve the predictive value of the classification. Such qualifiers include the femoral head dislocation/subluxation and the presence of chondral lesions, osteochondral and impacted fractures.

10.4 Conservative Treatment

For many decades the management of acetabular fractures was purely conservative. Operative management was initiated by the fundamental studies of Judet et al., reinforced by improvements in radiologic interpretations and established following long follow-up studies demonstrating that even small residual incongruency in the weight-bearing surface of the acetabulum leads to arthritis in contrast to similar fractures where anatomical reduction was achieved with internal fixation [26, 27].

The indications for conservative management of acetabular fractures are shrinking. Undisplaced fractures or those displaced up to 2 mm can be treated conservatively. The patient has to remain non-weight-bearing for a period of 6–8 weeks with X-rays obtained at regular intervals to assess that articular congruency is maintained. Similar management can be utilized for fractures sparing the anatomic biomechanical weight-bearing surface of the acetabulum. The criteria, however, vary. In the study of Oslon and Matta, the criteria used were (1) intact superior 10 mm of the articular acetabular surface on CT (equivalent to roof arc measurements of 45°), (2) congruency of the femoral head with the superior acetabulum out of traction on anteroposterior and Judet views, and (3) more than 50% of posterior wall intact [28]. With regard to the minimal roof arc measurements, subsequent experimental studies have reported different angle values. In the biomechanical study on cadaveric pelvises, Vrahas et al. suggested that operative management is required with less than 45°, 25°, and 55° of medial, anterior, and posterior acetabular roof arc angles [29]. Other clinical and experimental studies have reported comparative measurements with the exception of anterior angle which reported between 42° and 52° [30, 31]. As far as the posterior wall fractures are concerned, several authors have proposed that fractures involving up to 20% of the posterior wall are stable, while in those involving more than 40% dynamic clinical instability can exist [32, 33]. Fluoroscopic stress views while the hip comes into flexion can be acquired to rule out instability (joint space widening suggests instability).

Conservative management has been previously proposed for some both column fracture configurations [13, 34–36]. In these fractures, the labrum and articular capsule remained intact allowing the molding of the fragments over the femoral head. Medial displacement of the femoral head and gaps without stem between the fragments are known to occur. This phenomenon is referred to as "secondary congruency" but is rarely found to occur in 5% of both column fractures [34]. Magu et al. reported good to excellent functional outcome in 88.8% of both column fractures with secondary congruence despite medial subluxation [36].

Patient related factors play a vital role in the decision between operative and conservative management. In many cases the severity of the associated injuries mandates the delay of surgery while medical contraindications to surgery are not uncommon. Some authors advocate early percutaneous fixation in severely injured patients. Skeletal traction can be used in such cases to protect the articular cartilage. Other factors include condition that disrupts or threatens the soft tissue envelope including the presence of open fractures, infected wounds, and soft tissue lesions from blunt trauma. In some patients the presence of Morel-Lavallee (closed degloving injury associated with a hemolymphatic mass) can significant delay surgery as operating through it increases the infection rate significantly. The presence of a suprapubic catheter is anecdotally considered a contraindication through the ilioinguinal approach due to the potential bacterial colonization of the catheter. Finally, patient's age was long considered a defining factor for the choice of surgery with patients over 60 years old to be allocated to conservative management. Current literature supports the view that older patients should not be precluded from a fixation, but instead, factors including the comorbidities, the presence of symptomatic arthritis, the activity level, poor bone stock with high risk for loss of reduction should be considered in the decision-making process [7].

10.5 Operative Treatment

The achievement of anatomical reduction of the articular surface combined with a rigid internal fixation, which will allow early mobilization, is the rationale behind the surgical treatment of acetabular fractures. Fractures resulting in more than 2 mm displacement of the weight-bearing surface and those resulting in subluxation of the femoral head should be treated surgically. Posterior wall fractures involving more than 40% of the wall do require fixation [28, 32, 33]. Injuries resulting in trapped bony fragments in the hip joint or those associated with avulsion of the ligamentum teres lodged between the articular surfaces generally require excision. Another indication of operative management in severely comminuted fractures is the preservation of adequate bone stock and avoidance of non-union that will improve the chances of a favorable outcome following a subsequent hip reconstructive surgery.

10.5.1 Choice of Surgical Approach

The type and configuration of the fracture determines the choice of the surgical approach (Table 10.1). The Kocher-Langenbeck, ilioinguinal, and modified Stoppa are most commonly used. Combined approaches can be performed for more complex and comminuted fractures.

Table 10.1 Approaches for the management of acetabular fractures

Fracture type	Approach
Posterior wall	Kocher-Langenbeck
Posterior column	Kocher-Langenbeck or mod. Stoppa or Pararectus
Anterior wall	Ilioinguinal or Iliofemoral or mod. Stoppa or Pararectus
Anterior column	Ilioinguinal or Iliofemoral or mod. Stoppa or Pararectus
Both columns	Ilioinguinal or extensile or combined
Transverse or T-type (posterior wall or displacement)	Kocher-Langenbeck
Transverse or T-type (anterior displacement)	Ilioinguinal or Stoppa
Hemitransverse	Ilioinguinal
Quadrilateral plate	Ilioinguinal or Iliofemoral or mod. Stoppa or Pararectus

10.5.1.1 Kocher-Langenbeck Approach

The Kocher-Langenbeck approach is indicated for posterior wall and column injuries. Structures at risk with this approach include the sciatic nerve, medial circumflex femoral artery, and superior gluteal artery and nerve. The superior gluteal artery can be a significant source of bleeding when injured. In such cases packing can control it, however, direct ligation or even embolization is required. The incidence of heterotopic ossification with the Kocher-Langenbeck approach is higher compared to the other approaches used to fix acetabular fractures.

A trochanteric osteotomy or a trochanteric flip osteotomy can increase the access provided by the Kocher-Langenbeck approach. These osteotomies provide better access to the dome and some limited access to the anterior column. Detaching the greater trochanter carries a high non-union rate, can result in abductor weakness, and requires experience and additional implants to reattach the trochanter. To overcome these problems the flip osteotomy has been popularized. A slice of the greater trochanter is created that leaves intact the tendinous attachment of the gluteus muscles and the tendinous origin of the vastus lateralis. Therefore, a neutralizing force is created keeping the trochanteric slice in place and preventing any proximal migration of the trochanter.

10.5.1.2 Iliofemoral Approach

The iliofemoral approach provides access to the iliac wing, anterior aspect of sacroiliac joint, and the entire internal iliac fossa. It also provides digital access to the quadrilateral surface and greater sciatic notch. The structures at risk include the superior gluteal neurovascular bundle, sciatic nerve, lateral femoral cutaneous nerve, and the perforating branches of the femoral artery.

10.5.1.3 Ilioinguinal Approach

The ilioinguinal approach allows exposure to the internal iliac fossa, pelvic brim, anterior wall and column and quadrilateral plate and sacroiliac joint. Thus, fractures of the anterior wall, anterior column, anterior column with posterior hemitransverse and some both column fractures can be treated through this approach. Structures at risk include the femoral nerve, femoral and external iliac blood vessels, the lateral cutaneous nerve of the thigh, the obturator nerve, and spermatic cord. Also, the corona mortis (vascular anastomosis between the external iliac artery or deep inferior epigastric artery with the obturator artery) should be identified and ligated otherwise can be a significant source of bleeding if accidentally damaged.

10.5.1.4 Modified Stoppa Approach

An alternative to the ilioinguinal approach is the modified Stoppa approach [37]. It is an anterior intrapelvic extraperitoneal approach though the rectus abdominis [38]. It provides access to the pubis, posterior aspect of ramus, pubic eminence, sciatic buttress, and notch as well as the anterior aspect of the sacroiliac joint [37–39]. Structures at risk include the obturator nerve and vessels, corona mortis, external iliac vessels, and urinary bladder.

10.5.1.5 Pararectus Approach

The pararectus approach is an alternative to the Stoppa approach [40]. The indications include fractures involving the anterior column and the quadrilateral plate. The pararectus approach is versatile and can be extended without an additional incision in cases where the fixation of the posterior pelvis is required. Structures at risk include the peritoneum, inferior epigastric vessels, spermatic cord, and external iliac vessels.

10.5.2 Techniques of Open Reduction and Fixation

The reduction of acetabular fractures is often the most difficult element of their surgical management. When possible, surgery should be performed early as fracture reduction can be difficult or even impossible if surgery is delayed for three or more weeks. A thorough preoperative plan with provisions for the difficulties, materials, and instruments that may be required during the fixation of the fracture is essential. Intraoperatively, several strategies can be employed to restore the anatomy and fix the fractures. Such techniques include cerclage wiring, special reduction tools and implants, traction, and disimpaction techniques for depressed osteochondral fragments.

Reduction tools designed specifically for pelvic and acetabular surgery exist and they play a vital role in the reduction of the fragments. Pointed reduction clamps with their tips introduced in drill holes or on washers can facilitate stronger fixation. Farabeuf or Jungbluth clamps attached on bi-cortical screws is an alternative option. Surgeon's armamentarium includes offset clamps for the posterior column fracture reduction or single- or double-pronged clamps for both column fracture reduction. Cerclage wires placed on the greater or lesser sciatic notch can facilitate reduction and could be even retained to improve fixation.

Traction is often essential intraoperatively. Traction can be applied on the extremity through the traction table. The traction table should allow application of traction in every direction. Instead of a traction table, manual traction can be applied by the use of assistants. Direct traction to the femoral head or pelvis can be applied during reduction maneuvers. A Schanz screw placed directly into the femoral head or a hook over the greater trochanter can assist the distraction of the joint. In addition, the use of Schanz pins could provide strong lever to reduce fracture and derotate large bony fragments.

The restoration of the articular surface congruency often requires the disimpaction of osteochondral fragments (Fig. 10.6). Once such

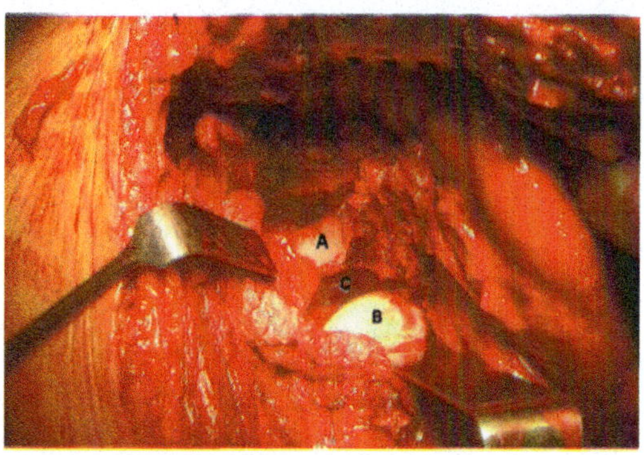

Fig. 10.6 Marginal impaction of acetabulum exposed via a Kocher-Langenbeck posterior approach. (A) Impaction articular fragment; (B) Femoral head; (C) Acetabulum joint

fragments are lifted, subchondral voids are created which could require grafting. Autologous tricortical bone graft harvested from the iliac crest is currently the gold standard, however, synthetic void filling materials can also be used like hydroxyapatite granules or calcium phosphate. Often the disimpaction of the articular fragments can be performed through the preexisting fracture. In cases where the direct visualization of the fragment is not feasible, reduction can be achieved through a cortical window or balloon osteoplasty followed by bone grafting. In complex circumscribed impacted fractures, fragment elevation and molding over the intact femoral head can be implemented.

The fixation of the acetabular fracture requires an array of screw sizes and lengths together with reconstruction plates that can be contoured in all three dimensions. The AO principles of anatomic reduction and stable fixation with interfragmentary lag screw and neutralizing plates apply. Alternatively, plates can be used to secure or buttress fragments (most commonly a posterior wall fracture) or as a "spring plate" (modified one-third tubular plate, cut through distal hole, tines bent 90 degrees and used to secure the fragment) (Figs. 10.7 and 10.8) [41]. The 3.5 mm reconstruction plate (straight or curved) fixed with 3.5 mm cortical screws is the implant of choice. Great care should be taken to ensure that the screws do not penetrate into the joint space.

10.5.3 Minimal Invasive Techniques and Navigation

Intraoperative navigation has been implemented in the management of acetabular fractures. It requires a specific image intensifier, which allows 3D reconstruction. This technology has several advantages over conventional approaches. Firstly, it can provide advanced resolution that could facilitate a better understanding and control of the quality of articular reduction during and after fracture fixation [42]. Secondly, the use of screw navigation allows the insertion of "high risk" screw safely in the periarticular space. Thirdly, it allows percutaneous or minimally invasive metalwork placement. These advantages were shown in cases of percutaneous iliosacral screw place-

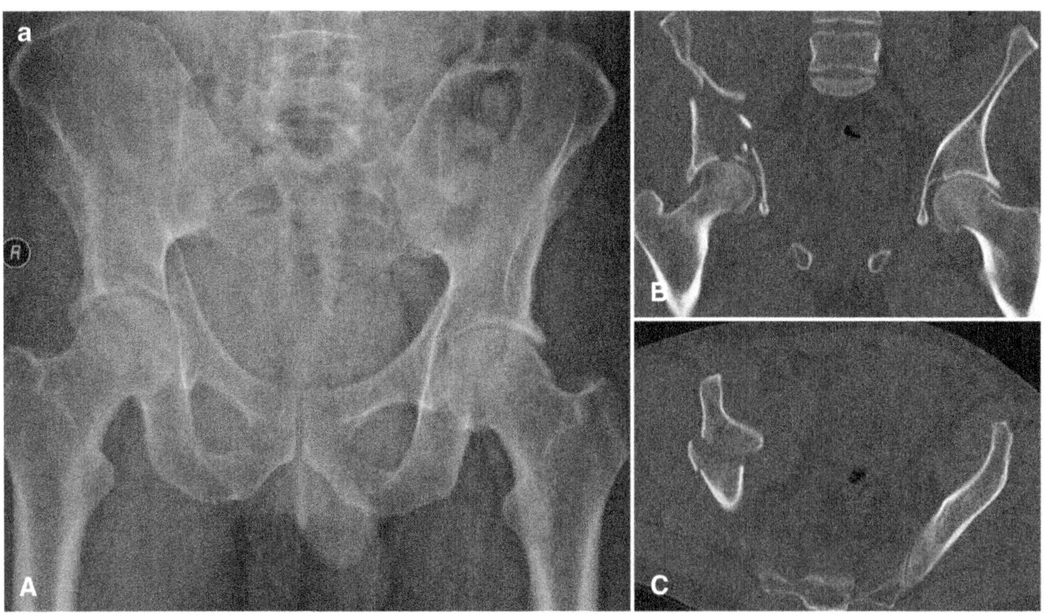

Fig. 10.7 (**a**) Pre-operative radiographs (A: AP pelvis; B: CT coronal, C: CT axial cuts) of a two-column right acetabulum fracture. (**b**) Postoperative radiographs following reconstruction (A: Pelvic inlet view, B: Obturator oblique, C: Iliac oblique)

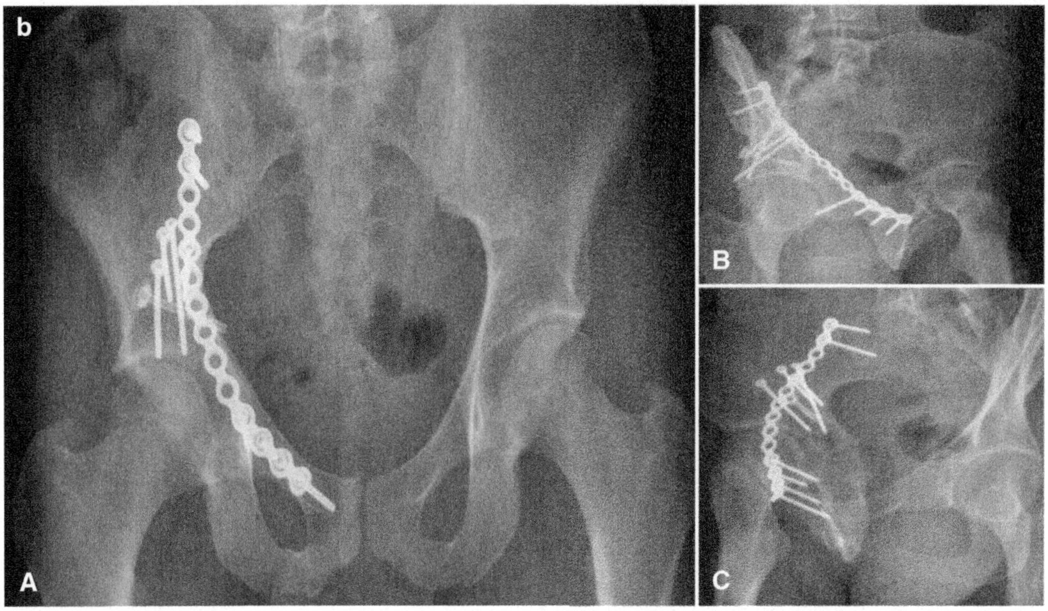

Fig. 10.7 (continued)

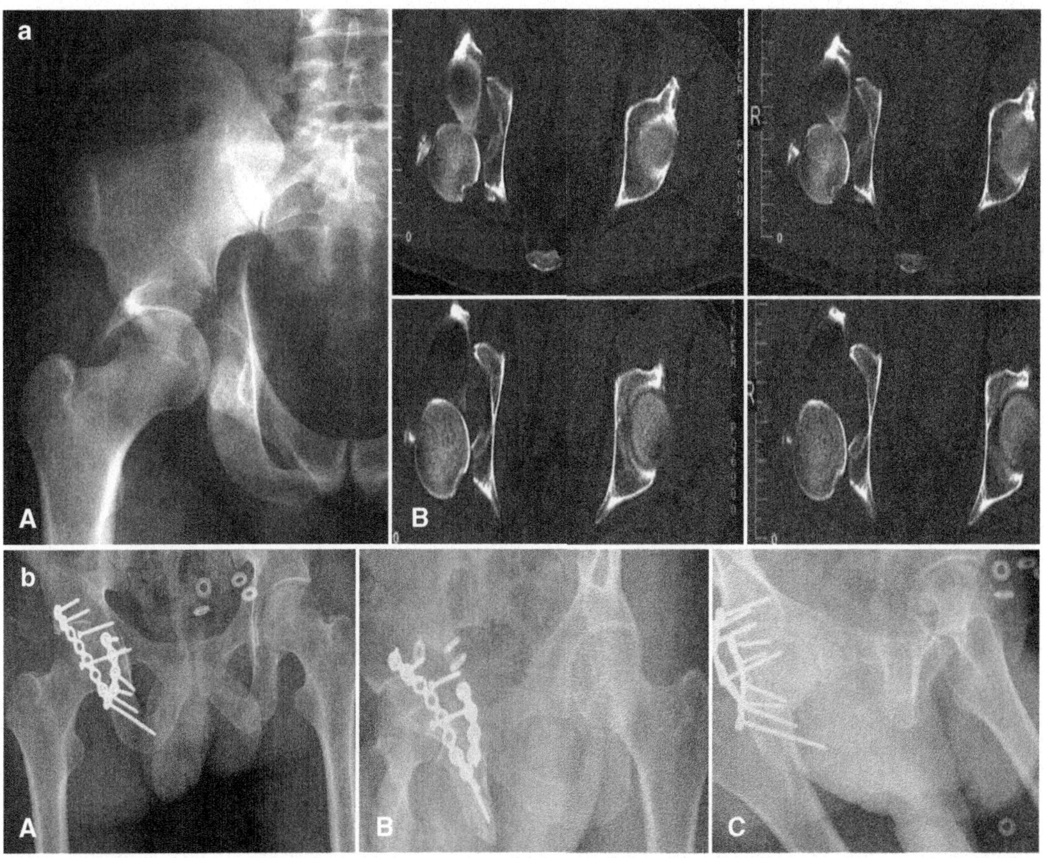

Fig. 10.8 (**a**) Pre-operative AP pelvis (A) and CT images (B) of a transverse posterior wall left acetabulum fracture. (**b**) Postoperative images (A) AP pelvis, (B) Obturator oblique, and (C) Iliac oblique view demonstrating reconstruction of the fracture

ment and percutaneous acetabular fracture fixation and the reported results were favorable [43–46]. In regards to the radiation exposure, available studies suggest that is comparable or even lower to that of conventional fluoroscopy [43, 44]. The main limitation of navigation is the need of a substantial financial investment in the operating room, in addition to the mobile imaging system, the navigator and ancillary [43].

Arthroscopic techniques for the fixation of acetabular fractures exist. Arthroscopy is minimally invasive, offers superior visualization of the hip joint, facilitates the diagnosis, and even allows fracture reduction. The removal of loose osteochondral fragments, joint debridement or lavage can be performed reducing the risk of osteoarthritis [47]. It is however technically demanding, so significant experience in both hip arthroscopy and acetabular fracture management is essential. Several authors have reported good to excellent results following arthroscopic reduction of acetabular fractures even in cases of femoral head fractures or dislocations [48–50]. Yamamoto et al. reported, through a case series study, that arthroscopy was capable of detecting small free osteochondral or chondral fragments that were not detectable on either plain radiographs or computed tomography scans in 70% of the cases [50]. Similar finding were reported when arthroscopy was used to evaluate symptomatic hip pathologies following injury. Loose bodies, labral tears, step deformities, and osteochondral lesions were injuries difficult to diagnose with CT or MRI scans, but can be easily identified and managed with arthroscopy [51]. Complications of hip arthroscopy are rare. Reported complications include venous thromboembolism, peripheral nerve injury, septic arthritis, instrument failure, and extravasation of fluid leaking in the abdomen or causing compartment syndrome [52].

10.5.4 Operative Results

The outcomes of the surgical management of acetabular fractures are good to excellent in the majority of the cases (Table 10.2) [26, 53–62]. A recent meta-analysis has shown that 79% of the patients report a favorable outcome [62]. This figure, however, varies according to the specific outcome instrument used [62]. Factors that are associated with poor outcome included delays in treatment, the presence of articular incongruence, the presence of associated injuries and osteonecrosis [54]. Complications are not uncommon. They include iatrogenic nerve palsy, infection, DVT, and avascular necrosis of the femoral head [26, 54, 56]. The incidence of heterotopic ossification varies between the studies and is associated with the surgical approach as well as the fracture configuration [56]. The clinical and radiologic outcomes are favorable in the majority of the patients. Gait analysis studies highlight that although the walking velocity of the patients will recover, the gait, muscle strength, and outcome will deteriorate [53, 63]. Similarly, the forward tilt of the pelvis and the peak hip abduction moment show incomplete recovery [53]. It is recommended that with maximizing muscle strength early, the gait and functional recovery are likely to improve further [53, 63].

10.5.5 Influence of Associated Pelvic and Femoral Fractures

A combination of pelvic and acetabular injury is a devastating dyad. Such patients are polytraumatized and present with a high injury severity score, which often represents a resuscitative challenge. Patients with combined injury have higher transfusion requirements and lower systolic blood pressure at presentation [64]. Their incidence vary, however, reported incidence can be as high as 16% [64]. The fracture patterns differ from those observed in isolated injuries; posterior acetabular fractures are less common and anterior–posterior compression pelvic injuries seem much more frequent in cases of combined injuries [65]. Mortality rates are high ranging from 1.5 to 13% between different studies [64, 65]. Once the patient is stable, a detailed analysis of the injuries is required together with the formulation of an overall treatment strategy to address the injuries [64]. Ideally, an initial accurate reduction of the pelvic injuries is required,

Table 10.2 Selected recent studies presenting the outcome of the operative management of acetabular fractures

Study	Patient Nrs (gender)	Age (range)	Fracture type	Conclusions and outcomes
Ochs et al. [26]	858	49.4 (range 12–92 years)	Elementary fracture patterns 42.5% and associated fracture patterns 57.5%	• Complications occurred in 20% of patients • Complications included nerve palsy (5.6%), infection (2.3%), thrombosis (2.7%), hematoma (1.9%), and multiple organ failure (0.7%)
Kubota et al. [53]	19 (15 M)	52.5 (range, 26–77 years)	Twelve partial articular 1-column fractures Two partial articular, transversely oriented fractures; Five both column fractures	• Pelvic forward tilt and peak hip abduction moment showed incomplete recovery at 12 months after ORIF • Improvement of hip abductor muscle strength in the early postoperative period could improve the functional outcome
Dunet et al. [54]	72 (56 M)	41.6 (range 16–75 years)	Simple fractures is 45 (62.5%) patients, complex 27 (37.5%)	• 25 THRs were performed, with a mean time to surgery of 3.7 years • Factors associated with poor outcome included no functional treatment, initial traction, anterior and posterior congruency defect, initial traction, VAS, osteoarthritis, and osteonecrosis
Meena et al. [55]	118 (99 M)	38.75 (range 16–65 years)	Elementary fracture patterns 45.8% and associated fracture patterns 54.2%	• The clinical outcome was good-excellent in 79 (67%), good in 52 (33%) • Poor reduction, associated injuries, fracture displacement of >20 mm, joint dislocation and late surgery definitely carry poor prognosis
Anizar-Faizi et al. [56]	30 (23 M)	39.9 (range 14–81 years)	17 (56.7%) were elementary fractures and 13 cases (43.3%) associated type fractures	• 20 (66.7%) patients had excellent/good results (Harris hip score > 80) • Postoperative complications were deep infection (6.7%), iatrogenic sciatic nerve injury (10.0%), avascular necrosis (16.7%), heterotopic ossification (3.3%), degenerative changes in hip joint (43.3%) and loss of reduction (3.3%)
Bhat et al. [57]	59 (45 M)	38.35 (range 18–60 years)	Associated in 15 (60%) and elementary in 35 (40%)	• Radiological evaluation revealed excellent outcome in 16% hips, good in 54% hips, fair in 20% hips, and poor in 10% hips • Good to excellent results were achieved in 42 cases (70%) • Complications included implant back-out, postoperative dislocation, iatrogenic nerve palsy, superficial wound infection, intraoperative bleeding and osteoarthritis
Borg and Hailer [58]	101 (76 M)	49, (range 17–83 years)	Associated in 61 (60%) and elementary in 40 (40%)	• Postoperative complications included deep infections in four patients, and thromboembolic complications in six • The hip joint was preserved in 78 (77%) patients whereas 21 patients received a THA and the remaining two had a Girdlestones
Iqbal et al. [59]	50 (36 M)	44.20 ± 11.65 years	Elementary fracture patterns 84% and associated fracture patterns 16%	• The clinical outcome was good to excellent in 35 (70.0%) • The radiological outcome was anatomical in 39 (78.0%) cases, congruent in 5 (10.0%) cases, incongruent in 6 (12.0%) cases

(continued)

Table 10.2 (continued)

Study	Patient Nrs (gender)	Age (range)	Fracture type	Conclusions and outcomes
Clarke-Jenssen et al. [60]	253 (197 M)	42 years (12–78 years).	Elementary fracture patterns in 99 (39%) and 154 (61%) associated fracture types	• THR in 36 patients (14%) • The presence of injury to the femoral head and acetabular impaction proved to be strong predictors of failure
Negrin and Seligson [61]	167 (111 M)	41.8 (range, 14–85 years)	Sixty five posterior wall (38.9%), 34 posterior column (20.4%), 51 transverse (30.5%), and 17 T-shaped (10.2%)	• Posttraumatic arthritis was found in 36 patients (21.6%) and THR in17 patients • Nine cases of iatrogenic damage (three permanent), eight patients (4.8%) sustained an infection, postoperative hemorrhagic shock was detected in 26 patients (15.6%) • Revision surgery due to secondary loss of reduction was indicated in five patients

followed by the reconstruction of the acetabulum [66]. The amount of residual pelvic displacement, patient's age, and the presence of T-shaped acetabular fractures are predictors of residual acetabular displacement [66, 67].

Femoral head fractures occur frequently with acetabular fractures. Beckmann et al. quantified this incidence to approximately 18% of acetabular fractures [68]. Most commonly occur with posterior wall fractures (56.3%), while their incidence with anterior and posterior hip dislocation is 66.7% and 71.9%, respectively [68]. Acetabular fractures occurring in association with femoral fractures carry a poor prognosis [68, 69]. It was previously suggested that even the mildest grade of femoral head fracture carries a greater than 10% risk for poor outcome [68]. Devastating results are also known to occur with combination of acetabular fracture combined with ipsilateral femoral neck fracture. Such injury combination carries a 93% risk of avascular necrosis of the femoral head [1]. This incidence is much higher to that of Garden III and IV that is known to range between 30–40% [70]. It has been hypothesized that there is extensive damage to the vasculature at the time of injury, preventing revascularization even with good reduction [71].

10.5.6 Primary Arthroplasty

Total hip replacement (THR) after an acetabular fracture can be indicated in two distinct scenarios; firstly, acutely in acetabular fractures deemed to conclude in a poor outcome following fixations and secondly in patients that develop osteoarthritis from either conservative or surgical management.

The indications of THR in the acute setting are placed in the context of the severity of the injury and the reported outcomes following ORIF. It allows early full weight bearing and eliminates the need of a second procedure for THR. Reported indications include complex or non-reconstructable fractures, concurrent hip osteoarthritis, associated femoral head fractures, and poor bone quality (Table 10.3) [72–79]. Studies have reinforced THR with cable fixation, reinforcement rings, bone grafting, and antiprotrusion cages [72, 73, 75, 77–79]. In one study THR prosthesis was used alone [76].

The indications of THR in the management of post-traumatic arthritis are similar to those of end-stage hip disease. Pain and stiffness that interfere with daily activities together with radiologic signs are the cardinal findings. Challenges are anticipated and pre-operative preparations are essential. Such challenges include bone loss, retained material, prominent metalwork, pelvic deformity, and osteonecrosis. Dealing with bone loss during a THR can be daunting. Voids or even total absence of the anterior or posterior walls or defect of the acetabular roof could require extensive grafting. Special THR revision implants (rings, cages, meshes), impaction grafting or structural grafts fixed with

Table 10.3 Selected studies presenting the outcomes and complications of THR after acetabular fractures

Author	Nr of patients	Outcome	Complications	Revision rate	Authors comments
Mears and Velyvis [72]	57	Good to excellent in 79%	• DVT 5% • Heterotopic ossification 10%	5%	• Substantial experience in both acetabular trauma and hip arthroplasty required
Tidermark et al. [73]	10	Good to excellent 60%	• DVT 10% • Heterotopic ossification 40%	10%	• All patients able to walk independently (three with walking aids)
Mouhsine et al. [74]	18	Good outcome in 17/18 patients	• Dislocation 6%	0%	• Cable fixations and early THR provides good primary fixation, stabilizes acetabular fractures, and permits early mobilization
Sarkar et al. [75]	19	n/a	• Infection 16% • Cup loosening 16% • Stem loosening 5% • Dislocation 10% • Ceramic head fracture 5%	42%	• Complications are not infrequent and a solid buttress is crucial
Sermon et al. [76]	54	Good to excellent results in 58%	• Heterotopic ossification 28%	8%	• Acute THR resulted in a lower revision rate and incidence of heterotopic ossifications
Herscovici et al. [77]	22	Average Harris hip score 74 (range 42–86)	• Heterotopic ossification 18% • Wound dehiscence 4% • Hip dislocation in six patients (27%)	22%	• Combined ORIF and THR is valid option in elderly patients
Enocson and Blomfeldt [78]	15	Average Harris hip score 88	• No complications	0%	• Primary reinforcement ring, bone graft and acute THR is a safe option with good functional outcome

plates and screws can be used [80]. In addition to bone loss, pelvic deformity can distort normal anatomy and can jeopardize the correct placement of the acetabular component leading to early wear or dislocation. A detailed pre-operative planning is essential and intraoperative X-rays are helpful to determine the ideal cup abduction and anteversion angles.

One scenario with potential devastating consequences is the presence of low-grade infection in cases of previous open reduction and internal fixation (ORIF). This should be strongly suspected in cases of rapid deterioration of the joint space or in cases of mismatch between radiologic and clinical symptoms. Baseline investigations include blood tests (white cell count, neutrophils, C-reactive protein, and erythrocyte sedimentation rate) followed by a joint aspiration if the suspicion is strong. In cases where infection is confirmed, removal of the implants and joint debridement is required. A two-stage reconstruction, following the eradication of the infection, can be then performed.

The results of delayed THR following an acetabular fracture vary significantly. Romnes et al. reported a revision rate of 13.7% with radiologic acetabular loosening of 53% at the 7.3-year follow-up. Subsequent studies have shown survival rates ranging from 70 to 97% [76, 81–84]. The most common complications included the development of heterotopic ossification, infection, early loosening, and dislocation [81].

References

1. Mears DC, Velyvis JH, Chang CP. Displaced acetabular fractures managed operatively: indicators of outcome. Clin Orthop Relat Res. 2003;407:173–86.
2. Mauffrey C, Hao J, Cuellar DO 3rd, Herbert B, Chen X, Liu B, Zhang Y, Smith W. The epidemiology and injury patterns of acetabular fractures: are the USA

and China comparable? Clin Orthop Relat Res. 2014;472:3332–7.
3. Giannoudis PV, Grotz MR, Papakostidis C, Dinopoulos H. Operative treatment of displaced fractures of the acetabulum. A meta-analysis. J Bone Joint Surg Br. 2005;87:2–9.
4. Al-Qahtani S, O'Connor G. Acetabular fractures before and after the introduction of seatbelt legislation. Can J Surg. 1996;39:317–20.
5. Ferguson TA, Patel R, Bhandari M, Matta JM. Fractures of the acetabulum in patients aged 60 years and older: an epidemiological and radiological study. J Bone Joint Surg Br. 2010;92:250–7.
6. Toro JB, Hierholzer C, Helfet DL. Acetabular fractures in the elderly. Bull Hosp Jt Dis. 2004;62:53–7.
7. Guerado E, Cano JR, Cruz E. Fractures of the acetabulum in elderly patients: an update. Injury. 2012;43(suppl 2):S33–41.
8. Kregor PJ, Templeman D. Associated injuries complicating the management of acetabular fractures: review and case studies. Orthop Clin North Am. 2002;33:73–95.
9. Culemann U, Holstein JH, Köhler D, Tzioupis CC, Pizanis A, Tosounidis G, Burkhardt M, Pohlemann T. Different stabilisation techniques for typical acetabular fractures in the elderly--a biomechanical assessment. Injury. 2010;41:405–10.
10. Magnussen RA, Tressler MA, Obremskey WT, Kregor PJ. Predicting blood loss in isolated pelvic and acetabular high-energy trauma. J Orthop Trauma. 2007;21:603–7.
11. Kaur P, Basu S, Kaur G, Kaur R. Transfusion protocol in trauma. J Emerg Trauma Shock. 2011;4:103–8.
12. Jouffroy P, Sebaaly A, Aubert T, Riouallon G. Improved acetabular fracture diagnosis after training in a CT-based method. Orthop Traumatol Surg Res. 2017;103:325–9.
13. Tornetta P 3rd. Displaced acetabular fractures: indications for operative and nonoperative management. J Am Acad Orthop Surg. 2001;9:18–28.
14. Geijer M, El-Khoury GY. Imaging of the acetabulum in the era of multidetector computed tomography. Emerg Radiol. 2007;14:271–87.
15. Scheinfeld MH, Dym AA, Spektor M, Avery LL, Dym RJ, Amanatullah DF. Acetabular fractures: what radiologists should know and how 3D CT can aid classification. Radiographics. 2015;35:555–77.
16. Garrett J, Halvorson J, Carroll E, Webb LX. Value of 3-D CT in classifying acetabular fractures during orthopedic residency training. Orthopedics. 2012;35:e615–20.
17. Kickuth R, Laufer U, Hartung G, Gruening C, Stueckle C, Kirchner J. 3D CT versus axial helical CT versus conventional tomography in the classification of acetabular fractures: a ROC analysis. Clin Radiol. 2002;57:140–5.
18. Chana-Rodríguez F, Mañanes RP, Rojo-Manaute J, Gil P, Martínez-Gómiz JM, Vaquero-Martín J. 3D surgical printing and pre contoured plates for acetabular fractures. Injury. 2016;47:2507–11.
19. Chen X, Chen X, Zhang G, Lin H, Yu Z, Wu C, Li X, Lin Y, Huang W. Accurate fixation of plates and screws for the treatment of acetabular fractures using 3D-printedguiding templates: an experimental study. Injury. 2017;48:1147–54.
20. Knight RA, Smith H. Central fractures of the acetabulum. J Bone Joint Surg Am. 1958;40-A:1–16.
21. Rowe CR, Lowell JD. Prognosis of fractures of the acetabulum. J Bone Joint Surg Am. 1961;43:30–59.
22. Judet R, Judet J, Letournel E. Fractures of the acetabulum: classification and surgical approaches for open reduction—preliminary report. J Bone Joint Surg Am. 1964;46:1615–46.
23. Kanakaris NK, Giannoudi MP. Fractures-dislocations of the hip. In: Lasanianos NG, Kanakaris NK, Giannoudis PV, editors. Trauma and orthopaedic classifications. A comprehensive overview. London: Springer; 2015. pp. 285, 289.
24. Harris JH Jr, Lee JS, Coupe KJ, Trotscher T. Acetabular fractures revisited: part 1, redefinition of the Letournel anterior column. AJR Am J Roentgenol. 2004;182:1363–6.
25. Harris JH Jr, Coupe KJ, Lee JS, Trotscher T. Acetabular fractures revisited. 2. A new CT-based classification. AJR. 2004;182:1367–75.
26. Ochs BG, Marintschev I, Hoyer H, Rolauffs B, Culemann U, Pohlemann T, Stuby FM. Changes in the treatment of acetabular fractures over 15 years: analysis of 1266 cases treated by the German Pelvic Multicentre Study Group (DAO/DGU). Injury. 2010;41:839–51.
27. Judet R, Judet J, Letournel E. Fractures of the acetabulum. Acta Orthop Belg. 1964;30:285–93.
28. Olson SA, Matta JM. The computerized tomography subchondral arc: a new method of assessing acetabular articular continuity after fracture (a preliminary report). J Orthop Trauma. 1993;7:402–13.
29. Vrahas MS, Widding KK, Thomas KA. The effects of simulated transverse, anterior column, and posterior column fractures of the acetabulum on the stability of the hip joint. J Bone Joint Surg Am. 1999;81:966–74.
30. Harnroongroj T, Suangyanon P, Tharmviboonsri T, Harnroongroj T. Posterior acetabular arc angle of the femoral head assesses instability of posterior fracture-dislocation of the hip. Int Orthop. 2013;37:1141–5.
31. Harnroongroj T, Wattanakaewsripetch M, Sudjai N, Harnroongroj T. Acetabular roof arc angles and anatomic biomechanical superior acetabular weight bearing area. Indian J Orthop. 2014;48:484–7.
32. Vailas JC, Hurwitz S, Wiesel SW. Posterior acetabular fracture-dislocations: fragment size, joint capsule, and stability. J Trauma. 1989;29:1494–6.
33. Keith JE Jr, Brashear HR Jr, Guilford WB. Stability of posterior fracture-dislocations of the hip. Quantitative assessment using computed tomography. J Bone Joint Surg Am. 1988;70:711–4.
34. Matta JM. Operative indications and choice of surgical approach for fractures of the acetabulum. Tech Orthop. 1986;1:13.

35. Sen RK, Veerappa LA. Long-term outcome of conservatively managed displaced acetabular fractures. J Trauma. 2009;67:155–9.
36. Magu NK, Rohilla R, Arora S. Conservatively treated acetabular fractures: a retrospective analysis. Indian J Orthop. 2012;46:36–45.
37. Cole JD, Bolhofner BR. Acetabular fracture fixation via a modified Stoppa limited intrapelvic approach. Description of operative technique and preliminary treatment results. Clin Orthop Relat Res. 1994;305:112–23.
38. Guy P. Evolution of the anterior intrapelvic (Stoppa) approach for acetabular fracture surgery. J Orthop Trauma. 2015;29(Suppl 2):S1–5.
39. Archdeacon MT, Kazemi N, Guy P, Sagi HC. The modified Stoppa approach for acetabular fracture. J Am Acad Orthop Surg. 2011;19:170–5.
40. Bastian JD, Savic M, Cullmann JL, Zech WD, Djonov V, Keel MJ. Surgical exposures and options for instrumentation in acetabular fracture fixation: Pararectus approach versus the modified Stoppa. Injury. 2016 Mar;47(3):695–701.
41. Richter H, Hutson JJ, Zych G. The use of spring plates in the internal fixation of acetabular fractures. J Orthop Trauma. 2004;18:179–81.
42. Wu X, Chen W, Zhang Q, Su Y, Guo M, Qin D, Wang L, Zhang Y. The study of plate-screw fixation in the posterior wall of acetabulum using computed tomography images. J Trauma. 2010;69:423–31.
43. Coste C, Asloum Y, Marcheix PS, Dijoux P, Charissoux JL, Mabit C. Percutaneous iliosacral screw fixation in unstable pelvic ring lesions: the interest of O-ARM CT-guided navigation. Orthop Traumatol Surg Res. 2013;99:S273–8.
44. He J, Tan G, Zhou D, Sun L, Li Q, Yang Y, Liu P. Comparison of isocentric C-arm 3-dimensional navigation and conventional fluoroscopy for percutaneous retrograde screwing for anterior column fracture of acetabulum: an observational study. Medicine (Baltimore). 2016;95:e2470.
45. Ruan Z, Luo CF, Zeng BF, et al. Percutaneous screw fixation for the acetabular fracture with quadrilateral plate involved by three-dimensional fluoroscopy navigation: surgical technique. Injury. 2012;43:517–21.
46. Jacob AL, Suhm N, Kaim A, et al. Coronal acetabular fractures: the anterior approach in computed tomography-navigated minimally invasive percutaneous. Cardiovasc Intervent Radiol. 2000;23:327–31.
47. Yang JH, Chouhan DK, Oh KJ. Percutaneous screw fixation of acetabular fractures: applicability of hip arthroscopy. Arthroscopy. 2010;26:1556–61.
48. Kim H, Baek JH, Park SM, Ha YC. Arthroscopic reduction and internal fixation of acetabular fractures. Knee Surg Sports Traumatol Arthrosc. 2014;22:867–70.
49. Park MS, Her IS, Cho HM, Chung YY. Internal fixation of femoral head fractures (Pipkin I) using hip arthroscopy. Knee Surg Sports Traumatol Arthrosc. 2014;22:898–901.
50. Yamamoto Y, Ide T, Ono T, Hamada Y. Usefulness of arthroscopic surgery in hip trauma cases. Arthroscopy. 2003;19:269–73.
51. Khanna V, Harris A, Farrokhyar F, Choudur HN, Wong IH. Hip arthroscopy: prevalence of intra-articular pathologic findings after traumatic injury of the hip. Arthroscopy. 2014;30:299–304.
52. Ladner B, Nester K, Cascio B. Abdominal fluid extravasation during hip arthroscopy. Arthroscopy. 2010;26:131–5.
53. Kubota M, Uchida K, Kokubo Y, Shimada S, Matsuo H, Yayama T, Miyazaki T, Takeura N, Yoshida A, Baba H. Changes in gait pattern and hip muscle strength after open reduction and internal fixation of acetabular fracture. Arch Phys Med Rehabil. 2012;93:2015–21.
54. Dunet B, Tournier C, Billaud A, Lavoinne N, Fabre T, Durandeau A. Acetabular fracture: long-term follow-up and factors associated with secondary implantation of total hip arthroplasty. Orthop Traumatol Surg Res. 2013;99:281–90.
55. Meena UK, Tripathy SK, Sen RK, Aggarwal S, Behera P. Predictors of postoperative outcome for acetabular fractures. Orthop Traumatol Surg Res. 2013;99:929–35.
56. Anizar-Faizi A, Hisam A, Sudhagar KP, Moganadass M, Suresh C. Outcome of surgical treatment for displaced acetabular fractures. Malays Orthop J. 2014;8:1–6.
57. Bhat NA, Kangoo KA, Wani IH, Wali GR, Muzaffar N, Dar RA. Operative management of displaced acetabular fractures: an institutional experience with a midterm follow-up. Ortop Traumatol Rehabil. 2014;16:245–52.
58. Borg T, Hailer NP. Outcome 5 years after surgical treatment of acetabular fractures: a prospective clinical and radiographic follow-up of 101 patients. Arch Orthop Trauma Surg. 2015;135:227–33.
59. Iqbal F, Taufiq I, Najjad MK, Khan N, Zia OB. Functional and radiological outcome of surgical management of acetabular fractures in tertiary care hospital. Hip Pelvis. 2016;28:217–24.
60. Clarke-Jenssen J, Røise O, Storeggen SAØ, Madsen JE. Long-term survival and risk factors for failure of the native hip joint after operatively treated displaced acetabular fractures. Bone Joint J. 2017;99-B:834–40.
61. Negrin LL, Seligson D. Results of 167 consecutive cases of acetabular fractures using the Kocher-Langenbeck approach: a case series. J Orthop Surg Res. 2017;12:66.
62. Dodd A, Osterhoff G, Guy P, Lefaivre KA. Assessment of functional outcomes of surgically managed acetabular fractures: a systematic review. Bone Joint J. 2016;98-B:690–5.
63. Engsberg JR, Steger-May K, Anglen JO, Borrelli J Jr. An analysis of gait changes and functional outcome in patients surgically treated for displaced acetabular fractures. J Orthop Trauma. 2009;23:346–53.
64. Halvorson JJ, Lamothe J, Martin CR, Grose A, Asprinio DE, Wellman D, Helfet DL. Combined ace-

tabulum and pelvic ring injuries. J Am Acad Orthop Surg. 2014;22:304–14.
65. Osgood GM, Manson TT, O'Toole RV, Turen CH. Combined pelvic ring disruption and acetabular fracture: associated injury patterns in 40 patients. J Orthop Trauma. 2013;27:243–7.
66. Suzuki T, Smith WR, Hak DJ, Stahel PF, Baron AJ, Gillani SA, Morgan SJ. Combined injuries of the pelvis and acetabulum: nature of a devastating dyad. J Orthop Trauma. 2010;24:303–8.
67. Hess AE, Johal HS, O'Toole RV, Nascone JW. Early postoperative displacement of combined pelvic ring injury with acetabular fracture. Orthopedics. 2017;40:163–8.
68. Beckmann NM, Chinapuvvula NR, Cai C. Association of femoral head and acetabular fractures on computerized tomography: correlation with the Judet-Letournel classification. Emerg Radiol. 2017;24(5):531–9.
69. Tannast M, Najibi S, Matta JM. Two to twenty-year survivorship of the hip in 810 patients with operatively treated acetabular fractures. J Bone Joint Surg Am. 2012;94:1559–67.
70. Asnis SE, Wanek-Sgaglione L. Intracapsular fractures of the femoral neck. Results of cannulated screw fixation. J Bone Joint Surg Am. 1994;76:1793–803.
71. Wei L, Sun JY, Wang Y, Yang X. Surgical treatment and prognosis of acetabular fractures associated with ipsilateral femoral neck fractures. Orthopedics. 2011;34:348.
72. Mears DC, Velyvis JH. Acute total hip arthroplasty for selected displaced acetabular fractures: two to twelve-year results. J Bone Joint Surg Am. 2002;84-A:1–9.
73. Tidermark J, Blomfeldt R, Ponzer S, Söderqvist A, Törnkvist H. Primary total hip arthroplasty with a Burch-Schneider antiprotrusion cage and autologous bone grafting for acetabular fractures in elderly patients. J Orthop Trauma. 2003;17:193–7.
74. Mouhsine E, Garofalo R, Borens O, Blanc CH, Wettstein M, Leyvraz PF. Cable fixation and early total hip arthroplasty in the treatment of acetabular fractures in elderly patients. J Arthroplast. 2004;19:344–8.
75. Sarkar MR, Wachter N, Kinzl L, Bischoff M. Acute total hip replacement for displaced acetabular fractures in older patients. Eur J Trauma. 2004;30:296.
76. Sermon A, Broos P, Vanderschot P. Total hip replacement for acetabular fractures. Results in 121 patients operated between 1983 and 2003. Injury. 2008;39:914–21.
77. Herscovici D Jr, Lindvall E, Bolhofner B, Scaduto JM. The combined hip procedure: open reduction internal fixation combined with total hip arthroplasty for the management of acetabular fractures in the elderly. J Orthop Trauma. 2010;24:291–6.
78. Enocson A, Blomfeldt R. Acetabular fractures in the elderly treated with a primary Burch-Schneider reinforcement ring, autologous bone graft, and a total hip arthroplasty: a prospective study with a 4-year follow-up. J Orthop Trauma. 2014;28:330–7.
79. Malhotra R, Singh DP, Jain V, Kumar V, Singh R. Acute total hip arthroplasty in acetabular fractures in the elderly using the Octopus System: mid term to long term follow-up. J Arthroplasty. 2013;28:1005–9.
80. Choplin RH, Henley CN, Edds EM, Capello W, Rankin JL, Buckwalter KA. Total hip arthroplasty in patients with bone deficiency of the acetabulum. Radiographics. 2008;28:771–86.
81. Makridis KG, Obakponovwe O, Bobak P, Giannoudis PV. Total hip arthroplasty after acetabular fracture: incidence of complications, reoperation rates and functional outcomes: evidence today. J Arthroplast. 2014;29:1983–90.
82. Berry DJ, Halasy M. Uncemented acetabular components for arthritis after acetabular fracture. Clin Orthop Relat Res. 2002;405:164–7.
83. Lizaur-Utrilla A, Sanz-Reig J, Serna-Berna R. Cementless acetabular reconstruction after acetabular fracture: a prospective, matched-cohort study. J Trauma Acute Care Surg. 2012;73:232–8.
84. Lai O, Yang J, Shen B, Zhou Z, Kang P, Pei F. Midterm results of uncemented acetabular reconstruction for posttraumatic arthritis secondary to acetabular fracture. J Arthroplast. 2011;26:1008–13.

Pipkin Fractures

11

Benedikt J. Braun, Jörg H. Holstein,
and Tim Pohlemann

Abstract

Femoral head fractures are rare, but associated with a high complication risk. Appropriate treatment can significantly reduce complications and improve outcome. Pearls and pitfalls of the entire treatment from diagnostics through therapy and aftercare are presented within this chapter and the effect on overall outcome discussed with the current literature.

In short:

- Younger patients (average around 40 years).
- Most commonly observed during automobile collisions (>80%).
- Fracture commonly results from posterior hip dislocation (10%).
- Fracture results from chiseling mechanism; pattern depending on hip position during trauma.
- Early closed reduction improves outcome (<6 h)
  - Immediate open reduction if closed reduction fails.
- Post-reduction/Preoperative CT scan recommended.
- Pipkin classification most common; Brumback classification also includes anterior dislocations.
- Nonsurgical treatment associated with improved outcome only in Pipkin I fractures
  - If <2 mm dislocation, stable hip joint, and no interposed fragments
- If closed reduction succeeds, surgery during delayed primary care phase recommended.
- Main blood supply to femoral head from medial femoral circumflex artery
  - Cave: posterior approaches.
- No significant outcome differences between approaches; should be tailored to fracture pattern.
  - Increased avascular necrosis in posterior approaches.
  - Increased rate of heterotopic ossification in trochanteric flip osteotomy.
- Decision fragment excision vs. fixation based on:
  - Residual fragment displacement <2 mm
  - Fragment outside weight bearing region
  - Free range of motion, no interposition
- Management/approach depends on fracture type
  - Pipkin I: non-operative/fragment excision.
  - Pipkin II: Fixation with either countersunk interfragmentary compression screws, headless self-compression screws, and bio-absorbable pins and screws.
  - Pipkin III: Emergency surgery, open reduction favored.

B. J. Braun · J. H. Holstein · T. Pohlemann (✉)
Department of Trauma, Hand and Reconstructive Surgery, Saarland University Hospital, Homburg, Germany
e-mail: tim.pohlemann@uks.eu

L. Büchler, M. J.B. Keel (eds.), *Fractures of the Hip*, Fracture Management Joint by Joint,
https://doi.org/10.1007/978-3-030-18838-2_11

- Pipkin IV: If fracture pattern allows trochanteric flip shows better outcome.
- Postoperative care: early functional treatment; minimum of 6 weeks partial weight bearing; avoid high degrees of hip flexion.
- Common complications are nerve injury (20% sciatic nerve in posterior dislocations), avascular necrosis, heterotopic ossification, and osteoarthritis.
- Depending on fracture type about 50% good to excellent results can be expected.

Keywords
Femoral head fractures · Epidemiology · Classification · Nonsurgical management · Operative treatment · Aftercare

11.1 Epidemiology, Mechanism of Injury

The fracture of the femoral head was first described in 1869 by Birkett who saw this injury during an autopsy of a patient who fell from the second story of a building [1]. These fractures are rare and almost exclusively occur after hip joint dislocations. The resulting femoral head shearing fractures are encountered in about 10% of all posterior hip dislocations and less frequently in anterior hip dislocations [2]. The exact frequency varies from study to study between 7% and 18% [3]. Apart from the complete shearing fractures, cortical depression fractures are described. Before the routine use of computed tomography, cortical depression fractures of the femoral head without fragment dislocation were virtually never detected. Due to improved imaging modalities the incidence rate for cortical depression fractures has been shown to be over 80% for anterior hip dislocations [4], 60% for posterior dislocations [5], and even to occur in patients without dislocations [6]. In a systematic review by Giannoudis et al. the average age for over 450 patients with femoral head fractures was reported as 38.9 years [7]. The most commonly observed injury mechanism was an automobile collision (84.3%), followed by motorcycle accidents (5.1%) and falls (4.3%).

While it was classically assumed that the typical fracture pattern in femoral head fractures was a result of the pull of the foveal ligament ("staying effect") newer studies have shown that the ligament can only pull out a small osteocartilaginous fragment. The typical fracture pattern is explained as a chiseling mechanism of the acetabular wall on the femoral head [8]. The exact fracture pattern during dorsal hip dislocation then depends on the hip position during the trauma: If the hip is flexed below 60° and adducted, typically a Pipkin type I injury results as the medial part of the femoral head is pressed against the very solid posterior acetabular wall. Abduction with the same flexion will likely result in a type II injury. If the hip is flexed >60° the femoral head is pressed against a thinner portion of the posterior acetabular wall more likely resulting in acetabular fractures and cartilaginous damage, or cortical depression fractures, of the femoral head [9]. Pipkin type III fractures usually occur in cases with prolonged exposure to different forces: The first impact dislocates the femoral head from the joint and causes a part of the femoral head to shear-off. Prolonged adduction force then leads to a femoral neck fracture with the posterior acetabular rim acting as a hypomochlion [10]. Occasionally the femoral neck fracture can also occur during the reduction maneuver. It is assumed however that the majority of mechanical damage to the femoral neck region results from the initial trauma, and initially non-displaced fractures that were simply not noted on the primary X-ray dislocate during the reduction maneuver [8].

11.2 Clinical and Radiographic Assessment

As the majority of femoral head fractures are associated with high-energy trauma and multiple injured patients it is important to identify the fracture amongst concomitant injuries. Especially in unconscious patients careful history taking and reports about the mechanism of injury from the emergency medical personnel present on the scene of the accident can assist in determining the risk for such fractures. While the clinical presentation can be misleading, fractures with posterior hip dislocation generally appear with the leg in flexion, adduction, and internal rotation giving the impression of an overall shortened extremity. In fractures with anterior dislocation the leg is generally abducted and externally rotated. These classic malpositions can be missing in the case of concomitant femoral neck fractures. Careful examination of the integument is needed to identify skin damages associated with high-energy trauma (Morel-Lavallée lesions). A detailed neurological examination should be performed in the conscious patient to determine sciatic nerve injuries associated with posterior dislocations or femoral nerve injuries associated with anterior dislocations. In the unconscious patient this examination should be performed as early as feasible; special attention needs to be paid to the neurovascular structures on the imaging.

Conventional radiographs are the primary means of determining the direction of dislocation and extent of gross bony injuries. The fracture dislocation of the hip is routinely recognized in anteroposterior (ap) radiographs by the disruption of Shenton's line (Fig. 11.1). In ap pelvic radiographs, the direction of dislocation can be determined by evaluating the size of the femoral head in relation to the contralateral, uninjured femur: Increased head size indicates that the femur is closer to the X-ray source, thus anteriorly dislocated; while posterior dislocations are closer to the radiographic film, thus appear smaller. Careful review of the femoral neck region is advisable to assess the existence of a Pipkin Type III situation that could dislocate during the reduction process. Furthermore oblique ala and obturator views can be used to determine acetabular fractures, while inlet and outlet views can be performed to detect pelvic ring injuries. Especially in the polytraumatized patient these views are commonly replaced by an immediate, pre-reduction computed tomography (CT).

CT is considered routine following closed reduction of the hip to correctly identify the fracture pattern and to decide upon the appropriate therapy (Fig. 11.1). In cases of irreducible hip dislocation, CT can be performed to determine the presence of intraarticular fragments that might prevent reduction before surgery. In general, CT can determine size, number, and location of fracture fragments as well as concomitant injuries. Some studies have recommended a special CT patient positioning to allow for CT-directed pelvic oblique conventional radiographs [11]. This has been shown to be an effective method to determine the extent of fracture displacement and congruity of the joint and is still recommended in current textbooks. However

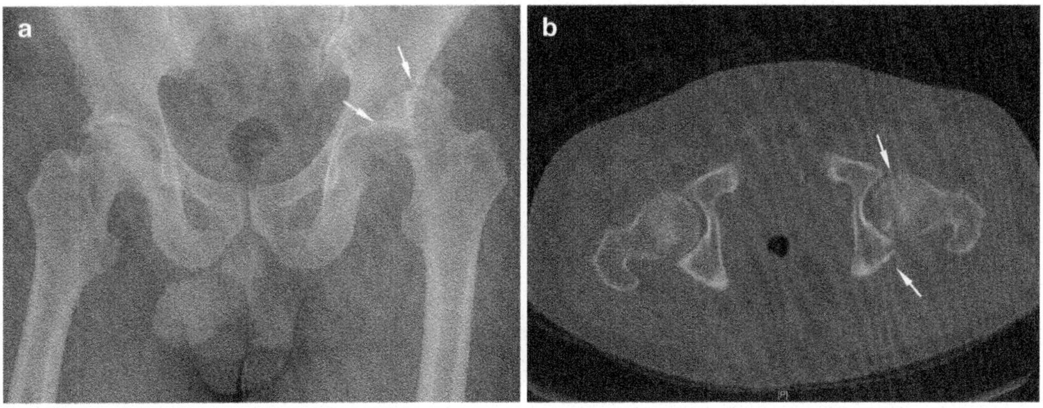

Fig. 11.1 The conventional ap radiograph shows a Pipkin IV fracture left with concomitant posterior hip dislocation (**a**). The CT scan after closed reduction shows fragment dislocation of the femoral head and associated posterior acetabular wall fracture (**b**)

with the available technical ability to manually adjust the CT plain and three-dimensional CT reconstructions, these radiographs have no added value during primary diagnostics and should be used for follow-up purposes only.

Magnetic resonance imaging (MRI) is primarily used to determine the cartilage and vascular integrity of the femoral head. As such it has been suggested during the initial examination. Due to time constraints during the emergency treatment however its main value is during follow-up visits in determining the existence of early forms of avascular necrosis (AVN) [12]. If an injury to the external obturator muscle is suspected MRI can discover injuries to the anatomically close medial femoral circumflex artery and determine future risk of AVN.

11.3 Classification

As femoral head fractures are commonly associated with hip dislocations this is represented in the existing classification systems. The most common classification system was introduced by Pipkin in 1957 [13] (Fig. 11.2): Type I fractures are fractures where the fracture line ends caudal to the Fovea capitis femoris, whereas in Type II fractures the line ends cranial to the Fovea. This helps distinguish between fractures outside (Type I) and within (Type II) the load-bearing portion of the femoral head. In Type III fractures the femoral head fracture of either kind is associated with a femoral neck fracture. In Type IV fractures it is associated with acetabular wall fractures.

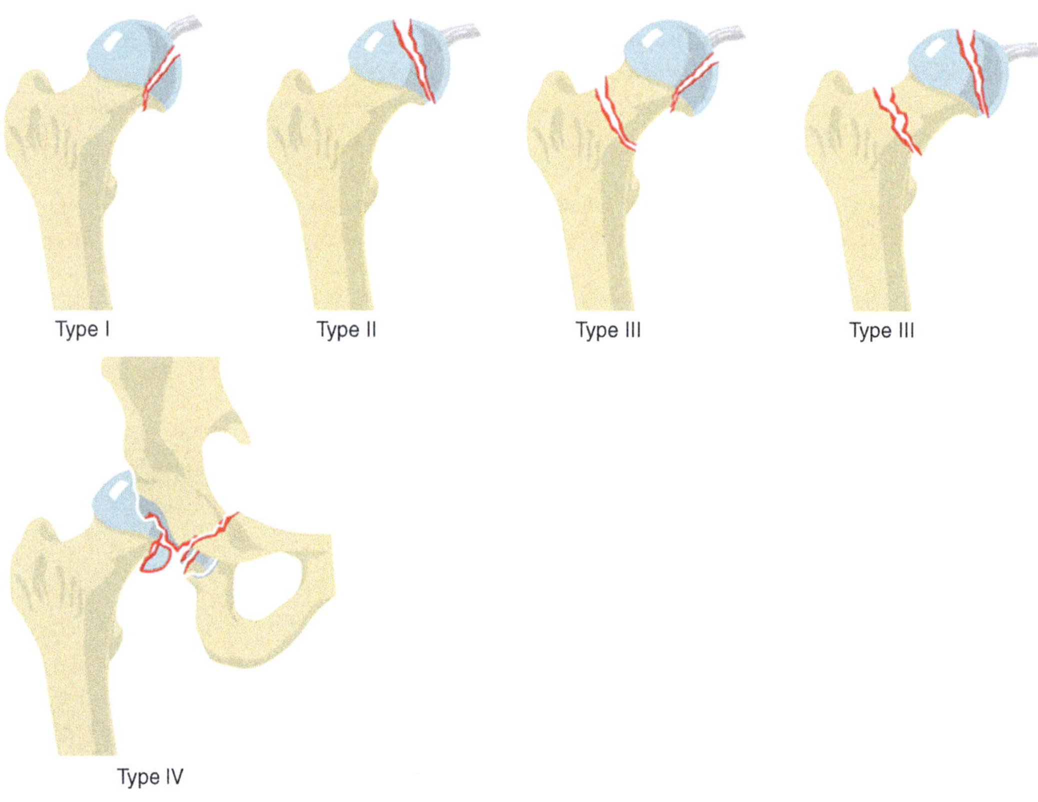

Fig. 11.2 Pipkin classification of femoral head fractures; Type I: Fracture line ends caudal to the Fovea capitis femoris; Type II: Fracture line ends cranial to the Fovea; Type III: Femoral head fracture of either kind associated with femoral neck fracture; Type IV: Femoral head fracture of either kind associated with acetabular wall fractures (Haas, Norbert P., and Christian Krettek, eds. Tscherne Unfallchirurgie: Hüfte und Oberschenkel. Springer-Verlag, 2011. Adapted and reproduced with permission and copyright © of Springer)

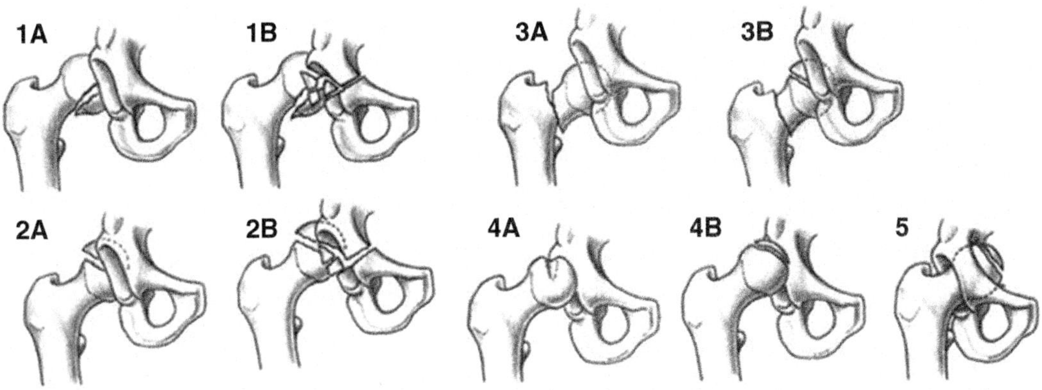

Fig. 11.3 Brumback classification of femoral head fractures. (Stannard JP, Harris HW, Volgas DA, Alonso JE: Functional outcome of patients with femoral head fractures associated with hip dislocations. Clin Orthop Relat Res 2000;377:44–56. Adapted and reproduced with permission and copyright © of Springer)

In this system, only the more common dorsocranial dislocations (90%) are classified. Brumback introduced a modification of the original classification 30 years later to incorporate all directions of dislocation and also therapeutic and prognostic estimations (Fig. 11.3) [14]: Type I and Type II fractures are defined like Pipkin I and II fractures, but divided into two subgroups. Subgroup A are fractures with minimal, or no acetabular rim damage and stable joint conditions after reduction. Subgroup B fractures show significant acetabular rim damage along with hip joint instability. Brumback III fractures are posterior hip dislocations with femoral neck fractures without (subgroup A) or with associated femoral head fractures (subgroup B). Type IV fractures result from anterior hip dislocations and either show an osteocartilaginous indentation (subgroup A), or a transchondral shear fracture (subgroup B). The final Type V fractures are central hip dislocations with femoral head fractures. While this classification system has been used in several larger studies [15, 16] and shown to be a valuable tool to assist outcome measurements, the clinical use of this classification is rare, in part due to its increased complexity when compared to the original Pipkin classification.

The AO fracture classification system accounts for femoral head fractures within the classification of proximal femoral fractures. All femoral head fractures are classified under 31-C. Pipkin Type I and II fractures are further classified as C1, osteochondral depression fractures as C2 and combined femoral head and femoral neck fractures as C3 (Fig. 11.4).

11.4 Conservative Treatment

11.4.1 General Considerations

The clinical and radiographic outcome of femoral head fractures with concomitant hip dislocation is directly linked to the time of reduction [17, 18] and should thus be considered as a true orthopedic trauma emergency. Several studies have shown superior results if the hip is reduced within 6 h [19], or even 3 h [20]. While many reduction maneuvers for hip dislocations have been proposed, they all incorporate common mechanisms for both anterior and posterior dislocations. In anterior dislocations, the reduction is generally performed by axial pull with the hip and knee in neutral flexion/extension. For posterior dislocations, knee and hip are flexed to around 90° and axial pull in the direction of the femur is applied. Adequate pain management and sedation/relaxation is required prior to reduction to keep the occurring stresses to the femoral head as low as possible. Post-reduction CT scan should be performed to guide the ensuing management. Closed reduction is contraindicated in patients with concomitant femoral neck fractures. If closed reduction is technically not possible, immediate open reduction is recommended. A CT scan should be

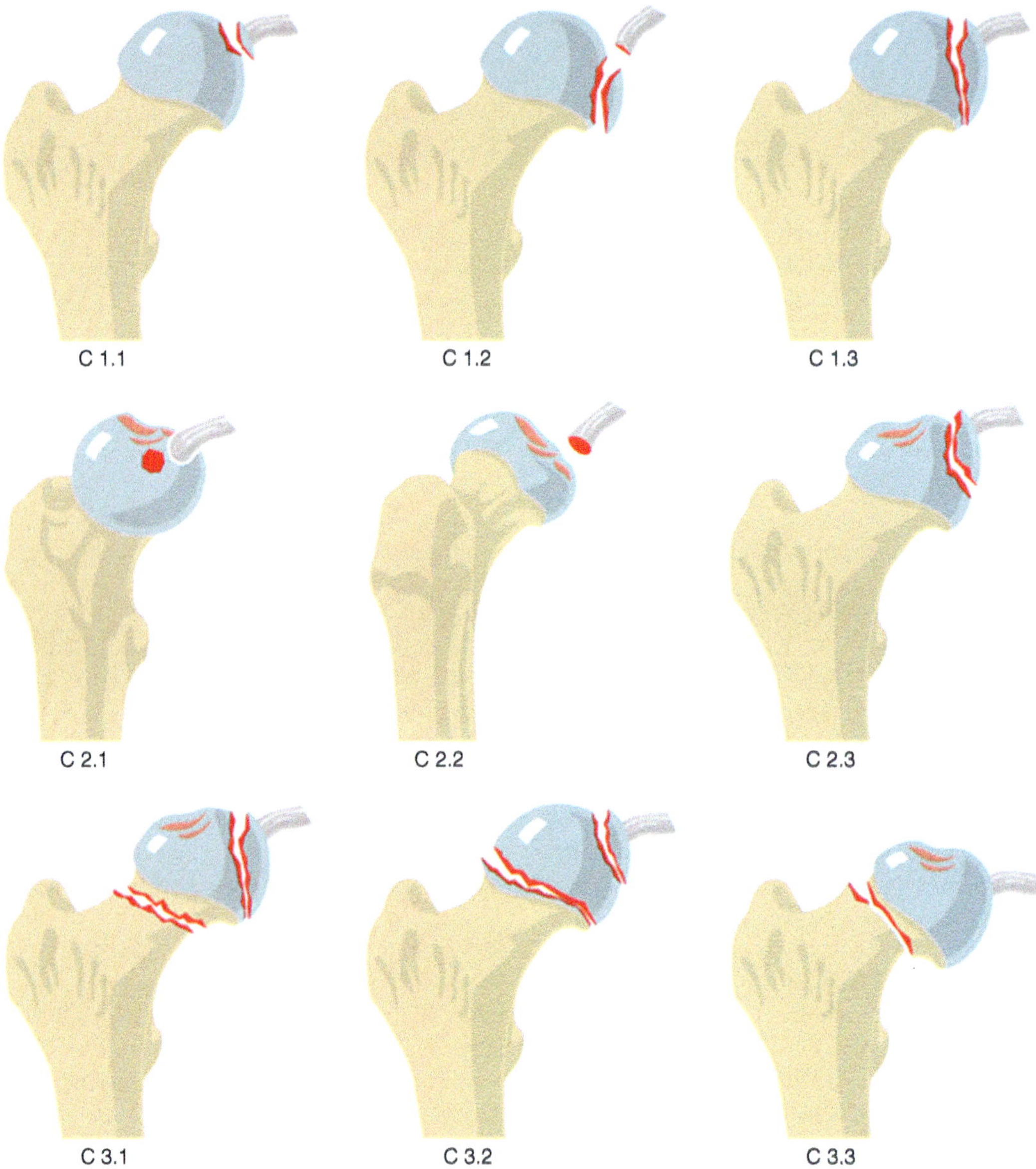

Fig. 11.4 AO classification system for femoral head fractures. (Haas, Norbert P., and Christian Krettek, eds. Tscherne Unfallchirurgie: Hüfte und Oberschenkel. Springer-Verlag, 2011. Adapted and reproduced with permission and copyright © of Springer)

performed beforehand to assess the fracture situation in detail if this does not lead to substantial delays until final reduction is achieved.

11.4.2 Nonsurgical Treatment

The historically predominant conservative fracture treatment with bed rest and traction has been largely abandoned due to relatively poor results [21] and the associated socioeconomic consequences. Non-operative treatment however can be considered especially in Pipkin I fractures under certain conditions: Near anatomic reduction with fragment dislocation below 2 mm, a stable hip joint and congruent joint surfaces without interposed fragments [22]. When applying these criteria studies with limited patient numbers have shown satisfactory outcomes [23]. Even if the fragment does not completely reduce after closed reduction, non-operative treatment can be performed if the hip range of motion is not compromised by it [24], as even necrotic changes to the fragment outside the weight bearing zone seem to have no effect on the clinical outcome [18]. The same criteria can be applied to Pipkin Type II fractures. However as they are located in the weight bearing portion of the femoral head surface these fractures are exposed to increased direct pressure and shear forces that can prevent adequate closed reduction [23]. Furthermore these fractures usually contain large areas of the femoral head, thus a high likelihood for an unstable hip joint and osteoarthritis in case of incongruity or osteonecrosis is given.

If nonsurgical treatment is chosen, the patient should be limited to partial weight bearing with crutches for at least 6 weeks. Adduction and excessive internal rotation of the hip should be avoided. Follow-up radiographs after 3 and 6 weeks should be performed to determine the maintenance of adequate reduction. The CT-directed pelvic oblique radiograph technique originally published by Moed et al. can be used to determine the positioning angle of the patient to allow for a standardized, perpendicular fracture line visualization [11].

11.5 Operative Treatment

11.5.1 Approaches

11.5.1.1 General Considerations: Time to Surgery

As with other fracture entities around the proximal femur the time to surgery can have significant implications on the long-term outcome. The most time sensitive and outcome predicting factor is early joint reduction. In cases of technically impossible reduction the time to surgery should thus ideally be below the 6 h threshold if comorbidities and concomitant injuries permit. Likewise in cases with a Pipkin III type injury early reduction and femoral neck fixation is needed especially if a head preserving therapy is planned. If closed reduction is accomplished current opinion is that the definitive surgery should be performed during the delayed primary care phase ideally between the sixth and tenth day [25]. If the definitive surgery is performed after the 14th day post reduction, significantly worse operative results have to be expected.

11.5.1.2 General Considerations: Vascular Anatomy

Before committing to any approach and treatment clear visualization of the approaches anatomy and associated vascular supply of the femoral head and neck is advisable to avoid iatrogenic damage to the important vessels. The most important blood supply of the femoral head weight bearing cartilage is provided by the terminal branches of the medial femoral circumflex artery [26]. The medial circumflex artery originates from the deep femoral artery and runs between the iliopsoas and pectineus muscles along the basal part of the femoral neck. From there it continues around the inferior border of the external obturator muscle, runs posterior to its tendon and anterior to the gemellus muscles and into the hip capsule just superior to the superior gemellus muscle insertion. From there the terminal branches of the artery lie within the periosteum and enter the bone postero-superiorly just lateral to the joint cartilage. As a result of this course the main risk of injuring the medial circumflex artery is during posterior approaches [27]. Important medial blood supply from the vessels within Weibrecht's ligament [28] is furthermore at risk during reduction of femoral head fractures and care should be taken not to injure the medial synovial fold, as it is often attached to the fragment. The lateral circumflex artery has barely any contribution to the femoral heads blood supply.

11.5.1.3 Anterior Approaches

Traditionally anterior approaches such as the Smith-Petersen approach were unpopular due to misinterpreted anatomical considerations. The believe was that the more common posterior hip dislocation injures the posterior blood supply so that an anterior approach with possible damage to the ascending branch of the lateral circumflex artery would then cut all blood supply from the femoral head [21]. With the above-mentioned anatomical considerations in mind however anterior approaches have gained considerably in popularity. Studies have shown that this approach is associated with decreased operating time and blood loss [23]. Furthermore the rate of avascular necrosis of the femoral head seems to be decreased [29]. In cases of isolated femoral head fracture the associated fragment is most commonly anteromedial. The Smith-Petersen approach thus offers direct visualization of most fragments in Pipkin I and II fractures without compromising the vascular integrity of the femoral head. A radial capsulotomy at the beginning of the acetabulum usually offers sufficient fracture visualization. If improved exposure is needed, the iliac rectus femoris origin can be released. Without dislocating the hip most fractures can then be visualized by extension, abduction, and external rotation. The anterolateral Watson Jones approach offers less soft tissue trauma, but also less adaptability when it comes to extending the approach. Pipkin III fractures can be addressed by an anterolateral approach to manage both the femoral neck fracture with open reduction and also the femoral head fracture through a single incision.

Some older studies have seen higher incidence for heterotopic ossifications for anterior approaches. Swiontkowski et al. have shown an increased overall (58% vs. 25%) rate of heterotopic ossifications when comparing anterior with posterior approaches in the treatment of Pipkin I and II fractures [23]. Of the ossifications 29% were functionally significant in anterior approaches while none were functionally significant in posterior approaches. In a follow-up study the author has thus recommended to only use the distal, gluteal musculature sparing part of the Smith-Petersen approach. Newer studies have thus shown not only similar, but lower incidence rates of heterotopic ossifications for the anterior approach [29, 30].

11.5.1.4 Posterior Approaches

Posterior fracture dislocations are often associated with posterior soft tissue damage to structures such as the piriformis tendon. These structures most commonly block closed reduction. To directly address the posterior structures in irreducible fracture dislocations as well as in cases with associated posterior acetabulum fractures (Pipkin IV) the Kocher-Langenbeck approach is recommended [31]. To manage femoral head damages through a posterior approach a combination of the approach with a trochanteric flip osteotomy surgical hip dislocation is suggested. The advantage of this approach was demonstrated in a cadaver study by Gautier et al. that provided insight into the femoral heads blood supply [27]. Through this technique the obturator externus muscle is kept intact, thus preserving blood supply to the femoral head through the medial femoral circumflex artery [32]. Patient positioning and initial exposure are performed analogue to the Kocher-Langenbeck approach, with the actual transmuscular approach going through the Gipson Interval. A trochanteric step cut osteotomy is then performed from the superior edge of the greater trochanter distally to the posterior end of the vastus ridge and mobilized anteriorly. Afterwards the capsule is incised and the foveal ligament transected and excised with the hip joint in a flexed and externally rotated position. The hip can now be anteriorly dislocated and the complete femoral head can be surgically addressed. To facilitate anatomical refixation of the greater trochanter with two cortical screws drilling should be performed prior to the osteotomy.

In their original study of patients with surgical anterior hip dislocation Ganz et al. experienced no cases of avascular necrosis in 213 patients [32]. In a further study Kloen et al. compared patients treated either with an anterior, anterolateral, isolated posterior, or trochanteric flip approach [30]. They found that around 80% of the patients with trochanteric flip osteotomy had either excellent or good results. Again they noticed no avascular necrosis but a high rate (60%) of functionally significant heterotopic ossification. As such the excellent exposure of this approach is limited by the extensive soft tissue trauma and should be used in cases with posterior bony acetabulum injury combined with anterior femoral head fractures. Careful operative technique is needed to protect the femoral heads vasculature.

Table 11.1 Common treatment options in relation to the Pipkin classification

Pipkin classification	Conservative option[a]	Surgical treatment	Approach
I	Yes	(1) Fragment excision (2) Internal fixation (3) Arthroplasty	Anterior preferred, depending on fragment location
II	Possible	(1) Internal fixation (2) Fragment excision (3) Arthroplasty	Anterior preferred, depending on fragment location
III	No	(1) (Open) Reduction internal fixation of the neck (2) Internal fixation of the head (3) Fragment excision (4) No head treatment[a] (5) Arthroplasty	Anterolateral/anterior
IV	Yes	(1) Internal fixation of the acetabulum (2) Internal fixation of the head (3) Fragment excision (4) Arthroplasty	Posterior/trochanteric flip Separate anterior Anterior with Smith-Petersen extension

[a]Conservative treatment if: closed reduction is possible, residual fragment dislocation <2 mm and fragment outside of weight bearing region

11.5.2 Techniques of Open Reduction and Fixation (Table 11.1)

As the surgical technique is dependent on the fracture morphology the treatment options are discussed using the more common Pipkin classification:

11.5.2.1 Pipkin Type I/II

If the above-mentioned criteria for nonsurgical management are not met (Sect. 11.4.2), the surgical treatment can be performed either by internal fixation or fragment excision. Earlier studies have generally advised for fragment excision as long as the fragment size was less than one third of the femoral head, as this has been shown to have a superior outcome compared to fragment fixation [33]. Further criteria advocating excision are the degree of fracture comminution and thus technical operability, exact fragment size, and fracture location in a non-weight bearing area of the femoral head. A cadaveric study by Holmes et al. showed that fragment excision in Pipkin Type I fractures does not change the peak load and load distribution on the acetabulum surface [34]. A recent randomized controlled trial has shown superior functional outcome scores in patients with Pipkin Type I fractures and fragment excision compared to nonsurgical treatment [35]. In light of these results Pipkin Type I fractures should mainly be treated with fragment excision. Pipkin Type II fractures and larger fragments have however been shown to significantly interfere with normal hip joint function if excised [34]. After excision the contact area was increased, mean pressures higher and displaced centrally. This is thought to increase the chance of chondral deterioration and ultimately osteoarthritis. If technical operability is given, these fracture fragments should be addressed by osteosynthesis. The approach should be tailored to the fragment location as determined on the preoperative CT scan and temporal fixation after open reduction can be achieved with Kirschner wires. Definitive fragment fixation then depends on fragment size and surgeon preference. In larger fragments extra-articularly introduced lag screws can be an option [36]. Most fractures however require fixation from within the joint. Treatment options are countersunk interfragmentary compression screws [37], headless self-compression screws [38], and bio-absorbable pins and screws [39]. Studies comparing the outcome between these treatment methods in a randomized, controlled fashion do not exist and all studies with these fixation methods suggest comparable outcomes. Only one study using 3-mm cannulated screws with washers has shown a high failure rate due to dissociation between screw and washer [29].

In cases of technically impossible anatomic fixation of fragments in the weight bearing region, as well as in older patients, hemi- and total hip arthroplasty is a treatment option [40]. Especially in the geriatric patient this enables early rehabilitation without the risk of secondary complications such as avascular necrosis or traumatic osteoarthritis.

11.5.2.2 Pipkin III

This rare fracture type has to be addressed by emergency surgery to allow for successful reduction and fixation of both the femoral neck and head with adequate outcome. Internal fixation of the femoral neck and hip reduction can be performed by the Watson Jones approach, or any approach of the surgeon's preference. Open reduction decreases the risk of vascular compromise [7]. If the Watson Jones approach is used the approach can subsequently serve as the approach to the femoral head in adequately located fracture situations. Whether or not surgical fixation of the femoral head is needed is dependent on the fragment size and position after reduction. In principle the same criteria apply as mentioned above (Sect. 11.4.2). Fragments smaller than 2 mm, outside the weight bearing region with near normal hip range of motion can be left untreated. Primary hemi- or total hip arthroplasty can be a treatment option in elderly patients and femoral neck fractures with large displacements [41].

11.5.2.3 Pipkin IV

The treatment and approach to these fractures is dictated by the location and severity of the acetabular fracture. Small, well-reduced fragments without interposed loose bodies can be treated conservatively in the same fashion as Pipkin I fractures. Especially in younger patients however fixation should be performed in larger and displaced fragments. The most common posterior wall fractures can be addressed through the Kocher-Langenbeck approach and possibly a separate anterior approach depending on the femoral head fragment location or through a single approach with a trochanteric flip osteotomy. This has been shown to improve outcome in Pipkin type IV fractures [16]. Pipkin IV fractures with anterior acetabular involvement can be addressed either by the ilioinguinal or the Stoppa approach with a Smith-Petersen extension [22]. The indications for hemi- or total hip arthroplasty are the same as for the previously reported Pipkin I-III fractures.

11.5.3 Results

11.5.3.1 Postoperative Care

Regardless of surgical or nonsurgical treatment several studies have shown that early mobilization yields equivalent, if not superior results to prolonged bed rest and extension treatment if the hip joint is stable [9, 30]. Early functional treatment with 20% body weight partial weight bearing with crutches is thus recommended for a minimum of 6 weeks. Early mobilization can be assisted by continuous passive motion devices as early as the first postoperative day. Especially in posterior hip dislocations flexion above 70–90° should be avoided, to decrease the load on the structurally weak part of the posterior acetabular rim. Careful, repeated physical therapy instructions on the correct postoperative behavior as well as aids such as wedge-shaped bolster should be used. If radiographic signs of fracture healing are evident after 6 weeks careful, assisted weight bearing increases combined with low impact training should be begun. Full weight bearing is generally achieved after 3 months.

11.5.3.2 Complications

The most common early complication associated with posterior hip dislocations is sciatic nerve injury (Fig. 11.5). This injury is seen in up to 20% of all fracture dislocations. The nerve damage is either caused by entrapment of the nerve between the femoral head or fracture fragments and the ischium, rupture on a fracture surface, or indirect pull and stretch [42]. In the majority of cases the damage results from direct compression through fracture fragments. The most commonly injured part of the sciatic nerve are the peroneal nerve fibers, as they are most susceptible to isch-

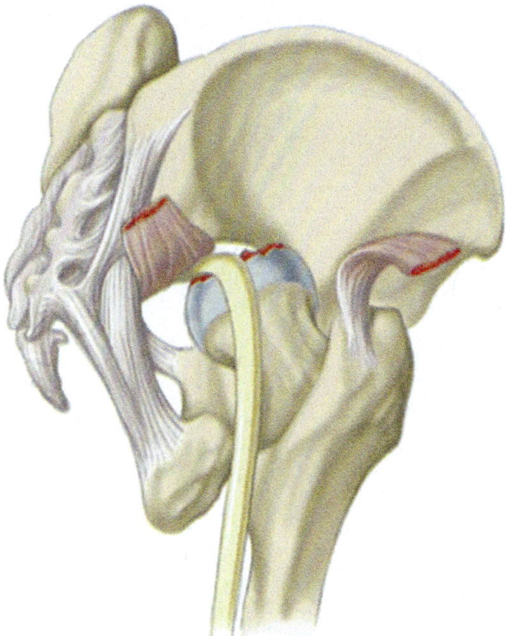

Fig. 11.5 Injury mechanism for sciatic nerve damages: Over-stretch and direct pressure damage. (Haas, Norbert P., and Christian Krettek, eds. Tscherne Unfallchirurgie: Hüfte und Oberschenkel. Springer-Verlag, 2011. Adapted and reproduced with permission and copyright © of Springer)

emic damage and have less stretching reserve due to the fixed course around the fibular head [43]. Immediate hip reduction is thus the most important method to reduce the pressure on the nerve. Letournel et al. have shown that in more than 2/3 of all patients with symptomatic sciatic nerve injuries no macroscopic injury can be observed [44]. Partial to total symptomatic recovery can be expected in about 70% of all patients [45].

In their 2009 meta-analysis Giannoudis et al. have shown that the postoperative infection rate for all femoral neck fractures is 3.2% [7]. They have furthermore shown that the three most common long-term complications after these fractures are femoral head necrosis (11.8%), heterotopic ossification (16.8%), and posttraumatic arthritis (20%).

Femoral head avascular necrosis typically occurs within the first 2 years after femoral head fractures. Long before conventional radiographic changes can be noticed, the MRI can determine early changes associated with avascular necrosis. Common signs are edema, wavy, low signal lines with fatty centers, the double line sign, and later on osteochondral fragmentation. Prolonged compromise of the initial vascularity of the femoral head is regarded as a main risk factor for osteonecrosis [46]. In this regard early reduction of an associated hip dislocation is the key element to reduce this risk. However several studies have shown that despite early reduction osteonecroses were seen [47], suggesting that the etiology is multifactorial. A major risk factor is direct osteochondral trauma from the initial injury, as well as the reduction [17]. Therefore multiple, unsuccessful closed reduction maneuvers have to be avoided. Current studies also suggest that the medial femoral circumflex artery can be damaged if the obturator externus muscle is injured. Older studies have suggested that anterior surgical approaches might compromise vascular integrity [17]. This was however soon refuted by newer studies [33].

The second most common long-term complication is heterotopic ossification (Fig. 11.6) which some authors have seen in as many as 80% of all cases [47]. Associated risk factors are pronounced muscle damage, traumatic brain injury, and insufficient soft tissue management. Furthermore fracture patterns requiring extensive approaches with long operating times seem to be associated with more heterotopic ossifications. Some studies report the incidence of heterotopic ossification to be higher in anterior approaches possibly due to aggressive muscle stripping from the ilium during this approach [22]. The underlying exact mechanism remains unknown. To prevent this complication either oral non-steroidal anti-inflammatory (NSAR) drugs or single dose radiation with seven Gray is suggested. Radiation is however hard to perform, especially in multiple injured, hemodynamically unstable patients. Radiation therapy has to be performed immediately preoperative, or within the first postoperative hours. Common oral NSAR regimes are either 50 mg twice daily or 25 mg of Indomethacin three times a day over 6 weeks postoperatively. It was shown that this effectively reduces the risk of severe heterotopic ossification [46]. As some studies have shown

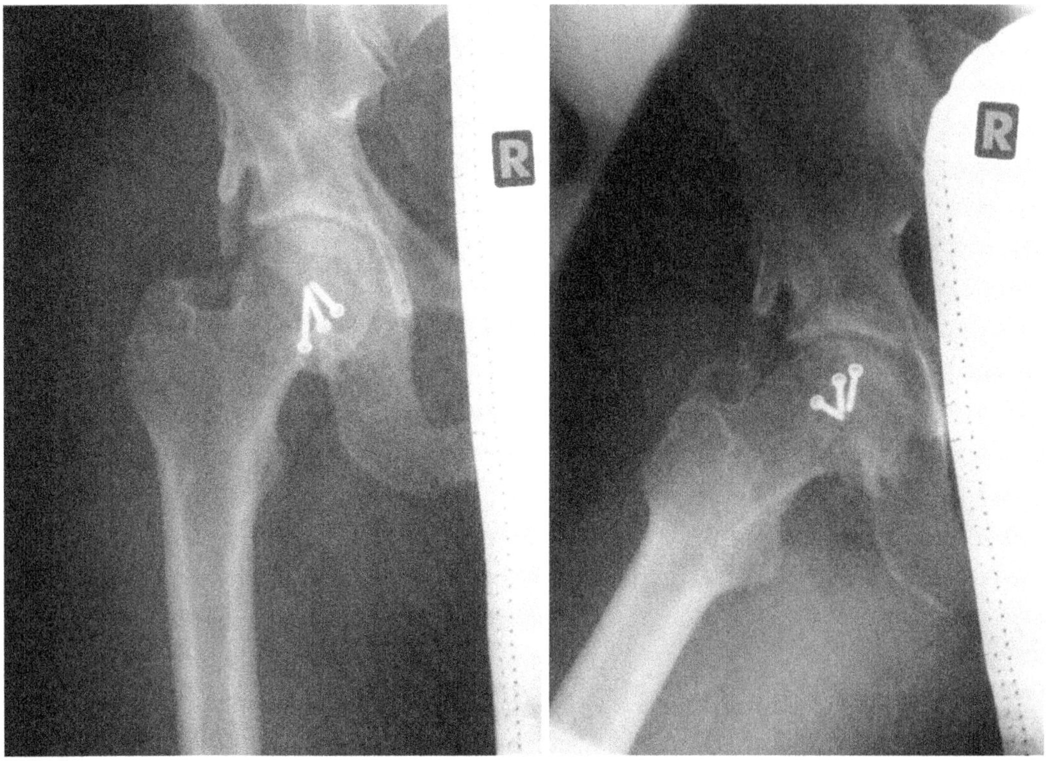

Fig. 11.6 Heterotopic ossification (Brooker III; <1 cm between ossifications) 10 years after treatment of a Pipkin II fracture through an anterior approach

that prolonged NSAR treatment can compromise bone healing [48], newer studies suggest this prophylaxis only in the presence of extensive muscle damage, traumatic brain injury, or prolonged mechanical ventilation [22].

By far the most common complication after hip dislocations with or without associated fractures is posttraumatic osteoarthritis. The development of posttraumatic osteoarthritis is associated with the severity of the initial trauma [49], the amount of direct injury to the joint cartilage [50], and the postoperative congruity of the articular surface [51]. Accordingly the risk of osteoarthritis development is different among the various fracture types: While some degree of osteoarthritis is seen in almost all patients with Pipkin III fractures, or ventral dislocations, only as much as 50% of patients with Pipkin I, II, or IV fractures show this complication [14, 46].

11.6 Results

Due to the rarity of the injury many of the published studies report case series with small patient numbers, different treatment options, inhomogeneous follow-up, non-standardized outcome measures and different classification systems, thus limiting the comparability of the reported results. In one of the earliest larger studies Thompson and Epstein reported <10% of good results in patients with femoral head fractures [5]. Within this article they introduced an outcome measure for radiographic, as well as clinical results that include gross radiographic appearance, as well as pain, range of motion, and walking ability. In order to achieve good or excellent results only minimal joint line narrowing and osteophyte formation is allowed radiographically while clinically at least 75% range of motion have to be achievable without any associated pain (Table 11.2).

Table 11.2 Outcome classification according to Thompson and Epstein [5]

Radiographic criteria	
Excellent (normal)	Good (minimal changes)
1. Normal relationship between head and acetabulum	1. Normal relationship between head and acetabulum
2. Normal articular cartilaginous space	2. Minimal narrowing of cartilaginous space
3. Normal density of the femoral head	3. Minimal de-ossification
4. No spur formation	4. Minimal spur formation
5. No calcification of the capsule	5. Minimal capsular calcification
Fair (moderate changes)	Poor (severe damages)
1. Normal relationship between head and acetabulum	1. Almost complete obliteration of cartilaginous space
Any one or more of the following	2. Relative increase in density of femoral head
1. Moderate narrowing of cartilaginous space	3. Subchondral cyst formation
2. Mottling of head, sclerotic areas, decreased density	4. Formation of sequestrate
3. Moderate spur formation	5. Gross deformity of femoral head
4. Moderate to severe capsular calcification	6. Severe spur formation
5. Depression of subchondral cortex of femoral head	7. Acetabular sclerosis
Clinical criteria	
Excellent (all of the following)	Good
1. No pain	1. No pain
2. Full range of hip motion	2. Free motion (75% of normal hip motion)
3. No limp	3. Not more than slight limp
4. No radiographic evidence of progressive changes	4. Minimal radiographic changes
Fair (any one or more of the following)	Poor (any one or more of the following)
1. Pain, but not disabling	1. Disabling pain
2. Limited motion of hip; no adduction deformity	2. Marked limitation of motion or adduction deformity
3. Moderate limp	3. Re-dislocation
4. Moderately severe radiographic changes	4. Progressive radiographic changes

This score is the most predominant score in the current literature and has been used to stratify the outcome in larger reviews. Studies applying the modern management principles mentioned above have shown some improvements in the clinical and radiographic outcome when compared to the earlier treatment results. Intermediate term follow-up studies (mean follow-up of 33 months) with sufficient patient numbers (>30 patients) have shown good and excellent results in over 55% of all patients [30, 33]. These numbers are confirmed by current reviews [7, 52]. In these studies the incidence of poor outcome increased with increasing fracture type (Pipkin I through IV). A non-significant tendency towards better outcome in surgically treated fractures was seen, however limited data suggest better outcome for Pipkin Type I fractures with conservative treatment. No statistically significant outcome differences were seen between anterior, posterior, and trochanteric flip approaches. Trochanteric flip osteotomy presented with an increased odds ratio for heterotopic ossification, while posterior approaches had a higher incidence of avascular necrosis. Due to this trend towards better outcome and less complication some authors favor the anterior approaches in the current literature [22]. It should be noted however that the primary decision on the approach is dictated by the fracture pattern. Interestingly only one study has used a validated, patient centered health status survey (SF-12) to quantify the outcome after femoral head fractures [29]. No relationship between the SF-12 score and time to surgery, surgical approach, or treatment method was seen, in part due to the low patient number ($n = 17$).

For future studies the use of validated, comparable outcome measures (Thompson Epstein score, Merle d'Aubigne and Postel Score, Harris Hip Score, SF-35, EQ 5d) paired with a multicenter approach is needed to generate sufficient statistical power required to truly evaluate treatment and fracture specific outcome.

References

1. Birkett J. Description of a dislocation of the head of the femur, complicated with its fracture; with remarks. Med Chir Trans. 1869;52:133–8.
2. Duquennoy A, Decoulx J, Capron JC, Torabi DJ. Les luxations traumatiques de la hanche avec fracture de la tête fémorale. À propos de 28 observations. Rev Chir Orthop. 1975;61:209–19.
3. Yang RS, Tsuang YH, Hang YS, Liu TK. Traumatic dislocation of the hip. Clin Orthop Relat Res. 1991;265:218–27.
4. DeLee JC, Evans JA, Thomas J. Anterior dislocation of the hip and associated femoral-head fractures. J Bone Joint Surg Am. 1980;62(6):960–4.
5. Thompson VP, Epstein HC. Traumatic dislocation of the hip; a survey of two hundred and four cases covering a period of twenty-one years. J Bone Joint Surg Am. 1951;33-A(3):746–78; passim.
6. Yoon PW, Jeong HS, Yoo JJ, Koo KH, Yoon KS, Kim HJ. Femoral head fracture without dislocation by low-energy trauma in a young adult. Clin Orthop Surg. 2011;3(4):336–41. https://doi.org/10.4055/cios.2011.3.4.336.
7. Giannoudis PV, Kontakis G, Christoforakis Z, Akula M, Tosounidis T, Koutras C. Management, complications and clinical results of femoral head fractures. Injury. 2009;40(12):1245–51. https://doi.org/10.1016/j.injury.2009.10.024.
8. Goulet JA, Levin PE. Hip dislocations. In: Skeletal trauma: basic science, management, and reconstruction, vol. 3. Philadelphia: Saunders; 2003. p. 1657–69.
9. Lang-Stevenson A, Getty CJ. The Pipkin fracture-dislocation of the hip. Injury. 1987;18(4):264–9.
10. Brumback RJ, Holt ES, McBride MS, Poka A, Bathon GH, Burgess AR. Acetabular depression fracture accompanying posterior fracture dislocation of the hip. J Orthop Trauma. 1990;4(1):42–8.
11. Moed BR, Maxey JW. Evaluation of fractures of the femoral head using the CT-directed pelvic oblique radiograph. Clin Orthop Relat Res. 1993;296:161–7.
12. Henle P, Kloen P, Siebenrock KA. Femoral head injuries: which treatment strategy can be recommended? Injury. 2007;38(4):478–88. https://doi.org/10.1016/j.injury.2007.01.023.
13. Pipkin G. Treatment of grade IV fracture-dislocation of the hip. J Bone Joint Surg Am. 1957;39-A(5):1027–42; passim.
14. Brumback RJ, Kenzora JE, Levitt LE, Burgess AR, Poka A. Fractures of the femoral head. Hip. 1987;1987:181–206.
15. Prokop A, Helling HJ, Hahn U, Udomkaewkanjana C, Rehm KE. Biodegradable implants for Pipkin fractures. Clin Orthop Relat Res. 2005;432:226–33.
16. Solberg BD, Moon CN, Franco DP. Use of a trochanteric flip osteotomy improves outcomes in Pipkin IV fractures. Clin Orthop Relat Res. 2009;467(4):929–33. https://doi.org/10.1007/s11999-008-0505-z.
17. Epstein HC, Wiss DA, Cozen L. Posterior fracture dislocation of the hip with fractures of the femoral head. Clin Orthop Relat Res. 1985;201:9–17.
18. Hougaard K, Thomsen PB. Traumatic posterior dislocation of the hip--prognostic factors influencing the incidence of avascular necrosis of the femoral head. Arch Orthop Trauma Surg. 1986;106(1):32–5.
19. Schweikert CH, Weigand H. Hüftkopfkalottenfrakturen. Hefte Unfallheilkd. 1979;140:188–200.
20. Schiedel F, Rieger H, Joosten U, Meffert R. Wenn die Hüfte nicht "nur" luxiert. Unfallchirurg. 2006;109(7):538–44.
21. Epstein HC. Posterior fracture-dislocations of the hip; long-term follow-up. J Bone Joint Surg Am. 1974;56(6):1103–27.
22. Droll KP, Broekhuyse H, O'Brien P. Fracture of the femoral head. J Am Acad Orthop Surg. 2007;15(12):716–27.
23. Swiontkowski MF, Thorpe M, Seiler JG, Hansen ST. Operative management of displaced femoral head fractures: case-matched comparison of anterior versus posterior approaches for Pipkin I and Pipkin II fractures. J Orthop Trauma. 1992;6(4):437–42.
24. Thannheimer A, Gutsfeld P, Buhren V. Current therapy options for fractures of the femoral head. Chirurg. 2009;80(12):1140–6. https://doi.org/10.1007/s00104-009-1738-4.
25. Pape HC, Rice J, Wolfram K, Gansslen A, Pohlemann T, Krettek C. Hip dislocation in patients with multiple injuries. A followup investigation. Clin Orthop Relat Res. 2000;377:99–105.
26. Harrison MH, Schajowicz F, Trueta J. Osteoarthritis of the hip: a study of the nature and evolution of the disease. J Bone Joint Surg. 1953;35-B(4):598–626.
27. Gautier E, Ganz K, Krugel N, Gill T, Ganz R. Anatomy of the medial femoral circumflex artery and its surgical implications. J Bone Joint Surg. 2000;82(5):679–83.
28. Gojda J, Bartonicek J. The retinacula of Weitbrecht in the adult hip. Surg Radiol Anat. 2012;34(1):31–8. https://doi.org/10.1007/s00276-011-0829-3.
29. Stannard JP, Harris HW, Volgas DA, Alonso JE. Functional outcome of patients with femoral head fractures associated with hip dislocations. Clin Orthop Relat Res. 2000;377:44–56.
30. Kloen P, Siebenrock KA, Raaymakers ELFB, Marti RK, Ganz R. Femoral head fractures revisited. Eur J Trauma. 2002;28(4):221–33.
31. McKee MD, Garay ME, Schemitsch EH, Kreder HJ, Stephen DJ. Irreducible fracture-dislocation of the hip: a severe injury with a poor prognosis. J Orthop Trauma. 1998;12(4):223–9.
32. Ganz R, Gill TJ, Gautier E, Ganz K, Krugel N, Berlemann U. Surgical dislocation of the adult hip a technique with full access to the femoral head and acetabulum without the risk of avascular necrosis. J Bone Joint Surg. 2001;83(8):1119–24.

33. Marchetti ME, Steinberg GG, Coumas JM. Intermediate-term experience of Pipkin fracture-dislocations of the hip. J Orthop Trauma. 1996;10(7):455–61.
34. Holmes WJ, Solberg B, Bay BK, Laubach JE, Olson SA. Biomechanical consequences of excision of displaced Pipkin femoral head fractures. J Orthop Trauma. 2000;14(2):149–50.
35. Chen ZW, Lin B, Zhai WL, Guo ZM, Liang Z, Zheng JP, et al. Conservative versus surgical management of Pipkin type I fractures associated with posterior dislocation of the hip: a randomised controlled trial. Int Orthop. 2011;35(7):1077–81. https://doi.org/10.1007/s00264-010-1087-4.
36. Mostafa MM. Femoral head fractures. Int Orthop. 2001;25(1):51–4.
37. Ross JR, Gardner MJ. Femoral head fractures. Curr Rev Musculoskelet Med. 2012;5(3):199–205. https://doi.org/10.1007/s12178-012-9129-8.
38. Murray P, McGee HM, Mulvihill N. Fixation of femoral head fractures using the Herbert screw. Injury. 1988;19(3):220–1.
39. Jukkala-Partio K, Partio EK, Hirvensalo E, Rokkanen P. Absorbable fixation of femoral head fractures. A prospective study of six cases. Ann Chir Gynaecol. 1998;87(1):44–8.
40. Roeder LF Jr, DeLee JC. Femoral head fractures associated with posterior hip dislocation. Clin Orthop Relat Res. 1980;147:121–30.
41. Kozin SH, Kolessar DJ, Guanche CA, Marmar EC. Bilateral femoral head fracture with posterior hip dislocation. Orthop Rev. 1994;Suppl:20–4.
42. Rehm KE. Acetabulumfrakturen–posttraumatische und postoperative Nervenschäden. Hefte Unfallheilkd. 1985;174:472–6.
43. Trojan E. Gefäß-und Nervenverletzungen bei Frakturen und luxationen im Beckenbereich. Hefte Unfallheilkd. 1979;140:44–8.
44. Letournel E, Judet R. Fractures ofthe acetabulum (Translated and edited by Elson RA). Berlin: Springer; 1981.
45. Cornwall R, Radomisli TE. Nerve injury in traumatic dislocation of the hip. Clin Orthop Relat Res. 2000;377:84–91.
46. Hougaard K, Thomsen PB. Traumatic posterior fracture-dislocation of the hip with fracture of the femoral head or neck, or both. J Bone Joint Surg Am. 1988;70(2):233–9.
47. Schwarzkopf SR, Dreinhofer KE, Haas NP, Tscherne H. Isolated hip dislocation of traumatic origin. Unfallchirurg. 1996;99(3):168–74.
48. Burd TA, Hughes MS, Anglen JO. Heterotopic ossification prophylaxis with indomethacin increases the risk of long-bone nonunion. J Bone Joint Surg. 2003;85(5):700–5.
49. Upadhyay SS, Moulton A. The long-term results of traumatic posterior dislocation of the hip. J Bone Joint Surg. 1981;63B(4):548–51.
50. Borrelli J Jr. Chondrocyte apoptosis and posttraumatic arthrosis. J Orthop Trauma. 2006;20(10):726–31. https://doi.org/10.1097/01.bot.0000249882.77629.5c.
51. Bhandari M, Matta J, Ferguson T, Matthys G. Predictors of clinical and radiological outcome in patients with fractures of the acetabulum and concomitant posterior dislocation of the hip. J Bone Joint Surg. 2006;88(12):1618–24. https://doi.org/10.1302/0301-620X.88B12.17309.
52. Akula M, Giannoudis P, Gopal S, Pagoti R. Pipkin fractures–clinical outcomes. J Bone Joint Surg Br. 2010;92(SUPP IV):543.

Femoral Neck Fractures

12

Govind S. Chauhan, Mehool Acharya, and Tim J. S. Chesser

Abstract

Fractures of the proximal femur, commonly termed hip fracture, is a devastating injury for any age of patient. The injury carries a high mortality as well as significant morbidity and impact of function. They can be divided into intracapsular (also called subcapital) fractures and extracapsular fractures. Extracapsular fractures are further subdivided into basicervical, trochanteric, and subtrochanteric fractures. In this chapter we will discuss the epidemiology, assessment, classification, management, and outcome for patients of intracapsular (subcapital) fractures.

Keywords

Intracapsular femoral neck fracture · Garden · Pauwels · Internal fixation · Hemiarthroplasty · Total hip replacement · Arthroplasty

12.1 Mechanism of Injury and Epidemiology

12.1.1 Mechanism of Injury

The vast majority of hip fractures present as a result of low energy trauma in elderly patients with weakened osteoporotic bone. These are termed fragility fractures and generally result from falls from a standing height. As well as having weaker bone, the elderly are at high risk of falls due to multiple factors including co-morbidities, side effects of medications, reducing mobility, and poorer balance and co-ordination [1, 2]. Femoral neck fractures usually occur from a direct fall onto the lateral aspect of the hip around the greater trochanter, and may also occur from a twisting injury with a planted, fixed foot. In some low energy hip fractures, there are pre-existing pathological lesions in the femoral neck, and these pathological fractures are covered in Chap. 13.

In patients with normal bone, a large force is required to fracture the femoral neck, and these patients present after high-energy trauma such as motor vehicle accidents and falls from heights. A femoral neck fracture in these cases usually occurs from axial loading of the femur with the hip in an abducted position. If the hip is adducted and flexed at the time of impact, dislocation of the hip is the commoner injury. These high-energy injuries occur in younger patients, and the

G. S. Chauhan
The Knowledge Hub, The Royal Orthopaedic Hospital, Birmingham, UK

M. Acharya · T. J. S. Chesser (✉)
Department of Trauma and Orthopaedics, Brunel Building, Southmead Hospital, Bristol, UK
e-mail: tim.chesser@nbt.nhs.uk

L. Büchler, M. J.B. Keel (eds.), *Fractures of the Hip*, Fracture Management Joint by Joint,
https://doi.org/10.1007/978-3-030-18838-2_12

principles for treating them differ from the elderly, and are described later in this chapter.

12.1.2 Epidemiology

Worldwide, with improvements in medical care, nutrition and quality of life, the population continues to live longer, and thus there are more patients living with diseases of the elderly, including osteoporosis. This has led to increasing numbers of patients with hip fractures. In 1990, there were approximately 1.66 million hip fractures, with projections for 2050 estimating over 6 million hip fractures, and over half of these are expected to be in Asia [3]. The current incidence of hip fracture in the Western world is approximately one per thousand, but there remains significant variation between studies, as well as between countries [4].

12.1.3 Risk Factors

The major risk factors for femoral neck fractures are falls and osteoporosis, which show an increasing prevalence with age [5]. Twenty-five percent of patients presenting with femoral neck fractures will have had a previous fragility fracture [6]. Women are at a significantly higher risk of hip fracture, making up 75% of the patients. A third of patients presenting with hip fractures have been shown to have a significant degree of cognitive impairment [7]. Other risk factors that have a higher incidence of hip fracture include lower socioeconomic status, cardiovascular disease, renal disease, diabetes, and polypharmacy. It is the significant frailty of the geriatric population, which increases the complexity of treatment.

12.2 Clinical and Radiological Assessment

12.2.1 Clinical Assessment: Low Energy Trauma

Patients who have fractured their hip following a low energy fall will complain of pain in the affected hip and the majorities are unable to mobilize. On examination, these patients may have a shortened, externally rotated limb if the fracture has displaced. There may or may not be any signs of external bruising, particularly with intracapsular fractures as the hematoma is contained within the capsule of the hip joint. Due to the high prevalence of cognitive impairment in the geriatric population, an accurate clinical assessment is often difficult, and thus a low threshold for radiological investigation is required. Both anteroposterior and lateral views should be obtained and displacement in either plane can influence treatment [2]. Between 5% and 10% have an occult fracture that is not recognized on initial radiological screening. Any elderly patient who suffers a fall and has pain on weight bearing, with negative initial radiographs, requires further imaging. Magnetic resonance scans are thought to be the gold standard [8, 9], yet many will perform CTs due to ease of access. This imaging should be performed within 24 h of admission in order to prevent delay to surgery should it be required [2].

A key part of the assessment of the elderly patient with low energy trauma is identifying potential causes for the fall. Medical emergencies, such as myocardial infarction, sepsis, stroke, etc., must be considered and promptly treated if present. As well as a thorough history, a full systemic examination must be performed. It is well recognized that the majority of falls in the elderly are multifactorial, and these should be addressed during the patient's admission. Early evaluation of the patients' hydration status is also vital, and a proportion of the patients will have spent a significant amount of time on the floor before being able to obtain help. The assessing doctor must also actively look for any other injuries, in particular associated osteoporotic fractures, commonly distal radius or proximal humeral fractures.

Most units have developed fast track services allowing rapid radiological diagnosis and early medical optimization of the patients so not to delay surgical treatment [7]. Appropriate investigations should be undertaken on admission with the aim of immediate optimization, ensuring surgery is not delayed by anemia, volume depletion, electrolyte imbalance, correctable cardiac arrhythmias, uncontrolled diabetes, uncontrolled heart failure, acute chest infections, nor exacerbation of chronic chest conditions. All units should have policies in place for the reversal of anticoagulants, and in particular, surgery should not be delayed because of antiplatelet therapy [2]. A balance must be sought between avoiding excessive delays and inadequate optimization. Prolonged delays to surgery causing ongoing pain and greater time to weight bearing, which in turn is associated with the complications of inactivity such as pressure ulcers, respiratory tract infections, thromboembolism, etc. Conversely, inadequate optimization places the patient at risk of perioperative complications. To date, there remains a paucity of good evidence regarding the impact of timing of surgery; however no study has shown an advantage by delaying surgery [2]. Early surgery has been shown to result in reduced mortality, reduced pain, shorter length of stay, and reduced incidence of significant complications. Acute medical physicians or specialist orthogeriatricians, and anesthetists are increasingly being involved preoperatively to provide assistance and support to optimize what is often a long, complex list of co-morbidities. Surgery should be performed as soon as possible, ideally on the day of, or day after injury.

Structured multidisciplinary management and pathways have shown to significantly reduce mortality and improve patient outcomes whilst reducing complications and length of stay [2, 7].

12.2.2 Clinical Assessment: High-Energy Trauma

The assessment of patients with high-energy trauma differs greatly from that in the elderly described above. The initial assessment of these patients is guided by resuscitation and lifesaving interventions, with the help of a trauma team [10].

Once the patient has been resuscitated and stabilized, the orthopedic surgeon can then assess the injured hip. It is important to accurately assess and document the neurovascular status of the injured limb. The motor and sensory functions of the sciatic nerve should be assessed through both its tibial and common peroneal branches. Additional CT imaging is now routinely performed as part of the initial trauma assessment, allowing better understanding of the fractures.

It is also important to undertake imaging of the femoral neck in patients who have femoral shaft fractures as a result of high-energy trauma, with up to 6% patients having ipsilateral femoral neck fractures [11].

12.3 Classification

There are numerous classification systems which exist for proximal femoral fractures, however the most important things to determine are whether the fracture is intracapsular or extracapsular, and whether it is displaced or undisplaced (Fig. 12.1).

This is of importance due to the retrograde blood supply to the femoral head. At the base of the femoral neck, retinacular vessels branch off the medial femoral circumflex artery and penetrate the head at the 11 o'clock position to supply it [13]. As well as this, the intracapsular femoral neck has little cancellous bone and a thin periosteum. Displaced intracapsular fractures are at

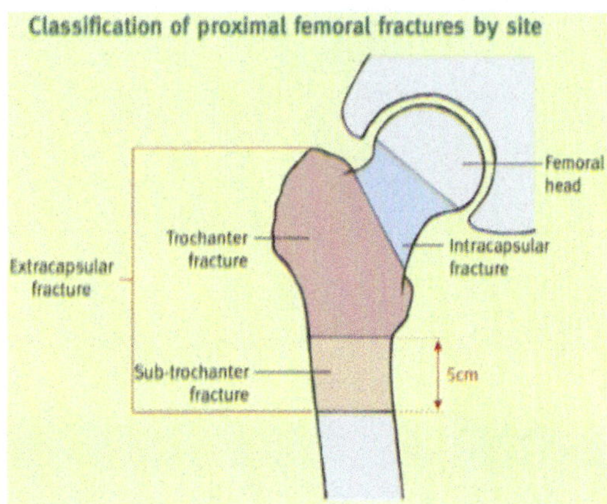

Fig. 12.1 Classification of proximal femoral fractures by site. Reproduced with permission and copyright © of Elsevier [12]

high risk of disrupting the blood supply to the femoral head, thus putting it at risk of avascular necrosis. Intracapsular fractures are also associated with higher rates of non-union and mal-union.

Commonly used classification systems include Garden, Pauwels, and AO/OTA, all of which have their own significant limitations. The simple classification into undisplaced and displaced is thought to help with surgical decision-making and prognosis.

12.3.1 Garden Classification (Intracapsular Fractures) [14]

The Garden classification is a widely used system based on the descriptions by British orthopedic surgeon Robert Symon Garden. It is based purely on the AP radiograph, and is divided into four categories based on fracture completeness and displacement. It can be useful in determining treatment strategies, but is flawed in that it does not consider the appearances on the lateral radiograph, nor does it consider the underlying quality of the bone (Fig. 12.2).

- Type 1—Incomplete fracture, with valgus impaction.
- Type 2—Complete fracture, but undisplaced.
- Type 3—Complete fracture with partial displacement.
- Type 4—Complete fracture with full displacement.

12.3.2 Intracapsular Fractures: Pauwels' Classification [16, 17]

Pauwels' classification of intracapsular fractures is a biomechanical classification system, dividing intracapsular fractures into three categories based on the angle between the fracture line and the horizontal on an AP radiograph. It was first described in 1935 by Friedrich Pauwels, a German orthopedic surgeon, with the original text in German. This was then republished in 1976 in English. Over the years, there have been misinterpretations of Type 3 in Pauwels' classification system which have been repeated and printed in multiple highly regarded texts [18]. The angle is measured between the fracture line of the distal fragment

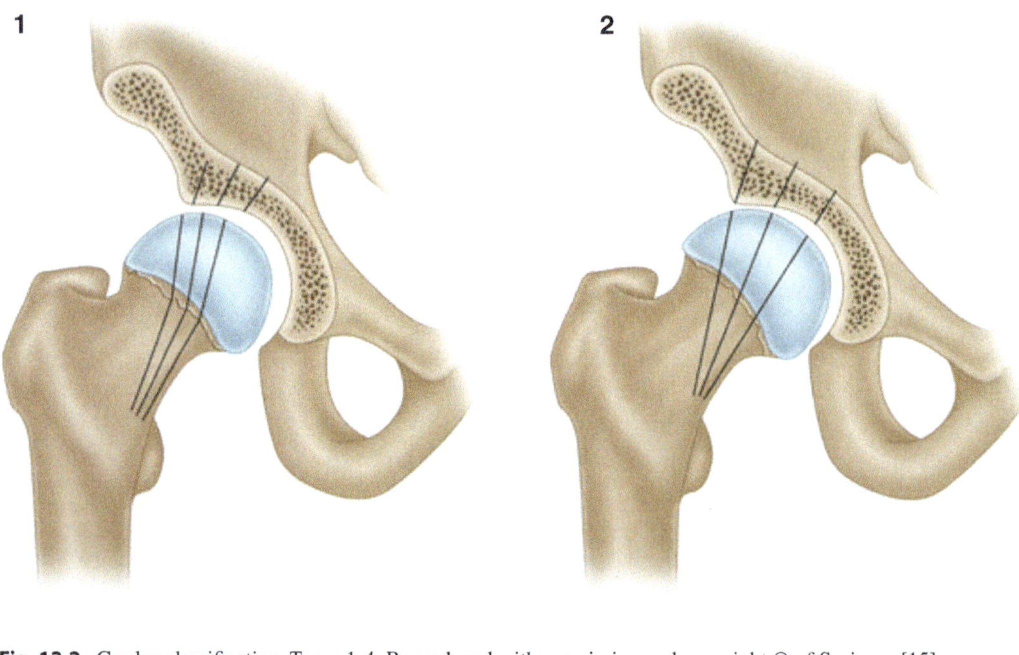

Fig. 12.2 Garden classification. Types 1-4. Reproduced with permission and copyright © of Springer [15]

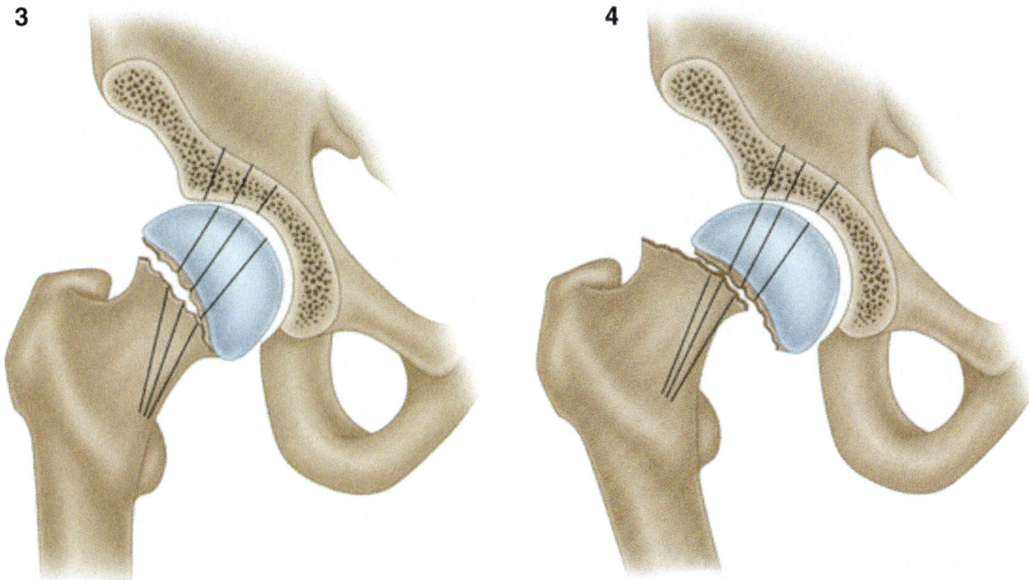

Fig. 12.2 (continued)

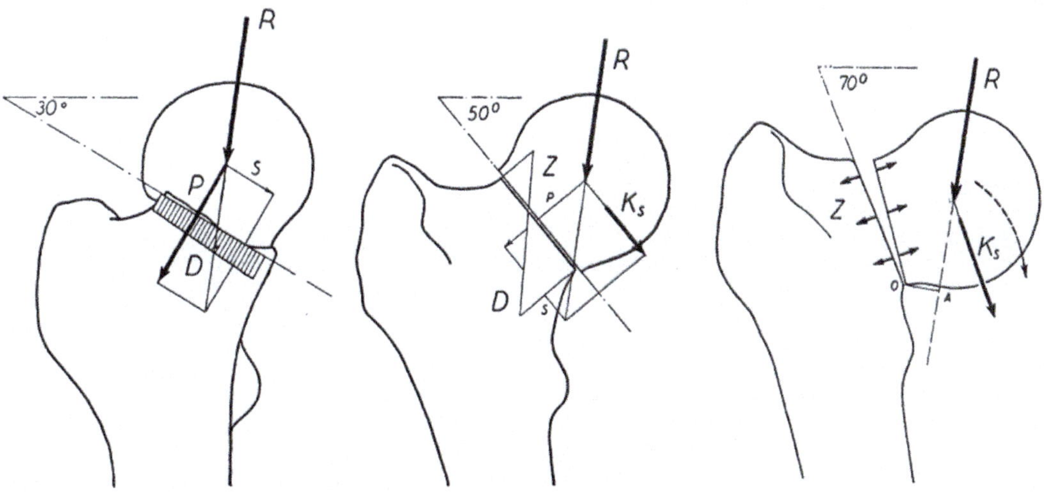

Fig. 12.3 Original images for Pauwels' classification. Type 1: Less than 30°; Type 2: Between 30° and 50°; Type 3: Greater than 50°. Reproduced with permission and copyright © of Springer [19]

and the horizontal line, to determine shearing stresses and compressive force. The correct system is described below (Fig. 12.3).

- Type 1—less than 30°
- Type 2—between 30° and 50°
- Type 3—greater than 50°

In Pauwels' Type 1, the forces are compressive across the fracture site. In Type 2 fractures, some shear forces are also present, having a negative impact on fracture healing. In Type 3 fractures, shear forces are dominant, causing varus collapse and displacement of the fracture. Again, similar to Garden's classification, Pauwels' system is limited by the fact that it too does not consider the lateral radiograph and nor the bone quality.

12.3.3 AO/OTA Classification [20]

The Arbeitsgemeinschaft für Osteosynthesefragen (AO)/Orthopaedic Trauma Association (OTA) has an extensive long bone classification system which includes hip fractures. These come under section 31 of the system (3 = femur, 1 = proximal). This has been updated in 2018. 31-B of the AO/OTA classification is for intracapsular fractures, and there are seven subtypes as described below (Fig. 12.4),

- 31-B1—subcapital with slight displacement
- 31-B1.1—Valgus impacted fracture
- 31-B1.2—Non-displaced fracture
- 31-B1.3—Displaced fracture
- 31-B2—Transcervical
- 31-B2.1—Simple fracture
- 31-B2.2—Multifragmentary fracture
- 31-B2.3—Shear fracture
- 31-B3—Basicervical fracture

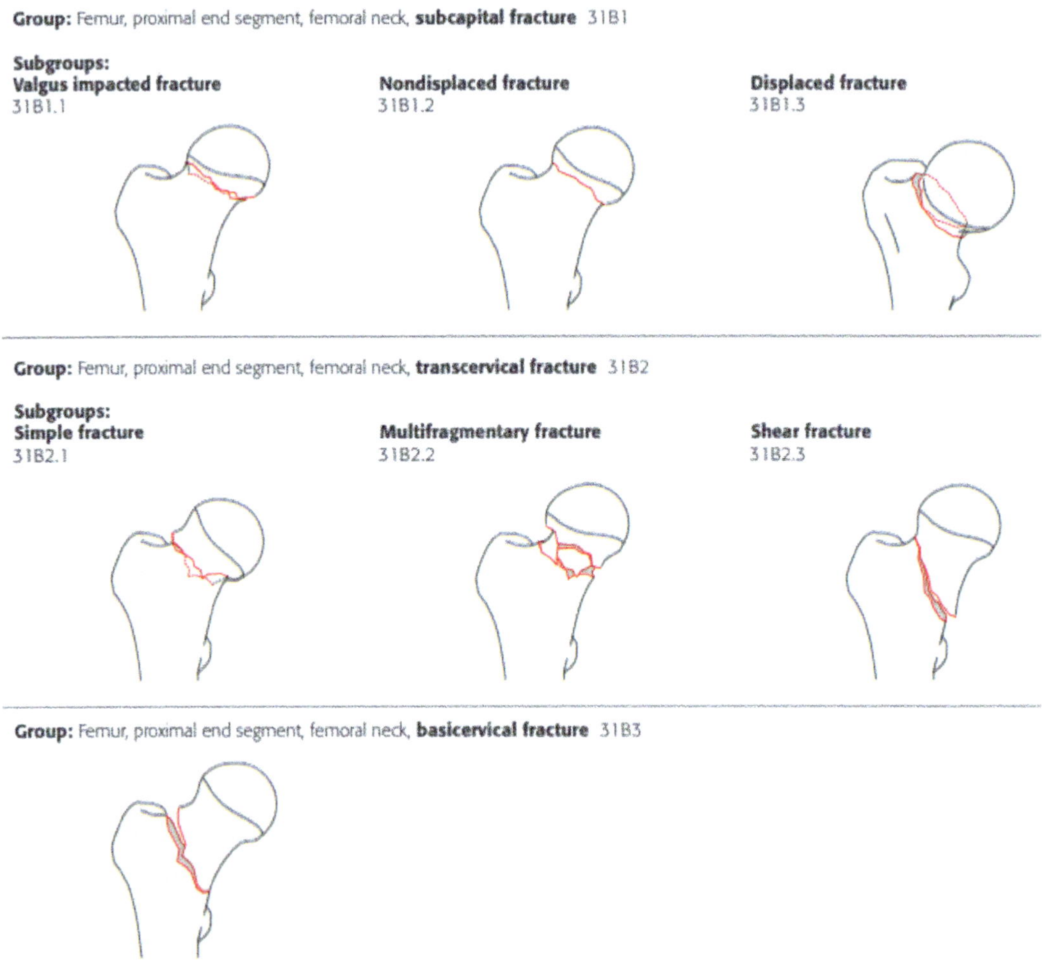

Fig. 12.4 AO/OTA Classification: 31-B. Reproduced with permission and copyright © of Wolters Kluwer Health, Inc. [20]

All three of these classification systems have significant limitations with intra-observer and inter-observer reliability. This is likely due to variation in identifying the angle of the primary fracture line, as there is often rotation and overlap of the fragments obscuring the view. Many surgeons opt to simply describe the fracture as either displaced or undisplaced, but there is widespread disagreement about what is defined an undisplaced intracapsular fracture [21, 22]. The Garden classification is the most widely used in literature.

12.4 Conservative Treatment

12.4.1 Initial Treatment

Once a hip fracture is suspected, patients must be provided with analgesia. This can often be overlooked, particularly in patients with cognitive impairment who are unable to communicate their pain. The majority of these patients will require opiate analgesia, and this can be provided in oral, intramuscular, or intravenous form, taking care to avoid potential complications such as respiratory depression and delirium. Following diagnosis, analgesia can also be supplemented with regional nerve blocks, such as fascia iliaca block or femoral nerve block [2].

12.4.2 Definitive Non-Operative Treatment

Definitive, non-operative treatment of hip fractures is reserved for a very small minority of patients (less than 2%) [7]. It should only be considered in either patients who are not expected to survive 24 h, those at extremely high risk from surgical intervention, non-ambulatory patients who are not in pain, or those who present late with partially healed fractures not affecting function. Patients in the terminal stages of illness should not be denied surgery if it can help to improve their quality of life by providing pain relief, ease of nursing and mobility, even if only temporarily [2].

12.5 Operative Treatment

The main aims of surgical intervention differ between the high and low energy trauma groups of patients with hip fractures, and this must be considered when assessing the patient and determining the surgical plan.

For the young patient with a high-energy hip fracture, the aim is to preserve the femoral head if at all possible. These patients can usually tolerate restrictions on mobility for a period of time whilst the fracture heals.

For the elderly patient with a low energy hip fracture, the primary aim is to restore mobility as quickly as possible. These patients should have one definitive surgical procedure to treat their injury allowing them to mobilize weight bearing without restrictions [2].

In any surgical approach where fixation is to be undertaken, the critical step is reduction. An accurate reduction will restore the mechanics of the hip joint, promote fracture healing, and distribute the forces to avoid excess stress on the implant.

12.5.1 Undisplaced Subcapital Fractures

Undisplaced, subcapital fractures are generally treated with internal fixation. There is significant variation in what surgeons classify as undisplaced. With more tilt and valgus collapse there is more of a tendency to replacement, though the evidence for this is currently lacking. The two commonest fixation methods available to the surgeon are either cannulated screw fixation or sliding hip screw. Recently, more fixed angle implants have been introduced, but with limited published evidence comparing them against traditional separate screw or sliding hip screw fixation [23–25]. A recent large randomized trial studied 1108 patients with low-energy femoral neck fractures, who were randomized to internal fixation with a sliding hip screw or cancellous screws.

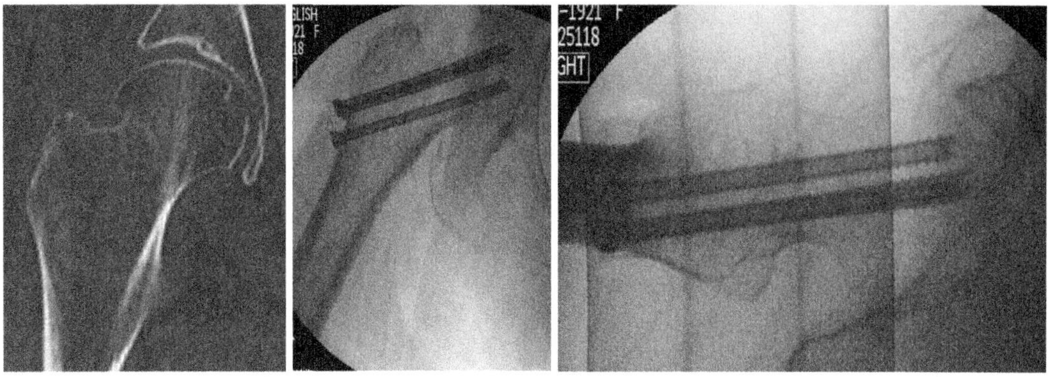

Fig. 12.5 Cannulated screw fixation of a marginally displaced fracture of the femoral neck (Garden Type 1)

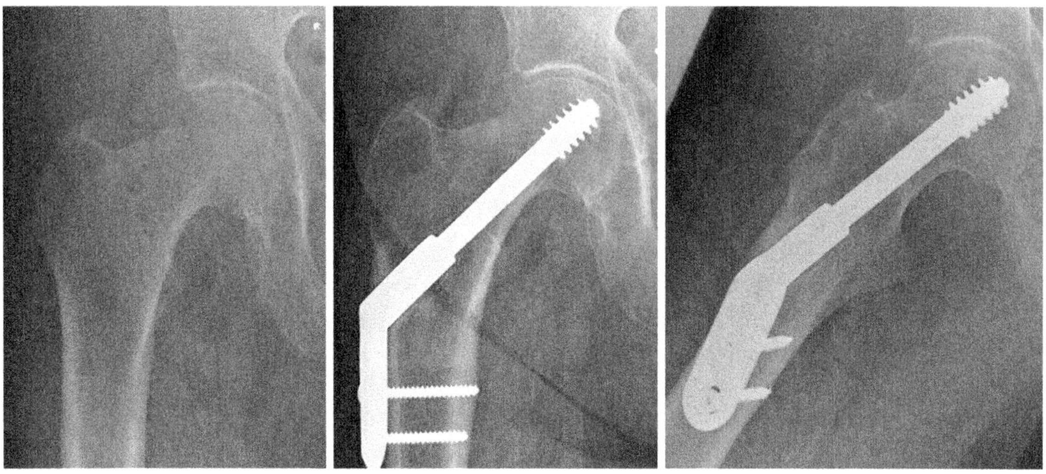

Fig. 12.6 Sliding hip screw fixation of a varus displaced femoral neck fracture (Pauwels Type 3)

The results show no significant difference in the rate of re-operation between the sliding hip screw (19.7%; 107/542) and the cancellous screw (21.8%; 117/537), groups ($p = 0.18$), and no difference in any measure of quality of life up to 2 years [26]. This suggests either technique can be used (Figs. 12.5 and 12.6).

For fixation, the patient can be positioned either supine or in the lateral position. In the supine position, the patient is carefully positioned on the traction table with the contralateral leg flexed and abducted. It is important to remember that as the fracture is undisplaced, no traction should be applied to the limb, and great care should be taken on transferring the patient to ensure the fracture is not displaced iatrogenically. Alternatively, these fractures can be fixed with the patient in the lateral position, again taking care not to displace the fracture.

Following internal fixation of undisplaced fractures, there remains great variation in re-operation rates reported in the literature (4–19%). The commonest causes for re-operation are fracture non-union (0.7–11%), avascular necrosis of the femoral head (2.5–10.8%), localized pain from metalwork prominence (1.3–5%), and peri-prosthetic fracture (0.3–1.7%) [27–33].

12.5.2 Displaced Intracapsular Fractures in the Elderly

Internal fixation of displaced intracapsular fractures is associated with a significant re-operation rate (14–53%) when compared to initial arthroplasty (0–16%) [33–37]. Complication rates following fixation of intracapsular fractures also remain high, with literature reporting 10–38% non-union, 0–19% avascular necrosis, and 4–6% localized pain [35, 36, 38]. Studies have also shown improved functional recovery and less pain with arthroplasty compared to fixation [37–39].

Given the level 1 evidence and meta-analysis that is available for this topic, arthroplasty is the treatment of choice recommended by most guidelines for displaced intracapsular fractures in the elderly [34, 35].

Internal fixation does however have a lower blood loss, length of surgery, and risk of deep wound infection [35].

The anterolateral approach has been shown to have a lower dislocation rate compared to a posterior approach, and in this frail group where the aim is to avoid complications, this is the approach recommended for UK surgeons [2]. The anterior approach provides another alternative. Both unipolar and bipolar hemiarthroplasty have been recommended, yet there is no evidence that bipolar heads give any improvement in any measured outcomes and function, hence unipolar hemiarthroplasty is advised, due to lower costs [40].

12.5.2.1 Hemiarthroplasty or Total Hip Replacement

The published literature to help surgeons decide which of these two operations is best for the patient has not yet clearly defined which population of patients will benefit from total hip replacement over hemiarthroplasty. It is accepted that those with pre-existing symptomatic osteoarthritis and patients with rheumatoid arthritis should be considered for a total hip replacement.

The evidence for total hip replacement remains relatively limited. In the selected patient groups studied, total hip replacement is found to be associated with improved functional status at 3 months and 1 year, more cost effective and have a lower re-operation rate (2–8% versus 0–24%) than hemiarthroplasty [34, 41, 42].

Total hip replacement does however have a higher rate of dislocation than hemiarthroplasty for displaced intracapsular fractures in the elderly (9–23% vs. 0–13%) [35, 39, 43]. More recent studies suggest this dislocation rate can be reduced with anterior and anterolateral approaches.

Guidelines in the UK advise offering total hip replacement to those who were able to walk independently out of doors with no more than the use of one stick prior to the fall, who are not cognitively impaired, and who are medically fit [2]. There remains concern regarding the more elderly patient, and currently many patients are not offered total hip replacement for logistical reasons, with a lack of experienced surgeons [7].

12.5.2.2 Cemented or Uncemented

There remains worldwide variation in the use of cement in replacement arthroplasty for hip fractures, usually depending on the individual countries practice. Most larger studies and database publications have shown advantages with cement with decreased mortality, improved function, and lower peri-prosthetic fracture rate. Many of these studies looked at older type prosthesis, such as the Austin-Moore and Thompsons implants, now not commonly used. There have been reports of bone cement implantation syndrome, or a dropping of blood pressure, associated with cement insertion and implantation of the femoral stem. Strategies to avoid this include adequate resuscitation and medical optimization of the patient, lavage of the femoral canal and not to overpressurize in those as risk [44–47].

12.5.3 Displaced Intracapsular Fractures in the Young

The aim of surgery in the young patient is to preserve the femoral head. This is achieved by reduction, either closed or open, and internal fixation, with either cannulated screws or sliding hip screw [48].

12.5.3.1 Time to Surgery

The urgency of theater for the treatment of displaced femoral neck fractures remains a topic of debate, with inconclusive, poor quality evidence in the literature. The advantages of early surgery are argued as by allowing early reduction and capsular decompression, it allows vessels to unkink and relieves the pressure on them, giving the femoral head the best chance of revascularization. Some studies have shown delays in fixation beyond 12 h to be associated with higher rates of osteonecrosis, whilst others have shown no difference when comparing delays of 24 h [48].

12.5.3.2 Closed Reduction

An initial closed reduction can be attempted by using the Leadbetter technique [49]. The hip is flexed whilst in abduction, and then traction applied. The hip is then slightly internally rotated and then extended whilst traction is maintained. Reduction is then checked with image intensifier on AP and lateral views. If an adequate closed reduction cannot be achieved, multiple reduction attempts should be avoided as they have been reported to show increased rates of avascular necrosis [48].

12.5.3.3 Open Reduction

Open reduction of the femoral neck can be achieved through a number of different techniques and approaches. One technique is to position temporary wires or pins into the proximal fragment by passing them anteriorly, utilizing them as a joystick to mobilize the fragment and achieve reduction, before then passing further lateral wires to maintain the reduction (Fig. 12.7).

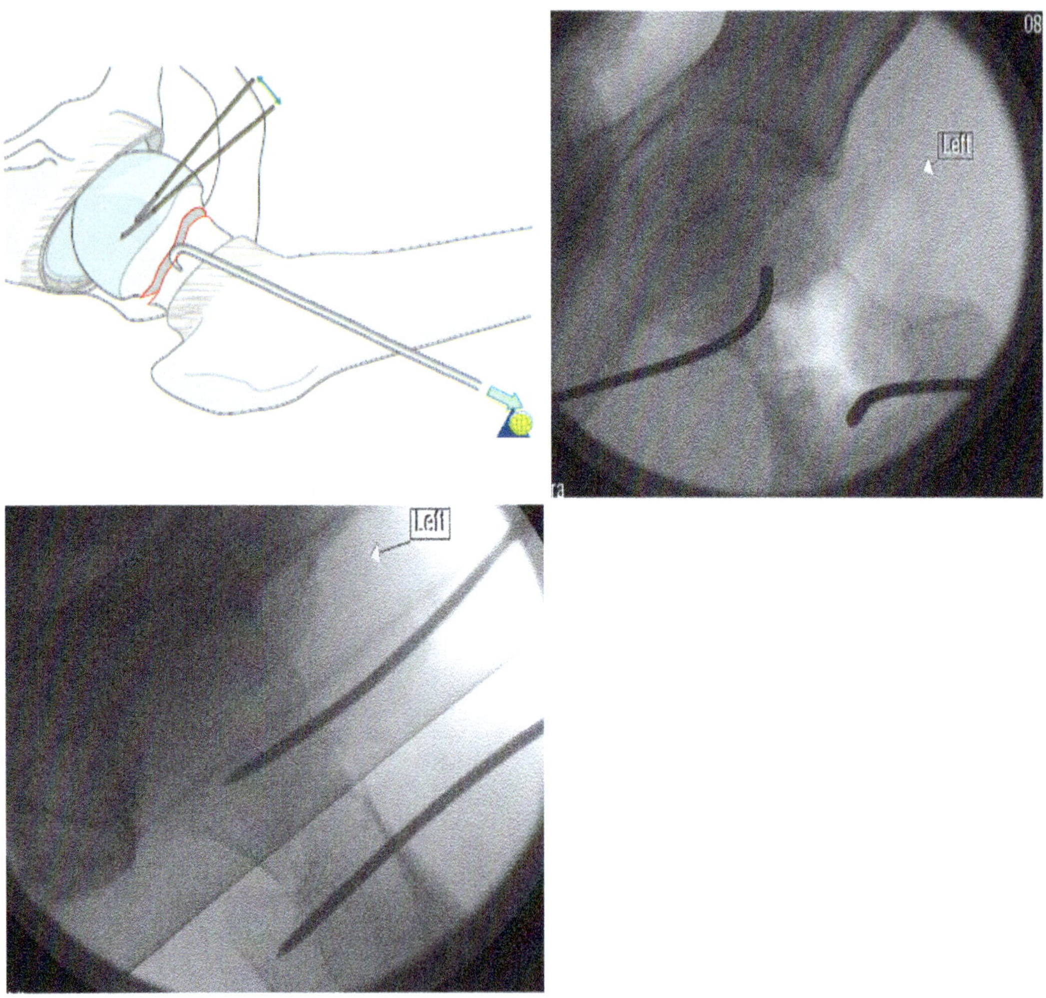

Fig. 12.7 Open reduction of intracapsular fracture with k-wires and bone hook [50]

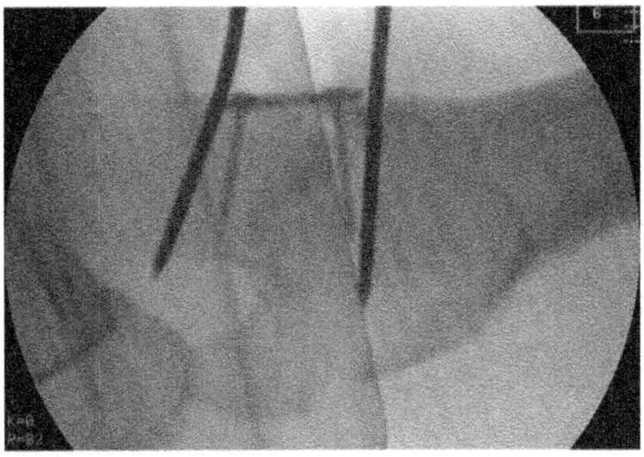

Fig. 12.8 Temporary bridging plate to maintain femoral neck reduction

Alternatively, reduction can be achieved following direct visualization of the femoral neck through either a Smith-Petersen or a Watson-Jones approach [51]. The approach chosen is usually dependent on the surgeons' experience, but care must be taken to prevent injury to the vessels supplying the femoral head, in particular the medial femoral circumflex artery.

Achieving reduction, especially rotationally, can be difficult and various strategies are employed including joystick wires, clamps or temporary plates bridging the fracture (Fig. 12.8) [50].

12.5.3.4 Capsulotomy

Some surgeons advocate performing a capsulotomy to decompress the hip and reduce the tamponade effect. An alternative is to perform an aspiration. Studies however have only been on small scales, and to date have failed to show a significant impact on clinical outcome. No study has shown a disadvantage to performing capsulotomy, and it can be performed during open surgery, or percutaneously under image guidance in closed procedures [48].

12.5.3.5 Internal Fixation Techniques

Once an anatomical reduction has been achieved, the fracture is fixed with either a dynamic hip screw or cannulated screws. When positioning cannulated screws, there should be parallel and as wide a spread in the femoral neck as possible, and an inverted triangle distribution along the calcar provides a stronger fixation with higher loads to failure [52]. Three screws should be utilized as a minimum, though no advantage has been shown from utilizing four or more screws.

Following internal fixation in these healthy patients, the majority of surgeons would advocate limiting weight bearing for up to 12 weeks post-operatively in order to allow healing without excessive collapse or displacement of the fracture. Whilst the traditional teaching has been to allow compression of the fracture, evidence in younger patients shows that collapse greater than 10 mm can start to affect function [53].

A 2015 meta-analysis of the available research analyzed the complications of re-operation, avascular necrosis, non-union, implant failure, and infection following internal fixation of intracapsular fractures in young (aged 16–60 years old) patients. It reported an 18% overall re-operation rate from 28 studies, with displaced fractures (17.8%, 95% CI 12.4–24.9) having a much higher incidence of re-operation than undisplaced fractures (6.9%, 95% CI 2.6–17.1%), however this was not statistically significant. For avascular necrosis, there was an overall 14.3% incidence, with displaced fractures (14.7%, 95% CI 12.3–17.5%) at greater risk than undisplaced fractures (6.4%, 95% CI 3.4–11.8%). Non-union occurred in 9.3% of patients, and again the point estimates showed a large difference between displaced (10.0%, 95% CI 6.9–14.3%) and undisplaced (5.2%, 95% CI 2.0–13.1%) fractures, but not demonstrating statistical significance due to wide confidence intervals. The authors noted that there were few studies which reported mal-union, implant failure and infection rates, thus only providing an overall incidence rate without comparing undisplaced and displaced fractures. The incidence of mal-union was 7.1%, implant failure 9.7%, and infection 5.1% [54].

A previous 2005 meta-analysis of the available research analyzed the complications of avascular necrosis and non-union following internal fixation of intracapsular fractures in young (aged 15–50 years old) patients. It reported a 23% incidence of avascular necrosis, with displaced fractures having a significantly higher incidence than undisplaced fractures. After excluding an outlying study, they could not identify a statistically significant difference in avascular necrosis incidence between those treated with open and closed reductions. The incidence of non-union was 8.9%, and again a higher incidence was observed in the displaced fracture group. For non-union, those patients treated with open reduction had a higher incidence than those treated by closed reduction. There was no difference in incidence of avascular necrosis, or non-union, between early (less than 12 h) and late (after 12 h) reduction [55].

12.5.3.6 Arthroplasty

Should reduction be unachievable due to the fracture pattern or severity, arthroplasty should be considered as the primary treatment [56]. For the active patient, total hip replacement is the procedure of choice, as it has lower re-operation rates and improved functional scores than hemiarthroplasty [41, 57]. The other advantage of arthroplasty over fixation is that patients are able to mobilize fully weight bearing from day one post-operatively.

It must be acknowledged, however, that total hip replacement in trauma is associated with a significantly higher risk of dislocation than hemiarthroplasty [39], and measures must be taken to reduce this, such as using larger head sizes, and the anterolateral or direct anterior approach.

12.6 Post-Operative Treatment

Post-operatively, the importance of the multidisciplinary approach to hip fracture care becomes even more prominent [2]. The team are vital in identifying and meeting the patients' medical, cognitive, analgesic, nutritional, social, and rehabilitation needs as early as possible. These patients should no longer be managed by trauma surgeons acting alone. Ideally, hospitals should have a tailored orthopedic hip fracture program, and especially in the Western world, we are increasingly seeing specialist orthogeriatricians taking the lead for the post-operative management of these complex patients [2].

12.7 Results

12.7.1 Morbidity

Outcomes following hip fractures remain poor, with those who survive the injury faced with significant morbidity. When quality of life was looked at, the majority of patients recovered to their optimum at 4 months, but all suffered approximately a 20% loss of quality of life [58]. In the elderly population, up to a third of patients require a change of residence on discharge, with even more being unable to perform all activities of daily living independently. Also, the majority require a mobility aid following their recovery and there is also a significant rate of hospital re-admission in the first 6 months following hip fracture [7, 59, 60].

12.7.2 Mortality in the Elderly

The implementation of national audits and standards has seen the mortality rate following hip fracture improve, but the condition is still associated with one of the highest death rates amongst orthopedic patients. Latest data puts the 30-day mortality rate in the Western world around 7.5%, rising to around 20% at 1 year. Excess mortality following hip fracture has been shown to persist for at least 10 years following the injury, with males having higher mortality rates than females at all intervals following hip fracture [61–63]. The relative hazard for death following hip fracture at 3 months post-injury was calculated at 5.75 in females and 7.95 in males in a meta-analysis [62]. The risk of death following hip fracture is also higher in those admitted from an institution, significant cognitive impairment, multiple medical co-morbidities, an admission hemoglobin <100 g/l, and age over 85. Of these, age over 85 is the single biggest risk factor [64].

12.7.3 Recurrent Fracture (Falls and Bone Health)

A key part in femoral neck fracture care for elderly patients is falls prevention and bone health [2].

Over a third of over 65s in the community suffer a fall each year, with the frequency increasing with age [65]. Epidemiological studies have shown that up to a quarter of elderly patients who fall suffer either a fracture or an injury that requires admission to hospital [66]. In the elderly, the cause for these falls is seldom a solitary finding, and is more often due to multiple causative factors. One of the greatest contributors to falls risk is disability of the lower limbs [65], such as when in the recovery phase from hip fracture. As well as this added risk, these patients have presented as a result of a fall, and investigations and assessment must be carried out to identify all reducible risks. Polypharmacy is one such risk which can be addressed during the inpatient stay, together with therapy assessment of the patient's mobility and living environment, highlighting the importance of a multidisciplinary approach to the care of hip fracture patients [2, 7].

It is well evidenced that patients with fragility fractures are at high risk of future fractures [67, 68], and the opportunity to identify these vulnerable patients and reduce their risk should be utilized when they present with femoral neck fractures. This increased fracture risk is greatest during the first year after the injury, but is still present 10 years later [69]. To reduce the risk of future osteoporotic fractures, these patients should have their Vitamin D and Calcium levels corrected, and be assessed for anti-resorptive therapy.

References

1. Grisso JA, Kelsey JL, Strom BL, Chiu GY, Maislin G, O'Brien LA, Hoffman S, Kaplan F. Risk factors for falls as a cause of hip fracture in women. The Northeast Hip Fracture Study Group. N Engl J Med. 1991;324(19):1326–31.
2. National Institute for Health and Care Excellence (NICE). Hip fracture; the management of hip fracture in adults CG124. NICE, London. 2011. https://www.nice.org.uk/guidance/cg124. Accessed Dec 2018.
3. Cooper C, Campion G, Melton LJ. Hip fractures in the elderly: a world-wide projection. Osteoporos Int. 1992;2:285–9.
4. Dhanwal DK, Dennison EM, Harvey NC, Cooper C. Epidemiology of hip fracture: worldwide geographic variation. Indian J Orthop. 2011;45(1):15–22.
5. Melton LJ, Wahner HW, Richelson LS, O'Fallon WM, Riggs BL. Osteoporosis and the risk of hip fracture. Am J Epidemiol. 1986;124(2):254–61.
6. Kanis JA. Diagnosis of osteoporosis and assessment of fracture risk. Lancet. 2002;359:1929.
7. The National Hip Fracture Database (NHFD) Annual Report 2015. http://www.nhfd.co.uk/nhfd/nhfd2015reportPR1.pdf. Accessed Apr 2016.
8. Cannon J, Silvestri S, Munro M. Imaging choices in occult hip fracture. J Emerg Med. 2009;37(2):144–52.
9. Lubovsky O, Liebergall M, Mattan Y, Weil Y, Mosheiff R. Early diagnosis of occult hip fractures: MRI versus CT scan. Injury. 2005;36(6):788–92.
10. ATLS. Advanced trauma life support (ATLS) student course manual. 10th ed. Chicago: American College of Surgeons; 2018.
11. Tornetta P, Kain MS, Creevy WR. Diagnosis of femoral neck fractures in patients with a femoral shaft fracture. J Bone Joint Surg Am. 2007;89(1):39–43.
12. Chesser T, Chauhan G, Kelly M. Management of hip fractures in the elderly. Surgery (Oxford). 2016;34(9):440–3.
13. Gautier E, Ganz K, Krügel N, Gill T, Ganz R. Anatomy of the medial femoral circumflex artery and its surgical implications. J Bone Joint Surg Br. 2000;82(5):679–83.
14. Garden RS. Low-angle fixation in fractures of the femoral neck. J Bone Joint Surg Br. 1961;43(4):647–63.
15. Bandeira-Rodrigues E, Vasta S, Leitão JC, Monllau JC. Femur fractures. In: Espregueira-Mendes J, et al., editors. Injuries and health problems in football. Berlin: Springer; 2017. p. 247.
16. Pauwels F. Der schenkelhalsbruch ein mechanisches problem. Z Orthop Ihre Grenzgeb. 1935;63:1–135.
17. Pauwels F, Furlong RJ, Maquet P. Biomechanics of the normal and diseased hip, theoretical foundation, technique and results of treatment an atlas. Berlin: Springer; 1976.
18. Bartonicek J. Pauwels' classification of femoral neck fractures: correct interpretation of the original. J Orthop Trauma. 2001;15:358–60.
19. Pauwels F. Der Schenkelhalsbruch. In: Gesammelte Abhandlungen zur funktionellen Anatomie des Bewegungsapparates. Berlin: Springer; 1965. p. 28.
20. Meinberg E, Agel J, Roberts C, et al. Fracture and dislocation classification compendium. J Orthop Trauma. 2018;32(1):S1–S10.
21. Blundell CM, Parker MJ, Pryor GA, Hopkinson-Woolley J, Bhonsle SS. Assessment of the AO classification of intracapsular fractures of the proximal femur. J Bone Joint Surg Br. 1998;80(4):679–83.
22. Zlowodzki M, Bhandari M, Keel M, Hanson BP, Schemitsch E. Perception of Garden's classification for femoral neck fractures: an international survey of 298 orthopaedic trauma surgeons. Arch Orthop Trauma Surg. 2005;125(7):503–5.
23. Parker MJ, Blundell C. Choice of implant for internal fixation of femoral neck fractures: meta-analysis of 25 randomised trials including 4925 patients. Acta Orthop Scand. 1998;69(2):138–43.
24. Walsum AD, Vroemen J, Janzing HM, Winkelhorst T, Kalsbeek J, Roerdink WH. Low failure rate by means of DLBP fixation of undisplaced femoral neck fractures. Eur J Trauma Emerg Surg. 2016;19:1–6.
25. Parker M, Cawley S, Palial V. Internal fixation of intracapsular fractures of the hip using a dynamic locking plate. Bone Joint J. 2013;95(10):1402–5.
26. Fixation using Alternative Implants for the Treatment of Hip fractures (FAITH) Investigators.

Fracture fixation in the operative management of hip fractures (FAITH): an international, multicentre, randomised controlled trial. Lancet. 2017;389(10078):1519–27.
27. Lapidus LJ, Charalampidis A, Rundgren J, Enocson A. Internal fixation of garden I and II femoral neck fractures: posterior tilt did not influence the reoperation rate in 382 consecutive hips followed for a minimum of 5 years. J Orthop Trauma. 2013;27(7):386–90.
28. Murphy DK, Randell T, Brennan KL, Probe RA, Brennan ML. Treatment and displacement affect the reoperation rate for femoral neck fracture. Clin Orthop Relat Res. 2013;471(8):2691–702.
29. Conn KS, Parker MJ. Undisplaced intracapsular hip fractures: results of internal fixation in 375 patients. Clin Orthop Relat Res. 2004;421:249–54.
30. Gjertsen JE, Fevang JM, Matre K, Vinje T, Engesaeter LB. Clinical outcome after undisplaced femoral neck fractures. Acta Orthop. 2011;82:268–74.
31. Bjorgul K, Reikeras O. Outcome of undisplaced and moderately displaced femoral neck fractures. Acta Orthop. 2007;78(4):498–504.
32. Parker MJ, White A, Boyle A. Fixation versus hemiarthroplasty for undisplaced intracapsular hip fractures. Injury. 2008;39(7):791–5.
33. Rogmark C, Flensburg L, Fredin H. Undisplaced femoral neck fractures--no problems? A consecutive study of 224 patients treated with internal fixation. Injury. 2009;40(3):274–6.
34. Rogmark C, Johnell O. Primary arthroplasty is better than internal fixation of displaced femoral neck fractures: a meta-analysis of 14 randomized studies with 2,289 patients. Acta Orthop. 2006;77(3):359–67.
35. Parker MJ, Gurusamy KS. Internal fixation versus arthroplasty for intracapsular proximal femoral fractures in adults. Cochrane Database Syst Rev. 2006;4:CD001708.
36. Parker MJ, Pryor G, Gurusamy K. Hemiarthroplasty versus internal fixation for displaced intracapsular hip fractures: a long-term follow-up of a randomised trial. Injury. 2010;41(4):370–3.
37. Frihagen F, Nordsletten L, Madsen JE. Hemiarthroplasty or internal fixation for intracapsular displaced femoral neck fractures: randomised controlled trial. BMJ. 2007;335(7632):1251–4.
38. Johansson T, Jacobsson SA, Ivarsson I, Knutsson A, Wahlström O. Internal fixation versus total hip arthroplasty in the treatment of displaced femoral neck fractures: a prospective randomized study of 100 hips. Acta Orthop Scand. 2000;71(6):597–602.
39. Ravikumar KJ, Marsh G. Internal fixation versus hemiarthroplasty versus total hip arthroplasty for displaced subcapital fractures of femur—13 year results of a prospective randomised study. Injury. 2000;31(10):793–7.
40. Liu Y, Tao X, Wang P, Zhang Z, Zhang W, Qi Q. Meta-analysis of randomised controlled trials comparing unipolar with bipolar hemiarthroplasty for displaced femoral-neck fractures. Int Orthop. 2014;38(8):1691–6.
41. Baker RP, Squires B, Gargan MF, Bannister GC. Total hip arthroplasty and hemiarthroplasty in mobile, independent patients with a displaced intracapsular fracture of the femoral neck. J Bone Joint Surg Am. 2006;88(12):2583–9.
42. Hedbeck CJ, Enocson A, Lapidus G, Blomfeldt R, Törnkvist H, Ponzer S, Tidermark J. Comparison of bipolar hemiarthroplasty with total hip arthroplasty for displaced femoral neck fractures. J Bone Joint Surg Am. 2011;93(5):445–50.
43. Avery PP, Baker RP, Walton MJ, Rooker JC, Squires B, Gargan MF, Bannister GC. Total hip replacement and hemiarthroplasty in mobile, independent patients with a displaced intracapsular fracture of the femoral neck. J Bone Joint Surg Br. 2011;93(8):1045–8.
44. White SM, Moppett IK, Griffiths R. Outcome by mode of anaesthesia for hip fracture surgery. An observational audit of 65 535 patients in a national dataset. Anaesthesia. 2014;69(3):224–30.
45. Costa ML, Griffin XL, Pendleton N, Pearson M, Parsons N. Does cementing the femoral component increase the risk of peri-operative mortality for patients having replacement surgery for a fracture of the neck of femur? Data from the National Hip Fracture Database. J Bone Joint Surg Br. 2011;93(10):1405–10.
46. Gjertsen JE, Lie SA, Vinje T, Engesæter LB, Hallan G, Matre K, Furnes O. More re-operations after uncemented than cemented hemiarthroplasty used in the treatment of displaced fractures of the femoral neck: an observational study of 11,116 hemiarthroplasties from a national register. J Bone Joint Surg Br. 2012;94(8):1113–9.
47. Griffiths R, et al. Safety guideline: reducing the risk from cemented hemiarthroplasty for hip fracture 2015. Anaesthesia. 2015;70:623–6.
48. Ly TV, Swiontkowski MF. Treatment of femoral neck fractures in young adults: an instructional course lecture. JBJS Am. 2008;90-A(10):2253–66.
49. Leadbetter GW. Closed reduction of fractures of the neck of the femur. J Bone Joint Surg Am. 1938;20(1):108–13.
50. Hoffman R, Haas NP. Fractures of the femoral neck (31-B) in AO Principles of Fracture Management. Biel/Bienne: Arbeitsgemeinschaft für Osteosynthesefragen (AO) Foundation. https://www2.aofoundation.org/wps/portal/!ut/p/a0/04_Sj9CPykssy0xPLMnMz0vMAfGjzOKN_A0M3D2DDbz9_UMMDRyDXQ3dw9wMDAzMjfULsh0VAbWjLW0!/?bone=Femur&segment=Proximal&showPage=D&contentUrl=srg/popup/further_reading/PFxM2/31/661_32-Neck_fxs_surg_treat.jsp. Accessed Dec 2018.
51. Molnar RB, Routt ML Jr. Open reduction of intracapsular hip fractures using a modified Smith-Petersen surgical exposure. J Orthop Trauma. 2007;21(7):490.
52. Selvan VT, Oakley MJ, Rangan A, Al-Lami MK. Optimum configuration of cannulated hip screws for the fixation of intracapsular hip fractures: a biomechanical study. Injury. 2004;35(2):136–41.

53. Zlowodzki M, Brink O, Switzer J, Wingerter S, Woodall J, Petrisor BA, Kregor PJ, Bruinsma DR, Bhandari M. The effect of shortening and varus collapse of the femoral neck on function after fixation of intracapsular fracture of the hip. J Bone Joint Surg Br. 2008;90(11):1487–94.
54. Slobogean GP, Sprague SA, Scott T, Bhandari M. Complications following young femoral neck fractures. Injury. 2015;46(3):484–91.
55. Damany DS, Parker MJ, Chojnowski A. Complications after intracapsular hip fractures in young adults: a meta-analysis of 18 published studies involving 564 fractures. Injury. 2005;36(1):131–41.
56. McKinley JC, Robinson CM. Treatment of displaced intracapsular hip fractures with total hip arthroplasty: comparison of primary arthroplasty with early salvage arthroplasty after failed internal fixation. J Bone Joint Surg. 2002;84(11):2010–5.
57. Blomfeldt R, Törnkvist H, Eriksson K, Söderqvist A, Ponzer S, Tidermark J. A randomised controlled trial comparing bipolar hemiarthroplasty with total hip replacement for displaced intracapsular fractures of the femoral neck in elderly patients. J Bone Joint Surg Br. 2007;89(2):160–5.
58. Griffin XL, Parsons N, Achten J, Fernandez M, Costa ML. Recovery of health-related quality of life in a United Kingdom hip fracture population. Bone Joint J. 2015;97(3):372–82.
59. Van Balen R, Steyerberg EW, Polder JJ, Ribbers TL, Habbema JD, Cools HJ. Hip fracture in elderly patients: outcomes for function, quality of life, and type of residence. Clin Orthop Relat Res. 2001;390:232–43.
60. Wolinsky FD, Fitzgerald JF, Stump TE. The effect of hip fracture on mortality, hospitalization, and functional status: a prospective study. Am J Public Health. 1997;87:398–403.
61. The National Hip Fracture Database (NHFD) 2015 Annual report supplement—An analysis of 30-day mortality in 2014.
62. Haentjens P, Magaziner J, Colón-Emeric CS, et al. Meta-analysis: excess mortality after hip fracture among older women and men. Ann Intern Med. 2010;152:380.
63. Huddleston JM, Whitford KJ. Medical care of elderly patients with hip fractures. Mayo Clin Proc. 2001;76:295.
64. Moppett IK, Parker M, Griffiths R, Bowers T, White SM, Moran CG. Nottingham hip fracture score: longitudinal and multi-assessment. Br J Anaesth. 2012;109(4):546–50.
65. Tinetti ME, Speechley M, Ginter SF. Risk factors for falls among elderly persons living in the community. N Engl J Med. 1988;319(26):1701–7.
66. Campbell AJ, Borrie MJ, Spears GF, Jackson SL, Brown JS, Fitzgerald JL. Circumstances and consequences of falls experienced by a community population 70 years and over during a prospective study. Age Ageing. 1990;19(2):136–41.
67. Klotzbuecher CM, Ross PD, Landsman PB, Abbott TA, Berger M. Patients with prior fractures have an increased risk of future fractures: a summary of the literature and statistical synthesis. J Bone Miner Res. 2000;15(4):721–39.
68. Kanis JA, Johnell O, De Laet C, Johansson H, Odén A, Delmas P, Eisman J, Fujiwara S, Garnero P, Kroger H, McCloskey EV. A meta-analysis of previous fracture and subsequent fracture risk. Bone. 2004;35(2):375–82.
69. British Orthopaedic Association and British Geriatrics Society. The care of patients with fragility fracture 'blue book'. London: British Orthopaedic Association; 2007.

Pathologic Fractures

13

Frank M. Klenke, Attila Kollár,
and Christophe Kurze

Abstract

A bone fracture is termed pathologic when the fracture occurs through a region of a preexisting bone pathology weakening the bony architecture. Such pathologies include metabolic bone diseases such as Paget's disease, osteogenesis imperfecta, and osteoporosis as well as local alterations of the bone structure due to tumorous processes and tumor-like bone lesions.

This chapter discussed pathologic fractures of the hip caused by the processes leading to local bone destruction including tumor-like lesions as well as primary and secondary (i.e., metastases) bone tumors.

Keywords

Pathologic fracture · Bone · Tumor · Metastasis · Tumor-like lesion · Sarcoma · Surgery · Osteosynthesis · Arthroplasty

F. M. Klenke (✉) · C. Kurze
Department of Orthopaedic Surgery and Traumatology, Inselspital, Bern University Hospital, Bern, Switzerland
e-mail: frank.klenke@insel.ch

A. Kollár
Department of Medical Oncology, Inselspital, Bern University Hospital, Bern, Switzerland

13.1 Epidemiology

Metastatic bone disease is the most frequent cause for pathologic fractures of the acetabulum and the proximal end of the femur. It has been reported that 9–29% of patients with metastatic bone disease will develop pathological fractures out of which more than 90% require surgical intervention [1, 2]. Bone is the third most common site affected by metastatic disease, outnumbered only by metastases to the lung and the liver. Bone metastases may arise from any solid cancer. They are observed most frequently in prostate, breast, lung, kidney, and thyroid cancer [3]. Patients with prostate and breast cancer are affected by bone metastases and skeletal related events (SRE, i.e. bone pain, pathological fractures, spinal cord compression, palliative radiotherapy, and surgery) with particular frequency. This is due to the high incidence of bone metastases in these tumors and a relatively long survival time after diagnosis of bone metastases ranging between 7 and 28 months [3–6]. Within 5 years after the initial diagnosis 10–17% of patients with prostate and breast cancer will develop bone metastases and more than 70% of the patients with advanced prostate and breast cancer will develop bone metastases during the course of the disease.

Pathologic fractures associated with tumor-like bone lesions, benign bone tumors, and malignant bone tumors are markedly less frequent. Multiple myeloma, which is the most frequent

L. Büchler, M. J.B. Keel (eds.), *Fractures of the Hip*, Fracture Management Joint by Joint,
https://doi.org/10.1007/978-3-030-18838-2_13

primary bone tumor, accounts for 1% of all malignancies [7]. Approximately 30% of patients with multiple myeloma will be diagnosed with the disease due to a pathologic fracture and approximately 80% experience a pathologic fracture during the course of the disease [8, 9]. The vast majority of pathologic fractures occur at spine and ribs. Only 5% of the pathologic fractures associated with multiple myeloma involve the pelvis or the proximal femur [8]. In chondrosarcoma, the second most frequent primary malignancy of bone in adults, the rate of pathologic fractures of the proximal femur was shown to range between 25% and 28% [10, 11]. Although chondrosarcomas frequently involve the pelvis, pathologic fractures of the acetabulum are usually not observed [11, 12]. The rate of osteosarcoma or Ewing's sarcoma presenting with a pathological fracture is significantly lower and ranges between 4% and 13% [11, 13–15]. In contrast to multiple myeloma and chondrosarcoma, osteosarcoma and Ewing's sarcoma typically occur in children and young adults. The same is true for the majority of tumor-like lesions and benign bone tumors including solitary bone cysts (SBC), aneurysmal bone cysts (ABC), fibrous dysplasia (FD), eosinophilic granuloma (EG), and chondroblastoma. Thus, pathologic fractures associated with these bone lesions most often affect young patients. Solitary bone cysts show a specific risk of pathologic fractures. These lesions are the most common cause of pathologic fractures in children. Approximately 70% of these bone lesions are diagnosed due to a pathologic fracture [16]. The fracture rate at the proximal femur has been shown to be 52% [16]. In children under 18 years of age, pathologic fractures of the proximal femur account for approximately 35% of all fractures of the proximal femur [17].

Pathologic fractures around the hip are a result of a wide variety of underlying diseases. The causes of fracture have to be taken into consideration when deciding which type of fracture treatment needs to be applied in the individual situation.

13.2 Tumor-Like Lesions

Historically, tumor-like lesions have been defined as non-neoplastic bone lesions by Lichtenstein, which include non-ossifying fibroma (NOF), simple bone cysts (SBC), aneurysmal bone cysts (ABC), fibrous dysplasia (FD), osteofibrous dysplasia (OFD), and eosinophilic granuloma (EG). However, it is known today that some of these lesions are indeed neoplastic. For example, NOF has been classified as a benign fibrohistiocytic tumor by the World Health Organization (WHO). EG is a neoplastic proliferation of Langerhans cells and has been classified as a tumor of undefined neoplastic nature.

Due to their benign behavior, tumor-like lesions do not require surgical treatment per se but they often require surgical treatment due to pathological fractures. At the proximal femur and at the acetabulum, surgical treatment should also be considered when a lesion is discovered incidentally without fracture. This is due to the high risk of pathologic fractures and the severity of complications associated with the fractures such as femoral head necrosis, medial head migration, and persistent deformity [18]. It should be stressed that, in case of suspicion of ABC, biopsy should be performed prior to definitive treatment to rule out teleangiectatic osteosarcoma, which may resemble ABC on imaging studies [19].

Surgery for pathological fractures of tumor-like lesions has to address the fracture as well as the lesion itself in order to prevent persistence of the lesion and re-fracture [20–29]. Surgery involves open reduction and internal fixation using intramedullary nails, plates, and screws. To induce healing of the lesion, curettage plus high-speed burring followed by bone void filling with autogenous or allogeneic bone grafts or bone graft substitutes should be performed. In general, studies have shown equivalent results independent of whether bone grafts or bone graft substitutes were used. In fibrous dysplasia however, there is an increased risk of graft resorption. In adult patients with monostotic disease, bone grafting is indicated but the use of cortical

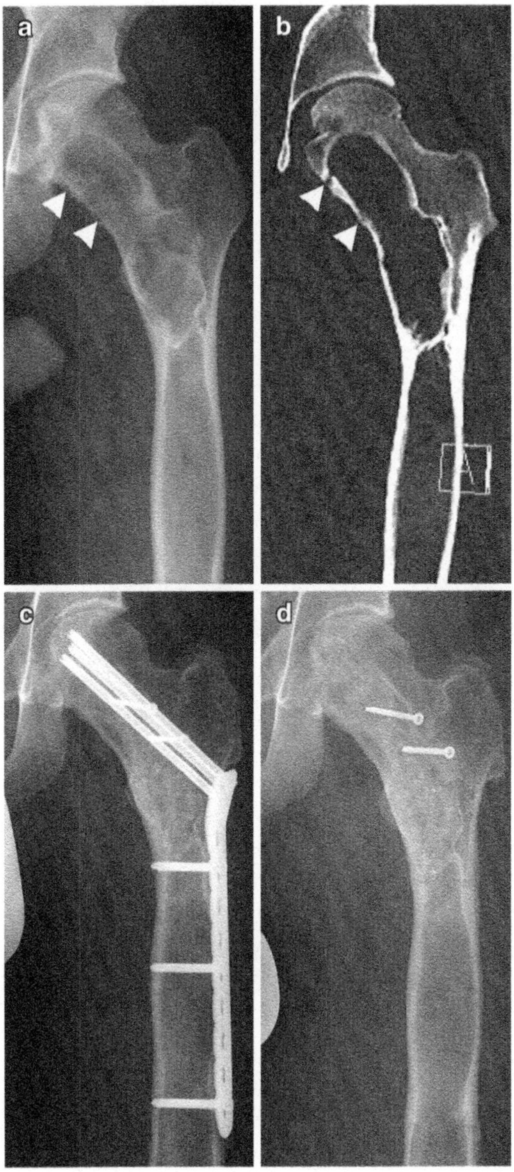

Fig. 13.1 25 year old male diagnosed with polyostotic fibrous dysplasia. The patient developed progressive hip pain with ambulation. X-ray and CT scans demonstrated an extensive osteolytic lesion and an un-displaced fracture at the calcar (marked with arrowheads, (**a**, **b**). The patient was treated with curettage through an anterior cortical window, bone grafting with impacted allogeneic bone and plate osteosynthesis of the proximal femur. The postoperative course was uneventful with complete bone reconstitution of the proximal femur after 2 years (**c**). Plate removal was performed 27 months after the index surgery (**d**)

instead of cancellous autologous bone grafts or impacted allogeneic bone has been recommended [24, 27, 28]. In young patients with polyostotic fibrous dysplasia, high graft resorption rates have been observed. Therefore, some authors have recommended abandoning bone grafting in this group of patients [30, 31]. We usually perform impacted allogeneic bone grafting in polyostotic fibrous dysplasia but have abandoned autologous bone grafting in these patients (Figure 13.1). In unicameral bone cysts, perforation of the inner cyst wall and creation of a communication with the bone marrow has been shown to stimulate cyst ossification and should be performed by standard [32, 33]. In non-ossifying fibroma, curettage of the lesion is not imperative because these lesions often heal after a fracture without specifically treating the lesion [20, 34]. However, the authors recommend curettage and grafting of the lesion in order to accelerate bony healing and prevent failure of the osteosynthesis.

13.3 Benign and Intermediate Bone Tumors

The vast majority of primary bone tumors are benign. Since many are not clinically apparent they usually remain undiscovered or are discovered incidentally at radiographic examinations for other reasons. Therefore, the true incidence of benign bone tumors has not been determined precisely. Despite their frequency, benign bone tumors are usually not associated with pathologic fractures [35]. Enchondroma, which is the second most frequent benign bone tumor carries the highest risk of pathologic fractures [36]. However, these fractures usually involve the small bones of the hand and feet [37, 38]. Enchondroma of the femoral neck or the acetabulum is extremely rare and may be associated with enchondromatosis, i.e. Ollier's disease or Maffucci syndrome [39, 40]. Furthermore, suspicion of a cartilaginous tumor necessitates the exclusion of chondrosarcoma, which is a much more common finding in the proximal femur and the pelvis [41]. Pathologic fractures of the acetabulum and the proximal femur are more frequently found in giant cell tumor of bone (GCTB). Histologically, GCTB is a benign neoplastic lesion. It has been classified as an intermediate tumor due to its clinically aggressive behavior and its potential to seed pulmonary metastases [36]. Approximately 11–15% of GCTB occur in the proximal femur and the pelvis [42, 43]. The rate of pathologic fractures ranges between 9% and 30% with fractures of the proximal femur being markedly more frequent than those of the acetabulum [44–49].

Surgical treatment of pathologic fractures due to benign and intermediate bone tumors is similar to that of tumor like lesions and involves removal of the tumor and open reduction and internal fixation of the fracture. The standard treatment protocol for tumor removal at our institution includes curettage and high-speed burring of the lesion plus thermocoagulation of the tumor void with argon beam as adjunctive therapy [50, 51]. We have omitted adjunctive local phenol application due to its limited therapeutic effect and the associated toxicity [52, 53]. Open reduction and fixation of pathologic fractures of the proximal femur and the acetabulum should be combined with autogenous or allogeneic bone grafts, or bone graft substitutes in order to fill the bone void created with the tumor removal. Polymethylmethacrylate (PMMA) bone cement has been recommended as bone void filler providing immediate structural stability and an effective adjunctive therapy for GCTB [42, 52, 54]. However, in case of a pathologic fracture the non-resorbable nature of PMMA may prevent biologic fracture healing and limit long-term mechanical stability of the fractured bone. It has been shown that joint salvage through curettage and internal fixation is a reasonable option for patients with pathologic fractures due to GCTB since functional outcomes and recurrence rates are similar GCTB without fracture [54–56]. On the other hand, extensive joint destruction or soft tissue extension may warrant wide resection and total hip arthroplasty.

13.4 Primary Malignant Bone Tumors

The treatment of primary malignant bone tumors such as osteosarcoma, chondrosarcoma, and Ewing sarcoma may be complicated by a pathologic fracture. Pathologic fractures through primary malignant bone tumors have been linked to an increased risk of local recurrences and decreased survival. However, the exact impact of pathologic fractures on local recurrence and survival is unclear. Some studies found a correlation between pathologic fracture and limited survival, whereas other studies failed to demonstrate such association [11, 15, 57–62]. Similarly, previous studies have shown conflicting results in finding an association of pathologic fracture and an increased risk of local recurrence [11, 15, 59, 60]. Around the hip, pathologic fractures through primary malignant bone tumors seem to be associated with a particular poor prognosis [15, 63]. This may be due to the lack of containment of the fracture hematoma resulting in widespread contamination of the surrounding soft tissues with tumor cells [63]. Furthermore, the pathologic fracture may be a sign for a more aggressive biologic behavior of sarcomas as demonstrated by the finding that such tumors are associated with a high rate of synchronous pulmonary metastasis [11, 63]. It is important to note that local recurrence and survival are not affected by the type of surgical treatment, viz. limb preserving surgery or amputation as long as adequate surgical margins can be obtained [11, 58, 62].

With this in mind, the general principles of tumor surgery apply to primary malignant bone tumors independent of whether they present with a pathologic fracture or not. Not recognizing a fracture as being of pathologic nature may result in inappropriate treatment, e.g. by open reduction and internal fixation. This again will result in local tumor spread necessitating a more extensive and morbid surgery for tumor removal and will worsen the prognosis of tumor treatment. As a standard of care, wide resection with negative surgical margins has to be aimed for in bone sarcoma with and without pathologic fracture [64]. The only exception is low-grade chondrosarcoma, which can be treated with intralesional surgery without worsening recurrence-free survival and overall prognosis [65–68]. However, in case of pathologic fracture, indicating a more aggressive local behavior we recommend wide resection also for low-grade chondrosarcoma [67, 68]. This is especially true for periacetabular tumors due to the dramatic consequence of a local recurrence in this location [69, 70].

Options for limb reconstruction after resection of primary malignant bone tumors around the hip include tumor endoprosthesis, allograft-prosthetic constructs, and extracorporeal irradiation and reimplantation [71–77]. The choice of the type of reconstruction should be individualized to the location and extent of the tumor resection but is independent of the presence of a pathologic fracture. For primary malignant bone tumors with the indication for neo-adjuvant chemotherapy (e.g., osteosarcoma, Ewing sarcoma), pathologic fractures should be treated by non-operative means whenever possible and wide tumor resection should be performed after completion of the preoperative portion of chemotherapy. This approach is feasible in stable pathologic fractures through bone tumors of the periacetabular region. However, in pathologic fractures of the proximal femur, immobilization is difficult if not impossible with non-surgical treatment. A joint spanning external fixator may achieve sufficient immobilization of the fracture site in such cases but is poorly tolerated and prone to secondary complications over the extended period of several cycles of preoperative chemotherapy. Therefore, adaption of the chemotherapy protocol should be considered. Adaption may consist in a curtailed preoperative induction chemotherapy or transition to an adjuvant setting allowing rapid surgical treatment of the local tumor disease and the fracture [63, 78].

Taken together, pathologic fracture through primary malignant bone tumors at the hip worsens prognosis but does not necessarily implicate amputation. If adequate surgical margins can be obtained, limb preserving surgery can be performed, especially when the tumor responds well to preoperative chemotherapy. Due to the severe consequences of a pathologic fracture through a primary malignant bone tumor around the hip, early surgery prior to chemotherapy should be considered if there is an extensive lytic process likely to lead to fracture following biopsy.

13.5 Bone Metastases

13.5.1 General Considerations

The primary goals of the treatment of metastases around the hip include sufficient and durable hip joint function, rapid return to full weight bearing, and immediate pain relief. Furthermore, local tumor control should be achieved to prevent progressive bone destruction, re-fracture, or implant failure [79, 80].

Bone metastases are classified into osteolytic and osteoblastic lesions. Invasion of the skeleton by cancer cells causes an imbalance in the activities of bone resorbing osteoclasts and bone forming osteoblasts resulting in pathologic bone destruction or bone formation [81]. Patients may exhibit osteolytic and osteoblastic lesions at a time and metastases are often heterogeneous containing both osteolytic and osteoblastic components [82]. Bone metastases without fracture, especially when located at the acetabulum may be treated non-surgically with local radiation and/or systemic therapy whereas the majority of pathologic fractures require surgical intervention.

Due to the dysregulation of bone (re-)modeling in bone metastases fracture healing of pathologic fractures is altered. In a study of 129 pathologic fractures originating from different tumor entities, Gainor and Buchert [83] showed that the overall fracture healing rate was only 35%. In those patients that survived longer than 6 months the healing rate was 74% indicating that fracture healing through metastases is prolonged but does occur in principle. Tumor entity, duration of survival, internal fracture fixation, postoperative irradiation, and chemotherapy correlated with fracture healing. Metastases originating from multiple myeloma, renal and breast carcinoma showed the highest fracture healing rates of 67%, 44% and 37%, respectively, whereas none of the fractures due to metastases from lung carcinoma healed and none of these patients survived longer than 6 months.

The major clinical challenges arising from skeletal metastases are pain and bone destruction, ultimately leading to pathologic fractures. Pain and bone destruction limit the patients' quality of life dramatically. During the past 25 years, improvements in cancer treatment have significantly increased the life expectancy of patients with bone metastases and thus, the treatment of bone metastases has gained increasing importance [84, 85]. According to a recent systemic review by Errani et al. the general indication for surgery of an impending or a pathologic fracture is a life expectancy of ≥6 weeks [86]. The type of the primary tumor and its response to chemo- and radiotherapy, the presence of visceral metastases and multiple skeletal metastases, abnormal laboratory data such as CRP and LDH levels or platelet count, and general health status, e.g. the ECOG performance score are the most important factors for survival [87–89]. In this regard, Katagiri et al. introduced a scoring system to predict survival of patients with bone metastases and help clinicians with their decision-making on the treatment of bone metastases and pathologic fractures [88].

Before initiating the surgical treatment of a pathologic fracture, a diagnosis needs to be established to rule out bone sarcoma, metabolic bone disease, and osteomyelitis. According to Rougraff et al. the standard diagnostic workup for patients without a definite primary tumor should include an X-ray of the affected limb, a whole-body bone scan, laboratory studies, and CT scans of the chest, abdomen, and pelvis [90]. If the diagnosis cannot be established despite adequate workup biopsy should be performed.

Surgical treatment options include intramedullary nailing, compound osteosynthesis, and prosthetic joint replacement. Besides the actual fracture treatment, the tumor tissue should be removed—usually by intralesional curettage—to improve local tumor control and the efficiency of postoperative adjuvant therapy. Adjuvant therapy most often includes local irradiation, which was shown to be effective in decreasing secondary surgical interventions due to local progression of metastases arising from breast, lung, prostate, and colorectal cancer [91]. In solitary metastases of tumors with slow and moderate progression including hormone (in)dependent breast and prostate cancer, thyroid cancer, multiple myeloma, malignant lymphoma, renal cell carcinoma, endometrial and ovarian cancer and in metastatic disease arising from tumors with poor radiation sensitivity, especially renal cell carcinoma wide resection of the metastasis may be recommended [86, 88, 92].

13.5.2 Metastases of the Proximal Femur

The femur is the most commonly affected long bone in metastatic bone disease [93]. Approximately 80% of femoral metastases are located in the proximal femur. Out of those, 35% involve the femoral neck and 65% the inter- and subtrochanteric region. Due to the immediate consequences on ambulation, surgical intervention is usually indicated in pathologic fractures of the proximal femur whereas bone metastases without fracture may be treated non-surgically [94]. Mirels introduced a scoring system to predict the pathologic fracture risk and guide physicians in their decision on how to treat femoral bone metastases [95]. The score is based on four variables: degree of pain, lesional size, lytic versus blastic nature, and anatomic location. Treatment recommendations generated by Mirels were prophylactic stabilization of patients with a total score of 9 points or more and consideration of prophylactic stabilization at a borderline score of 8 points. The Mirels' score has been shown to be reproducible and valid [96]. However, it seems to overestimate the actual occurrence of a pathological fracture. Thus, strict adherence to Mirels' recommendations would result in a large proportion of patients with a limited life expectancy to undergo unnecessary prophylactic stabilization [96, 97]. We therefore recommend to include additional factors into the decision making of whether to stabilize femoral metastases prophylactically such as the Katagiri score and an axial cortical involvement of greater than 30 mm [88, 97, 98].

Fractures involving the different regions of the proximal femur are addressed with different forms of stabilization or endoprosthetic replacement. Prior to selecting the type of treatment, imaging studies of the entire femur should be obtained to exclude additional sites of metastatic involvement in the same bone. If present, additional metastases should be addressed with the same surgery.

There is evidence that the treatment of pathologic or impending femoral neck fractures with endoprosthetic reconstruction is superior to that with internal fixation [99] (Figure 13.2). Advantages of endoprosthetic reconstruction over internal fixation include rapid return to full weight-bearing ambulation, reduced pain, and the ability to perform en-bloc resection minimizing the risk local recurrence [100]. Furthermore, the need of repeat surgical intervention is lower after endoprosthetic reconstruction. The rate of repeat surgeries has been reported to range from 16 to 42% after internal fixation and 3–8% after endoprosthetic reconstruction [101–103]. In a study including 142 patients with proximal femoral metastases Wedin and Bauer reported that the risk of re-surgery was twice as high in the osteosynthesis group (16%) compared to the arthroplasty group (8%). However, three periprosthetic pathologic fractures occurred in the arthroplasty group distal to the femoral component. To decrease the risk of secondary fractures, the use of a long femoral stem has been recommended [102]. There is no evidence in favor for or against using PMMA for fixation of the femoral component. However, one has to consider that cortical tumor growth may result in stem loosening when using uncemented implants [99]. Due to negative effects of radiation on bone ingrowth, cemented implants should be favored when postoperative radiotherapy is planned [104].

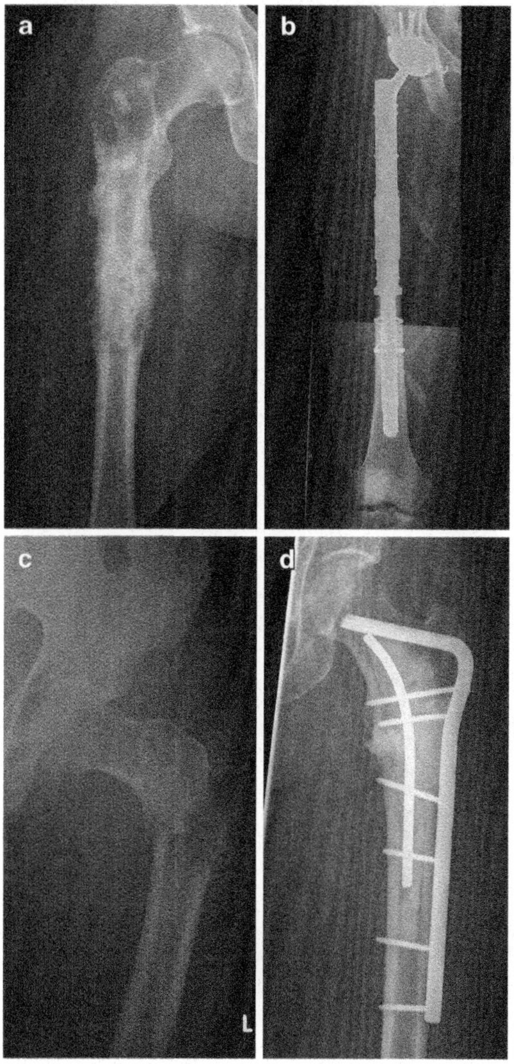

Fig. 13.2 Metastatic bone disease of the proximal femur with a pathologic femoral neck fracture through an extensive mixed osteoblastic/osteolytic prostate cancer metastasis in a 54 year old male (**a**). Resection of the affected bone and reconstruction with a modular tumor endoprosthesis was performed (**b**). Pathologic subtrochanteric fracture in a 39 year old male due to a previously unknown multiple myeloma (**c**). The fracture was treated with compound osteosynthesis (**d**) followed by local irradiation (total dose 30 Gy) and high-dose chemotherapy

Impending and pathologic inter-/subtrochanteric fractures may be treated with intramedullary nailing, plating, or arthroplasty. For successful intramedullary nailing, sufficient proximal nail fixation is essential. Furthermore, distal locking is mandatory. Usually, cephalomedullary nails have been recommended in order to avoid femoral neck fractures in case of progression of metastatic disease. However, there is no scientific evidence that a cephalomedullary nail would prevent femoral neck fracture or re-operation [105, 106]. In large defects, PMMA may be used to improve structural support and prolong implant survival [79]. Miller et al. found that hardware failure, non-union, tumor progression, and surgeon error were reasons for failure of intramedullary nailing of pathologic femoral fractures [107]. Due to the critical consequences of implant failure, arthroplasty should be preferred in case of poor bone stock of the proximal femur [99]. However, endoprosthetic reconstruction is associated with a longer surgery time as well as a higher rate of peri- and postoperative complications such as cardiac failure, cerebrovascular incidents, and dislocation [100, 102]. Alternatively, compound osteosynthesis, a PMMA augmented combination of an intramedullary placed small fragment plate and a condylar blade plate, may be used to address both pathologic and impeding femoral fractures [85, 108, 109]. The loading strength of a compound osteosynthesis equals the strength of an intact femur and has a higher mechanical strength than intramedullary nailing even if cement augmentation is used [108, 110–112]. Rompe et al. reported that the functional outcome was superior to endoprosthetic reconstruction with respect to range of motion and gait pattern [113]. The authors attributed this finding to the integrity of the gluteal insertion, which was not altered by the compound osteosynthesis. This technique has been used at our institution for over 30 years and has proven to be a viable option in cases with bone destruction where proximal locking of intramedullary nails is difficult to achieve [114].

13.5.3 Periacetabular Metastases

The pelvis is the second most frequent site of metastatic bone disease, only outnumbered by the spine [115]. According to the treatment of metastases of the femur, the treatment of periacetabular metastases should be adapted to the local situation, i.e. osteolytic versus osteoblastic lesions, single or multiple lesions, size of the lesion(s), as well as the stage and the overall prognosis of the tumor disease. Recently, Müller and Capanna [92] published a classification system for metastatic disease of the pelvis and a classification based treatment algorithm. Class 1 metastatic lesions stem from tumors with slow and moderate progression, class 2 lesions are metastases of the periacetabular region with pathologic fractures, class 3 are supra-acetabular osteolytic metastases with impending fractures (Fig. 13.3), and class 4 are metastatic lesions not compromising the mechanical stability in situations that cannot be classified under class 1. Surgical treatment has been recommended for classes 1–3, whereas situations that are classified as class 4 should be treated non-surgically by irradiation, systemic therapy, or with minimally invasive procedures including cryoablation and radiofrequency ablation [92]. For classes 1–3, the surgically treatment needs further stratification. In class 1 situations, wide resection viz. internal hemipelvectomy of a solitary metastasis and endoprosthetic reconstruction with saddle/socket endoprosthesis or custom-made triflange implants should be considered. Previous studies reported that curettage of single metastatic lesions is associated with decreased survival as compared to wide resection [80, 116]. Furthermore, wide resection of solitary periacetabular metastases may decrease the rate of secondary local complications such as local metastatic progression and implant failure [116]. Thus, wide resection seems to be justified to achieve local tumor control in class 1 situations despite the higher risk of surgical complications associated with internal hemipelvectomy. In cases of an impending or a pathologic fracture (class 2 and 3), the surgical treatment can be further stratified applying Harrington's criteria [117]. In Harrington group 1 lesions, without destruction of the subchondral bone of the acetabulum, curettage and void filling with bone cement (cementoplasty) provides a minimal invasive solution achieving rapid pain relief, ambulation, and improvement of quality of life [118–120]. Greater acetabular deficiencies (medial wall, Harrington group 2/acetabular roof and rim, Harrington group 3) require total hip arthroplasty with acetabular stabilization using reinforcement rings with or without cement/ Steinman pin augmentation (Harrington technique) [117, 121–124]. In cases of expected survival times greater than 24 months or metastatic

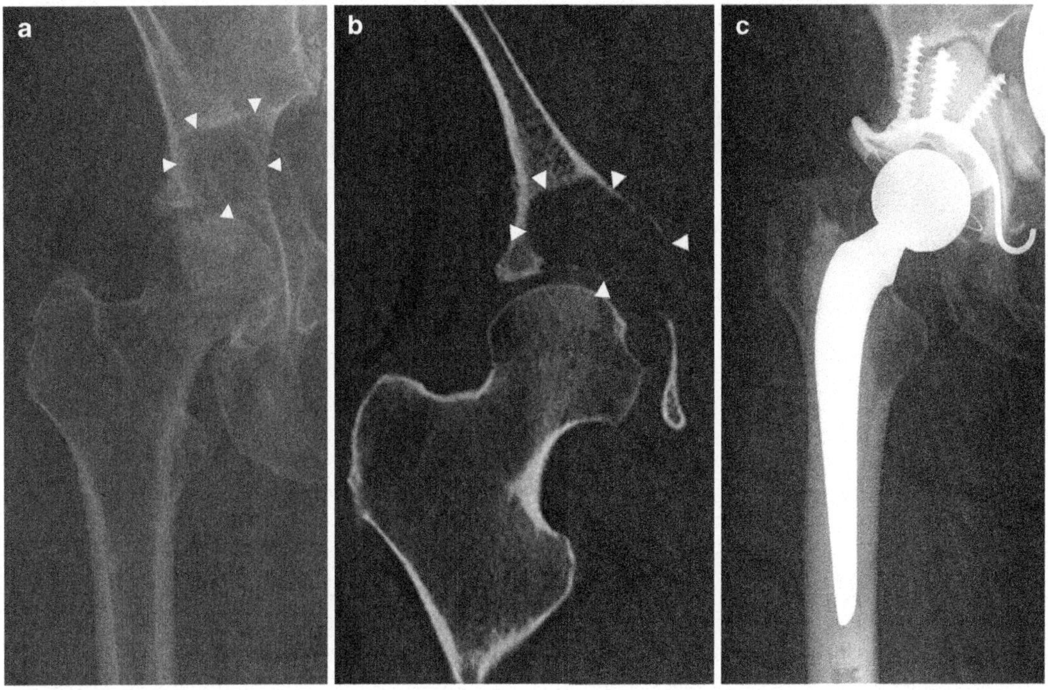

Fig. 13.3 51 year old female with metastatic lung cancer. An impending fracture due to a Harrington class 3 metastatic lesion of the right acetabulum (marked with arrowheads (**a**, **b**)) was treated with bone cement reinforced total hip arthroplasty with the use of a Ganz acetabular reinforcement ring (Zimmer Biomet Inc., Switzerland) (**c**)

disease with poor response to adjuvant therapy more extensive surgical procedures involving saddle/socket endoprosthesis or custom-made triflange implants should be considered [72, 92, 119, 125]. Similar treatment considerations apply to metastatic disease with unrestorable acetabular collapse (Harrington group 4).

13.6 Conclusion

The treatment options of impending and pathologic fractures around the hip are manifold and require careful analysis of the underlying disease. The treatment has to be individualized to the pathology of the bone lesion, the location, the extent of local bone destruction, the stage of the disease and its overall prognosis and involves a multidisciplinary team of radiologists, pathologists, radiation-oncologists, oncologists, and orthopedic surgeons familiar with the diagnosis and treatment of bone pathologies.

References

1. Aaron AD. Treatment of metastatic adenocarcinoma of the pelvis and the extremities. J Bone Joint Surg Am. 1997;79(6):917–32.
2. Harrington KD. Orthopaedic management of extremity and pelvic lesions. Clin Orthop Relat Res. 1995;312:136–47.
3. Coleman RE. Metastatic bone disease: clinical features, pathophysiology and treatment strategies. Cancer Treat Rev. 2001;27(3):165–76.
4. Harries M, Taylor A, Holmberg L, et al. Incidence of bone metastases and survival after a diagnosis of bone metastases in breast cancer patients. Cancer Epidemiol. 2014;38(4):427–34.
5. Jensen AO, Jacobsen JB, Norgaard M, Yong M, Fryzek JP, Sorensen HT. Incidence of bone metastases and skeletal-related events in breast cancer patients: a population-based cohort study in Denmark. BMC Cancer. 2011;11:29.
6. Norgaard M, Jensen AO, Jacobsen JB, Cetin K, Fryzek JP, Sorensen HT. Skeletal related events, bone metastasis and survival of prostate cancer: a population based cohort study in Denmark (1999 to 2007). J Urol. 2010;184(1):162–7.
7. Becker N. Epidemiology of multiple myeloma. Recent Results Cancer Res. 2011;183:25–35.

8. Melton LJ 3rd, Kyle RA, Achenbach SJ, Oberg AL, Rajkumar SV. Fracture risk with multiple myeloma: a population-based study. J Bone Miner Res. 2005;20(3):487–93.
9. Riccardi A, Gobbi PG, Ucci G, et al. Changing clinical presentation of multiple myeloma. Eur J Cancer. 1991;27(11):1401–5.
10. Albergo JI, Gaston CL, Jeys LM, et al. Management and prognostic significance of pathological fractures through chondrosarcoma of the femur. Int Orthop. 2015;39(5):943–6.
11. Bramer JA, Abudu AA, Grimer RJ, Carter SR, Tillman RM. Do pathological fractures influence survival and local recurrence rate in bony sarcomas? Eur J Cancer. 2007;43(13):1944–51.
12. Andreou D, Ruppin S, Fehlberg S, Pink D, Werner M, Tunn PU. Survival and prognostic factors in chondrosarcoma: results in 115 patients with long-term follow-up. Acta Orthop. 2011;82(6):749–55.
13. Bacci G, Ferrari S, Longhi A, et al. Nonmetastatic osteosarcoma of the extremity with pathologic fracture at presentation: local and systemic control by amputation or limb salvage after preoperative chemotherapy. Acta Orthop Scand. 2003;74(4):449–54.
14. Fuchs B, Valenzuela RG, Sim FH. Pathologic fracture as a complication in the treatment of Ewing's sarcoma. Clin Orthop Relat Res. 2003;415:25–30.
15. Scully SP, Ghert MA, Zurakowski D, Thompson RC, Gebhardt MC. Pathologic fracture in osteosarcoma : prognostic importance and treatment implications. J Bone Joint Surg Am. 2002;84-A(1):49–57.
16. Ahn JI, Park JS. Pathological fractures secondary to unicameral bone cysts. Int Orthop. 1994;18(1):20–2.
17. Azouz EM, Karamitsos C, Reed MH, Baker L, Kozlowski K, Hoeffel JC. Types and complications of femoral neck fractures in children. Pediatr Radiol. 1993;23(6):415–20.
18. Papagelopoulos PJ, Choudhury SN, Frassica FJ, Bond JR, Unni KK, Sim FH. Treatment of aneurysmal bone cysts of the pelvis and sacrum. J Bone Joint Surg Am. 2001;83-A(11):1674–81.
19. Mascard E, Gomez-Brouchet A, Lambot K. Bone cysts: unicameral and aneurysmal bone cyst. Orthop Traumatol Surg Res. 2015;101(1 Suppl):S119–27.
20. Arata MA, Peterson HA, Dahlin DC. Pathological fractures through non-ossifying fibromas. Review of the Mayo Clinic experience. J Bone Joint Surg Am. 1981;63(6):980–8.
21. Bali K, Sudesh P, Patel S, Kumar V, Saini U, Dhillon MS. Pediatric femoral neck fractures: our 10 years of experience. Clin Orthop Surg. 2011;3(4):302–8.
22. De Mattos CB, Binitie O, Dormans JP. Pathological fractures in children. Bone Joint Res. 2012;1(10):272–80.
23. Dormans JP, Hanna BG, Johnston DR, Khurana JS. Surgical treatment and recurrence rate of aneurysmal bone cysts in children. Clin Orthop Relat Res. 2004;421:205–11.
24. Guille JT, Kumar SJ, MacEwen GD. Fibrous dysplasia of the proximal part of the femur. Long-term results of curettage and bone-grafting and mechanical realignment. J Bone Joint Surg Am. 1998;80(5):648–58.
25. Krishnan H, Yoon TR, Park KS, Yeo JH. Eosinophilic granuloma involving the femoral neck. Case Rep Orthop. 2013;2013:809605.
26. Mankin HJ, Hornicek FJ, Ortiz-Cruz E, Villafuerte J, Gebhardt MC. Aneurysmal bone cyst: a review of 150 patients. J Clin Oncol. 2005;23(27):6756–62.
27. Ortiz EJ, Isler MH, Navia JE, Canosa R. Pathologic fractures in children. Clin Orthop Relat Res. 2005;432:116–26.
28. Tong Z, Zhang W, Jiao N, Wang K, Chen B, Yang T. Surgical treatment of fibrous dysplasia in the proximal femur. Exp Ther Med. 2013;5(5):1355–8.
29. Wai EK, Davis AM, Griffin A, Bell RS, Wunder JS. Pathologic fractures of the proximal femur secondary to benign bone tumors. Clin Orthop Relat Res. 2001;393:279–86.
30. Leet AI, Boyce AM, Ibrahim KA, Wientroub S, Kushner H, Collins MT. Bone-grafting in polyostotic fibrous dysplasia. J Bone Joint Surg Am. 2016;98(3):211–9.
31. Stanton RP, Ippolito E, Springfield D, Lindaman L, Wientroub S, Leet A. The surgical management of fibrous dysplasia of bone. Orphanet J Rare Dis. 2012;7(Suppl 1):S1.
32. Hou HY, Wu K, Wang CT, Chang SM, Lin WH, Yang RS. Treatment of unicameral bone cyst: surgical technique. J Bone Joint Surg Am. 2011;93(Suppl 1):92–9.
33. Kadhim M, Thacker M, Kadhim A, Holmes L Jr. Treatment of unicameral bone cyst: systematic review and meta analysis. J Child Orthop. 2014;8(2):171–91.
34. Easley ME, Kneisl JS. Pathologic fractures through nonossifying fibromas: is prophylactic treatment warranted? J Pediatr Orthop. 1997;17(6):808–13.
35. Hakim DN, Pelly T, Kulendran M, Caris JA. Benign tumours of the bone: a review. J Bone Oncol. 2015;4(2):37–41.
36. Fletcher CD. The evolving classification of soft tissue tumours - an update based on the new 2013 WHO classification. Histopathology. 2014;64(1):2–11.
37. Haase SC. Treatment of pathologic fractures. Hand Clin. 2013;29(4):579–84.
38. Sassoon AA, Fitz-Gibbon PD, Harmsen WS, Moran SL. Enchondromas of the hand: factors affecting recurrence, healing, motion, and malignant transformation. J Hand Surg Am. 2012;37(6):1229–34.
39. Khoo RN, Peh WC, Guglielmi G. Clinics in diagnostic imaging (124). Multiple enchondromatosis in Ollier disease. Singap Med J. 2008;49(10):841–845; quiz 846.
40. Singh P, Kejariwal U, Chugh A. A rare occurrence of enchondroma in neck of femur in an adult female: a case report. J Clin Diagn Res. 2015;9(12):RD01–3.
41. Murphey MD, Flemming DJ, Boyea SR, Bojescul JA, Sweet DE, Temple HT. Enchondroma versus chondrosarcoma in the appendicular skeleton: differentiating features. Radiographics. 1998;18(5):1213–37; quiz 1244-1215.

42. Balke M, Schremper L, Gebert C, et al. Giant cell tumor of bone: treatment and outcome of 214 cases. J Cancer Res Clin Oncol. 2008;134(9):969–78.
43. Klenke FM, Wenger DE, Inwards CY, Rose PS, Sim FH. Recurrent giant cell tumor of long bones: analysis of surgical management. Clin Orthop Relat Res. 2011;469(4):1181–7.
44. Balke M, Streitbuerger A, Budny T, Henrichs M, Gosheger G, Hardes J. Treatment and outcome of giant cell tumors of the pelvis. Acta Orthop. 2009;80(5):590–6.
45. Blackley HR, Wunder JS, Davis AM, White LM, Kandel R, Bell RS. Treatment of giant-cell tumors of long bones with curettage and bone-grafting. J Bone Joint Surg Am. 1999;81(6):811–20.
46. Campanacci M, Baldini N, Boriani S, Sudanese A. Giant-cell tumor of bone. J Bone Joint Surg Am. 1987;69(1):106–14.
47. Larsson SE, Lorentzon R, Boquist L. Giant-cell tumor of bone. A demographic, clinical, and histopathological study of all cases recorded in the Swedish Cancer Registry for the years 1958 through 1968. J Bone Joint Surg Am. 1975;57(2):167–73.
48. Sung HW, Kuo DP, Shu WP, Chai YB, Liu CC, Li SM. Giant-cell tumor of bone: analysis of two hundred and eight cases in Chinese patients. J Bone Joint Surg Am. 1982;64(5):755–61.
49. Turcotte RE, Wunder JS, Isler MH, et al. Giant cell tumor of long bone: a Canadian Sarcoma Group study. Clin Orthop Relat Res. 2002;397:248–58.
50. Benevenia J, Patterson FR, Beebe KS, Abdelshahed MM, Uglialoro AD. Comparison of phenol and argon beam coagulation as adjuvant therapies in the treatment of stage 2 and 3 benign-aggressive bone tumors. Orthopedics. 2012;35(3):e371–8.
51. Lewis VO, Wei A, Mendoza T, Primus F, Peabody T, Simon MA. Argon beam coagulation as an adjuvant for local control of giant cell tumor. Clin Orthop Relat Res. 2007;454:192–7.
52. Klenke FM, Wenger DE, Inwards CY, Rose PS, Sim FH. Giant cell tumor of bone: risk factors for recurrence. Clin Orthop Relat Res. 2011;469(2):591–9.
53. Mittag F, Leichtle C, Kieckbusch I, et al. Cytotoxic effect and tissue penetration of phenol for adjuvant treatment of giant cell tumours. Oncol Lett. 2013;5(5):1595–8.
54. van der Heijden L, Dijkstra PD, Campanacci DA, Gibbons CL, van de Sande MA. Giant cell tumor with pathologic fracture: should we curette or resect? Clin Orthop Relat Res. 2013;471(3):820–9.
55. Deheshi BM, Jaffer SN, Griffin AM, Ferguson PC, Bell RS, Wunder JS. Joint salvage for pathologic fracture of giant cell tumor of the lower extremity. Clin Orthop Relat Res. 2007;459:96–104.
56. Zheng K, Yu X, Hu Y, Wang Z, Wu S, Ye Z. Surgical treatment for pelvic giant cell tumor: a multi-center study. World J Surg Oncol. 2016;14:104.
57. Chung LH, Wu PK, Chen CF, Weng HK, Chen TH, Chen WM. Pathological fractures in predicting clinical outcomes for patients with osteosarcoma. BMC Musculoskelet Disord. 2016;17(1):503.
58. Moradi B, Zahlten-Hinguranage A, Lehner B, Zeifang F. The impact of pathological fractures on therapy outcome in patients with primary malignant bone tumours. Int Orthop. 2010;34(7):1017–23.
59. Schlegel M, Zeumer M, Prodinger PM, et al. Impact of pathological fractures on the prognosis of primary malignant bone sarcoma in children and adults: a single-center retrospective study of 205 patients. Oncology. 2018;94(6):354–62.
60. Sun L, Li Y, Zhang J, Li H, Li B, Ye Z. Prognostic value of pathologic fracture in patients with high grade localized osteosarcoma: a systemic review and meta-analysis of cohort studies. J Orthop Res. 2015;33(1):131–9.
61. Zeifang F, Sabo D, Ewerbeck V. [Pathological fracture in primary malignant bone tumors]. Chirurg. 2000;71(9):1121–5.
62. Zuo D, Zheng L, Sun W, Hua Y, Cai Z. Pathologic fracture does not influence prognosis in stage IIB osteosarcoma: a case-control study. World J Surg Oncol. 2013;11:148.
63. Chandrasekar CR, Grimer RJ, Carter SR, Tillman RM, Abudu A, Buckley L. Modular endoprosthetic replacement for tumours of the proximal femur. J Bone Joint Surg Br. 2009;91(1):108–12.
64. Kawaguchi N, Ahmed AR, Matsumoto S, Manabe J, Matsushita Y. The concept of curative margin in surgery for bone and soft tissue sarcoma. Clin Orthop Relat Res. 2004;419:165–72.
65. Chen X, Yu LJ, Peng HM, et al. Is intralesional resection suitable for central grade 1 chondrosarcoma: a systematic review and updated meta-analysis. Eur J Surg Oncol. 2017;43(9):1718–26.
66. Chen YC, Wu PK, Chen CF, Chen WM. Intralesional curettage of central low-grade chondrosarcoma: a midterm follow-up study. J Chin Med Assoc. 2017;80(3):178–82.
67. Meftah M, Schult P, Henshaw RM. Long-term results of intralesional curettage and cryosurgery for treatment of low-grade chondrosarcoma. J Bone Joint Surg Am. 2013;95(15):1358–64.
68. Weber KL, Raymond AK. Low-grade/dedifferentiated/high-grade chondrosarcoma: a case of histological and biological progression. Iowa Orthop J. 2002;22:75–80.
69. Deloin X, Dumaine V, Biau D, et al. Pelvic chondrosarcomas: surgical treatment options. Orthop Traumatol Surg Res. 2009;95(6):393–401.
70. Pring ME, Weber KL, Unni KK, Sim FH. Chondrosarcoma of the pelvis. A review of sixty-four cases. J Bone Joint Surg Am. 2001;83-A(11):1630–42.
71. Brown TS, Salib CG, Rose PS, Sim FH, Lewallen DG, Abdel MP. Reconstruction of the hip after resection of periacetabular oncological lesions: a systematic review. Bone Joint J. 2018;100-B(1 Supple A):22–30.

72. Bus MP, Szafranski A, Sellevold S, et al. LUMiC((R)) endoprosthetic reconstruction after periacetabular tumor resection: short-term results. Clin Orthop Relat Res. 2017;475(3):686–95.
73. Hong AM, Millington S, Ahern V, et al. Limb preservation surgery with extracorporeal irradiation in the management of malignant bone tumor: the oncological outcomes of 101 patients. Ann Oncol. 2013;24(10):2676–80.
74. Liang H, Ji T, Zhang Y, Wang Y, Guo W. Reconstruction with 3D-printed pelvic endoprostheses after resection of a pelvic tumour. Bone Joint J. 2017;99-B(2):267–75.
75. Sharma DN, Rastogi S, Bakhshi S, et al. Role of extracorporeal irradiation in malignant bone tumors. Indian J Cancer. 2013;50(4):306–9.
76. Sun W, Li J, Li Q, Li G, Cai Z. Clinical effectiveness of hemipelvic reconstruction using computer-aided custom-made prostheses after resection of malignant pelvic tumors. J Arthroplast. 2011;26(8):1508–13.
77. Thambapillary S, Dimitriou R, Makridis KG, Fragkakis EM, Bobak P, Giannoudis PV. Implant longevity, complications and functional outcome following proximal femoral arthroplasty for musculoskeletal tumors: a systematic review. J Arthroplasty. 2013;28(8):1381–5.
78. Goorin AM, Schwartzentruber DJ, Devidas M, et al. Presurgical chemotherapy compared with immediate surgery and adjuvant chemotherapy for nonmetastatic osteosarcoma: Pediatric Oncology Group Study POG-8651. J Clin Oncol. 2003;21(8):1574–80.
79. Choy WS, Kim KJ, Lee SK, et al. Surgical treatment of pathological fractures occurring at the proximal femur. Yonsei Med J. 2015;56(2):460–5.
80. Issack PS, Kotwal SY, Lane JM. Management of metastatic bone disease of the acetabulum. J Am Acad Orthop Surg. 2013;21(11):685–95.
81. Mundy GR. Metastasis to bone: causes, consequences and therapeutic opportunities. Nat Rev Cancer. 2002;2(8):584–93.
82. Roudier MP, Vesselle H, True LD, et al. Bone histology at autopsy and matched bone scintigraphy findings in patients with hormone refractory prostate cancer: the effect of bisphosphonate therapy on bone scintigraphy results. Clin Exp Metastasis. 2003;20(2):171–80.
83. Gainor BJ, Buchert P. Fracture healing in metastatic bone disease. Clin Orthop Relat Res. 1983;178:297–302.
84. Bohm P, Huber J. The surgical treatment of bony metastases of the spine and limbs. J Bone Joint Surg Br. 2002;84(4):521–9.
85. Jacofsky DJ, Haidukewych GJ. Management of pathologic fractures of the proximal femur: state of the art. J Orthop Trauma. 2004;18(7):459–69.
86. Errani C, Mavrogenis AF, Cevolani L, et al. Treatment for long bone metastases based on a systematic literature review. Eur J Orthop Surg Traumatol. 2017;27(2):205–11.
87. Forsberg JA, Eberhardt J, Boland PJ, Wedin R, Healey JH. Estimating survival in patients with operable skeletal metastases: an application of a Bayesian belief network. PLoS One. 2011;6(5):e19956.
88. Katagiri H, Okada R, Takagi T, et al. New prognostic factors and scoring system for patients with skeletal metastasis. Cancer Med. 2014;3(5):1359–67.
89. Ratasvuori M, Wedin R, Hansen BH, et al. Prognostic role of en-bloc resection and late onset of bone metastasis in patients with bone-seeking carcinomas of the kidney, breast, lung, and prostate: SSG study on 672 operated skeletal metastases. J Surg Oncol. 2014;110(4):360–5.
90. Rougraff BT, Kneisl JS, Simon MA. Skeletal metastases of unknown origin. A prospective study of a diagnostic strategy. J Bone Joint Surg Am. 1993;75(9):1276–81.
91. Wolanczyk MJ, Fakhrian K, Adamietz IA. Radiotherapy, bisphosphonates and surgical stabilization of complete or impending pathologic fractures in patients with metastatic bone disease. J Cancer. 2016;7(1):121–4.
92. Muller DA, Capanna R. The surgical treatment of pelvic bone metastases. Adv Orthop. 2015;2015:525363.
93. Nilsson J, Gustafson P. Surgery for metastatic lesions of the femur: good outcome after 245 operations in 216 patients. Injury. 2008;39(4):404–10.
94. Morishige M, Muramatsu K, Tominaga Y, Hashimoto T, Taguchi T. Surgical treatment of metastatic femoral fractures: achieving an improved quality of life for cancer patients. Anticancer Res. 2015;35(1):427–32.
95. Mirels H. Metastatic disease in long bones. A proposed scoring system for diagnosing impending pathologic fractures. Clin Orthop Relat Res. 1989;249:256–64.
96. Damron TA, Morgan H, Prakash D, Grant W, Aronowitz J, Heiner J. Critical evaluation of Mirels' rating system for impending pathologic fractures. Clin Orthop Relat Res. 2003;415:S201–7.
97. Van der Linden YM, Dijkstra PD, Kroon HM, et al. Comparative analysis of risk factors for pathological fracture with femoral metastases. J Bone Joint Surg Br. 2004;86(4):566–73.
98. Menck H, Schulze S, Larsen E. Metastasis size in pathologic femoral fractures. Acta Orthop Scand. 1988;59(2):151–4.
99. Issack PS, Barker J, Baker M, Kotwal SY, Lane JM. Surgical management of metastatic disease of the proximal part of the femur. J Bone Joint Surg Am. 2014;96(24):2091–8.
100. Peterson JR, Decilveo AP, O'Connor IT, Golub I, Wittig JC. What are the functional results and complications with long stem hemiarthroplasty in patients with metastases to the proximal femur? Clin Orthop Relat Res. 2017;475(3):745–56.
101. Steensma M, Boland PJ, Morris CD, Athanasian E, Healey JH. Endoprosthetic treatment is more

durable for pathologic proximal femur fractures. Clin Orthop Relat Res. 2012;470(3):920–6.
102. Wedin R, Bauer HC. Surgical treatment of skeletal metastatic lesions of the proximal femur: endoprosthesis or reconstruction nail? J Bone Joint Surg Br. 2005;87(12):1653–7.
103. Yazawa Y, Frassica FJ, Chao EY, Pritchard DJ, Sim FH, Shives TC. Metastatic bone disease. A study of the surgical treatment of 166 pathologic humeral and femoral fractures. Clin Orthop Relat Res. 1990;251:213–9.
104. Capanna R, Campanacci DA. The treatment of metastases in the appendicular skeleton. J Bone Joint Surg Br. 2001;83(4):471–81.
105. Alvi HM, Damron TA. Prophylactic stabilization for bone metastases, myeloma, or lymphoma: do we need to protect the entire bone? Clin Orthop Relat Res. 2013;471(3):706–14.
106. Scarborough MT. CORR Insights (R): Intramedullary nailing of femoral diaphyseal metastases: is it necessary to protect the femoral neck? Clin Orthop Relat Res. 2015;473(4):1503–4.
107. Miller BJ, Soni EE, Gibbs CP, Scarborough MT. Intramedullary nails for long bone metastases: why do they fail? Orthopedics. 2011;34(4):274.
108. Friedl W. [Double plate compound osteosynthesis. A procedure for primary stress-stable management of problem injuries of the subtrochanteric to supracondylar femoral area]. Aktuelle Traumatol. 1992;22(5):189–96.
109. Gruber G, Zacherl M, Leithner A, et al. [Surgical treatment of pathologic fractures of the humerus and femur]. Orthopade. 2009;38(4):324, 326–8, 330–4.
110. Friedl W, Ruf W, Mischkowsky T. [Compound double plate osteosynthesis in subtrochanteric pathologic fractures. A clinical and experimental study]. Chirurg. 1986;57(11):713–18.
111. Ganz R, Fernandez D. [Treatment of pathological fractures in metastases]. Ther Umsch. 1973;30(4):307–9.
112. Schottle H, Sauer HD, Jungbluth KH. [Measurements of stability of operative osteosynthesis on the proximal femur (author's transl)]. Arch Orthop Unfallchir. 1977;89(1):87–100.
113. Rompe JD, Eysel P, Hopf C, Heine J. Metastatic instability at the proximal end of the femur. Comparison of endoprosthetic replacement and plate osteosynthesis. Arch Orthop Trauma Surg. 1994;113(5):260–4.
114. Merckaert S, Siebenrock K, Tannast M. Compound osteosynthesis of the proximal femur as a choice for the treatment of pathological proximal femoral fractures. American Academy of Orthoppaedic Surgerons (AAOS) Annual Meeting, San Diego, USA; 2017.
115. Picci P, Manfrini M, Fabbri N, Gambarotti M, Vanel D. Atlas of musculoskeletal tumors and tumorlike lesions. Berlin: Springer; 2014.
116. Yasko AW, Rutledge J, Lewis VO, Lin PP. Disease- and recurrence-free survival after surgical resection of solitary bone metastases of the pelvis. Clin Orthop Relat Res. 2007;459:128–32.
117. Harrington KD. The management of acetabular insufficiency secondary to metastatic malignant disease. J Bone Joint Surg Am. 1981;63(4):653–64.
118. Cotten A, Deprez X, Migaud H, Chabanne B, Duquesnoy B, Chastanet P. Malignant acetabular osteolyses: percutaneous injection of acrylic bone cement. Radiology. 1995;197(1):307–10.
119. Guzik G. Treatment of metastatic lesions localized in the acetabulum. J Orthop Surg Res. 2016;11(1):54.
120. Scaramuzzo L, Maccauro G, Rossi B, Messuti L, Maffulli N, Logroscino CA. Quality of life in patients following percutaneous PMMA acetabuloplasty for acetabular metastasis due to carcinoma. Acta Orthop Belg. 2009;75(4):484–9.
121. Clayer M. The survivorship of protrusio cages for metastatic disease involving the acetabulum. Clin Orthop Relat Res. 2010;468(11):2980–4.
122. Ho L, Ahlmann ER, Menendez LR. Modified Harrington reconstruction for advanced periacetabular metastatic disease. J Surg Oncol. 2010;101(2):170–4.
123. Marco RA, Sheth DS, Boland PJ, Wunder JS, Siegel JA, Healey JH. Functional and oncological outcome of acetabular reconstruction for the treatment of metastatic disease. J Bone Joint Surg Am. 2000;82(5):642–51.
124. Tillman RM, Myers GJ, Abudu AT, Carter SR, Grimer RJ. The three-pin modified 'Harrington' procedure for advanced metastatic destruction of the acetabulum. J Bone Joint Surg Br. 2008;90(1):84–7.
125. Kitagawa Y, Ek ET, Choong PF. Pelvic reconstruction using saddle prosthesis following limb salvage operation for periacetabular tumour. J Orthop Surg (Hong Kong). 2006;14(2):155–62.

14 Acetabular and Femoral Neck Fracture Nonunion and Malunion

Robert C. Jacobs, Craig S. Bartlett, and Michael Blankstein

Abstract

Nonunion and malunion are uncommon complications following femoral neck fracture and even more rarely reported after a fracture of the acetabulum. These complications can be difficult to diagnose but can be successfully treated with a large number of patients experiencing good to excellent outcomes. Algorithmic approaches for each are included including the conversion to total hip arthroplasty after unsuccessful open reduction internal fixation of an acetabular fracture.

With respect to the acetabulum, malunion is likely more common than previously thought. Case examples for conversion to total hip arthroplasty after acetabular malunion and open reduction internal fixation after acetabular nonunion are included. Due to their bimodal demographics of young and old, fractures of the femoral neck have significant differences with respect to both their etiology and treatment. A case example for conversion of nonunion to total hip arthroplasty is included.

R. C. Jacobs (✉) · C. S. Bartlett · M. Blankstein
University of Vermont, Burlington, VT, USA
e-mail: robert.jacobs@uvmhealth.org

Keywords

Acetabular · Acetabulum · Nonunion · Malunion · Fracture · Femoral neck

14.1 Acetabular Fractures

14.1.1 Introduction

14.1.1.1 Incidence

Open reduction with internal fixation (ORIF) is the gold standard of treatment for most displaced acetabular fractures. Nonunion is a rare complication after ORIF with a rate less than 5% [1–4], occurring most commonly after transverse or associated transverse fracture patterns [1, 3, 5]. Malunion after an acetabular fracture is seen in less than 6% of cases [4]. The incidences of these two complications vary by the approach and the type of fracture as classified by Judet and Letournel [1]. Unfortunately, most large series presenting clinical and functional results of acetabular fractures do not elaborate on their occurrence or treatment [6–14].

The incidence of acetabular malunion may be loosely inferred using reported reduction quality after ORIF from post-operative or follow-up imaging as a surrogate measure. There are many subjective and different objective methods of reporting reduction quality. Most recent authors use the criteria of Matta [2] to define the reduction as anatomic (0–1 mm), imperfect (2–3 mm)

L. Büchler, M. J.B. Keel (eds.), *Fractures of the Hip*, Fracture Management Joint by Joint,
https://doi.org/10.1007/978-3-030-18838-2_14

or poor (>3 mm) based on the residual displacement noted on plain radiograph (AP and Judet views) [15]. If a malunion is defined as a healed fracture with >3 mm of residual displacement plain radiographs, then the real incidence of acetabular malunion is likely significantly higher with ranges between 4.0% and 32.6% [1–4, 6–8, 10–14, 16]. In his landmark paper, Letournel did not report specific measurements but did have "imperfect reductions" in 26% of 417 operatively treated cases [1].

Determining the incidence of malunion is further complicated by the fact that plain radiographs overestimate reduction quality due to the complex anatomy of the acetabulum, especially in fractures involving the posterior wall. In a study of 100 patients, Moed et al. noted 97 anatomic reductions by plain radiographs despite recognizing gaps of >3 mm intraoperatively in 41 cases [9].

The definitions of a malunion or nonunion can also be challenging as they are not universally agreed upon and are constantly evolving [17]. Unlike long bone fractures, obtaining quality imaging is more challenging and it is difficult to apply plain radiographic criteria to assess for multiple healed cortices.

14.1.1.2 Other Complications After ORIF of Acetabular Fractures

One of the most common complications following displaced acetabular fractures treated with ORIF is osteoarthritis. Giannoudis et al. reported a rate of severe osteoarthritis of almost 20% in a 2005 meta-analysis [18] with more recent authors reporting similar results [6]. There is also evidence that the rates of post-traumatic arthritis after ORIF of an acetabular fracture decrease with surgical specialization, increased experience and treatment in a tertiary referral setting [18]. Risk factors negatively affecting outcomes include: increasing patient age [2, 4, 6, 9, 10, 19], fracture pattern complexity [2, 6, 18, 19], increased time to surgery [1, 2, 6, 9, 16], local complications (including infection and avascular necrosis) [2, 10, 18], and heterotopic ossification (HO) [2, 3, 10, 18].

The use of indomethacin for prevention of HO following acetabular surgery has been commonplace for decades. Nevertheless, recent literature suggests that indomethacin treatment in posterior wall acetabular fractures may be associated with rates of nonunion approaching 62% [20]. The use of indomethacin may explain some of the of nonunions reported during conversion to total hip arthroplasty (THA), however the rates vary depending on the series and are subject to study design biases [5].

Despite anatomical reduction, rapid progression to arthritis can occur within the first few months following ORIF of a displaced acetabular fracture. Articular malreduction resulting in malunion or nonunion further compounds the significant damage to the osteochondral surface at the time of injury and is almost uniformly associated with poor functional outcomes [2, 4]. Studies have shown that THA after attempted ORIF occurs at rates at 6–35%, though this depends on fracture pattern [3, 11, 14]. It is interesting that younger patients frequently have more complicated fracture patterns, more severe injuries and worse radiographs but have similar or better functional outcomes [2]. They also tend to progress to THA more rapidly than the elderly patients, perhaps in part to the increased functional demands they place on their reconstructions [21, 22], however this is not born out in all studies [19].

14.1.2 Outcomes After Non-operative Treatment of Acetabular Fractures

Displaced acetabular fractures (>3 mm diastasis or step-off) have significantly decreased outcomes when treated nonoperatively when compared to those treated with modern techniques of open reduction and internal fixation [23]. This discrepancy in outcomes has limited non-operative treatment of acetabular fractures to those with near anatomic alignment, the elderly with secondary congruence, the severely poly traumatized patient who has significant medical comorbidities [23] and those with stable posterior wall fractures after exam under anesthesia [24]. Patients with minimally displaced acetabular fractures with ≤2 mm of step-off have reported 10-year hip survival rates of 94% without arthroplasty intervention and functional outcomes of good to excellent in 88% and 89% of patients [25].

14.1.3 Outcomes of ORIF of Acetabular Fractures

When operatively treated with an ORIF, reductions of ≤3 mm have been associated with good to excellent radiographic and functional outcomes in up to 70% of cases [2–4, 6, 9, 10, 18, 19]; even in the setting of extended approaches [13] and elderly patients [26]. Acetabular fractures with good to excellent functional outcomes after 2 years can usually expect to have good long-term outcomes at 10 and 20 years [6, 19, 25]. However, there are many fractures that progress rapidly to joint space loss, pain, and debilitating arthritis and require additional surgical intervention in an effort to provide a more functional joint [11, 19]. A predictive nomogram was developed based on the experience of Matta that helps predict the patients who will most likely need a THA after ORIF of acetabular fracture [19].

There are few select series that report on the delayed treatment of acetabular fractures and treatment of acetabular nonunions using ORIF [1, 16, 27]. These all report worse functional and radiographic outcomes of patients undergoing delayed ORIF compared to patients who receive operative intervention within 3 weeks of injury.

14.1.4 Outcomes of Revision ORIF of Acetabular Fractures

Less frequently reported in the literature are the results of revision ORIF of displaced acetabular fractures. If re-operated on within 3 weeks, 59% can still achieve good-excellent clinical results, however the outcomes are significantly worse for those treated beyond 12 weeks (29% good to excellent outcomes) [16, 27]. The need for surgery in most cases was the result of hardware failure with resulting redisplacement or surgical malreductions [5, 27].

Quality literature regarding revision ORIF for displaced acetabular fractures is scarce and often combines patients treated in both the acute and delayed fashion, the latter group overlapping with malunion and nonunion cohorts [5, 16]. In either case of revision or delayed ORIF, extensile approaches are often required and carry significant additional morbidity; with increased complications including infection, HO, avascular necrosis of the femoral head, and need for conversion to total hip arthroplasty [1, 2, 12, 13, 16, 19].

14.1.5 Evolution of the Conversion to THA

Conversion to total hip arthroplasty is the salvage operation of choice for most patients with arthritis of the hip joint following ORIF or non-operative treatment of a displaced acetabular fracture [28–30]. Some of the first efforts in this field met with poor results and high levels of morbidity. These studies showed significant rates of acetabular component failure and higher than expected revision rates of both acetabular and to a lesser extent, femoral components [21]. However, with improved understanding of the treatment of these complex patients, so have the results [22].

14.1.6 Outcomes After Conversion to THA

Short- and long-term outcomes of patients after conversion to THA after a displaced acetabular fracture show significant functional improvements with better functional scores in younger patients [29, 31–34]. Regarding outcomes, most results are not comparable to age matched patients undergoing primary THA [35] with complication rates more comparable to those expected after revision THA [28, 36]. However, there are some authors who report mid-term survivorship rates approaching the levels seen after primary THA with the only major differences being increased operative time, blood loss, and post-operative complications [22, 28, 31].

Overall, most recent studies report improved mid-term revision rates between 0 and 32% [28, 29]. The literature is relatively sparse regarding the long-term outcomes in these patients with 20-year acetabular survival rates at 57% [34]. Younger patients undergoing delayed arthroplasty after ORIF of an acetabular fracture can also expect a shorter time to revision THA [21, 35]. Regardless, patients requiring conversion to THA after ORIF of a displaced acetabular fracture are at increased risk for nerve injury, dislocation, infection, HO formation, loosening, and hardware failure [29, 35].

14.1.7 Preoperative Evaluation

When evaluating a patient for a potential nonunion or malunion following a previous acetabular fracture, care should be taken to spend adequate time on achieving a complete history and performing a detailed physical exam. The previous rationale for treatment of the acetabular fracture should be carefully reviewed. The course of initial recovery should also be scrutinized to help rule out additional hip pathology, especially infection.

If infection is on the differential diagnosis, then inflammatory markers should be drawn and repeated as necessary. If there is a high clinical suspicion, synovial fluid should be aspirated and sent for gram stain/culture, synovial cell count, differential and crystal analysis.

A thorough endocrine workup should also be considered as a part of the preoperative evaluation. In patients with an unexplained nonunion, Brinker et al. found that 84% had a treatable endocrine abnormality. Furthermore, 8/37 patients eventually healed their nonunion with correction of the abnormality and non-operative treatment [37]. Smoking cessation should also be attempted as it is associated with an increased time to union, as well as surgical complications, delayed healing, and need for multiple surgeries [38].

Regardless if a patient has undergone previous ORIF or non-operative treatment, complete imaging radiographs (AP and Judet views) of the pelvis are minimum requirements. Thin slice computed tomography (CT) scans are also generally recommended. Other helpful adjuncts are metal suppression CT scans with 3D reconstruction imaging. Magnetic resonance imaging (MRI) can also be considered to identify possible occult infection and femoral head avascular necrosis. This too can be performed with specific metal suppression sequences and imaging of the entire pelvis is helpful to allow comparison with the normal hip.

All operative notes should be obtained and the patient examined so that previous incisions and surgical intervals can be utilized when possible. This will also help develop an appropriate plan to address hardware for possible removal. Lastly, the expected outcomes of conversion THA after failed acetabular ORIF need to be weighed against the expected outcomes of revision ORIF. In most circumstances of nonunion or malunion, conversion to THA is recommended over revision ORIF due to its better overall outcomes in a wider selection of patients.

14.1.8 Surgical Planning of Revision ORIF

A successful surgical outcome starts with the development of a thorough surgical plan with contingencies in place for the major intraoperative hurdles. This is built upon a detailed history, physical exam, and discussions with the patient.

As mentioned previously, the surgeon should understand why the malunion or nonunion occurred and what critical steps will restore joint reduction and stability. Revision ORIF usually requires an extensile approach which carries significant morbidity [16]. The approach chosen should be matched to the nonunion or malunion deformity to be corrected and stabilized. Existing hardware should be evaluated for retention vs. removal and existing bone stock should be analyzed for quality and quantity. If multiple incisions will be required, the morbidity of these approaches should be weighed against the expected outcomes from a single approach conversion to THA.

An infectious and metabolic work-up should proceed as mentioned in the previous section. Previous operative reports, implant records, and skin incisions should be evaluated to see if revision ORIF is feasible. Specific plans for dealing with the location of hardware to be encountered, bone stock and instability should be in place, with backup options as needed.

The expectation of possible intraoperative complications and potential inability to achieve bony stability and/or anatomic acetabular joint congruence should be addressed. If the goals listed above of surgery cannot be achieved intraoperatively, then the procedure should be converted to a total hip arthroplasty. A non-anatomic reduction in the setting of delayed revision ORIF is associated with a poor outcome [16].

A separate preoperative plan for both revision ORIF and intraoperative conversion to THA should be prepared including under which conditions the procedure would be completed in a multi-approach or staged fashion. All necessary equipment for both procedures should be readily available before surgery. A surgical team with the appropriate skill set is critical. This will likely include an orthopedic traumatologist comfortable in treatment of complex acetabular fractures and an orthopedic reconstructive surgeon comfortable in revision of complex total hip arthroplasty if the primary surgeon is not facile in all portions of both procedures.

Case Example 1

A 19 year old male was the driver in a motor vehicle crash and sustained an isolated right hip posterior wall fracture dislocation. He was reduced successfully in the emergency department (Fig. 14.1a–e).

14.1.9 Surgical Planning of Conversion to THA

A successful surgical outcome starts with the development of a thorough surgical plan with contingencies in place for the major intraoperative hurdles. The most common patient to present for conversion to THA is one with a posterior wall component to the fracture pattern. These patients also have the worst outcomes amongst the 10 acetabular fracture patterns [1, 2, 11]. Fortunately most posterior wall patients have intact bone stock and do not require bone grafting. Restoration of native hip center should be a priority. Those patients with a hip center greater than 20 mm from normal after THA have increased rates of revision [22, 31].

In the setting of bone loss, bony stability can be achieved by several principles similar to those underlying revision total hip arthroplasty [39, 40]. Metal augments are increasingly being used in the revision arthroplasty setting to deal with large areas of bone loss, especially with a deficient posterior wall [33]. Other prosthetic considerations include porous titanium cups with multihole designs and cup/cage constructs [41]. These allow screw fixation through the acetabular component into the ilium, ischium, and even pubis. While they can be employed successfully with less than 50% native bony contact with the acetabular component, there is a trend to improved mid-term outcomes with more than 50% host bone contact [42].

There is still a role for using autograft and/or allograft to restore bone stock in the acetabular malunion or nonunion with bone loss [5, 28, 33, 43]. The stability of the grafts must be ensured with plate and screw fixation or incorporation into the final acetabular component [5, 43]. As discussed previously, cemented acetabular components can provide good outcomes in certain patients [22], however more recent uncemented revisions have been shown to have improved results [32].

The workhorse approach for addressing a conversion THA after acetabular fracture remains the Kocher-Langenbeck (KL) approach. If a previous posterior approach has been performed, then the original hardware the fracture will be more readily accessible should the need arise. Intra-articular hardware can be removed with the use of a metal-cutting burr and ultrasound gel in the setting of a buried screw [44].

Recreation of the hip center can be assisted with the use of computer navigation and preoperative computer assisted design templating. Additional methods for increasing stability after placement of the acetabular construct include the use of lipped liners and dual-mobility head components [28–31].

The Kocher-Langenbeck approach also allows for an easier extensile view of both the acetabulum and femoral shaft if needed. It can also accommodate partial or complete release of the gluteus maximus, digastric osteotomy, and an extended trochanteric osteotomy more easily than other approaches. As such, the subsequent operative plan and imaging will focus on the KL approach for treatment (Table 14.1).

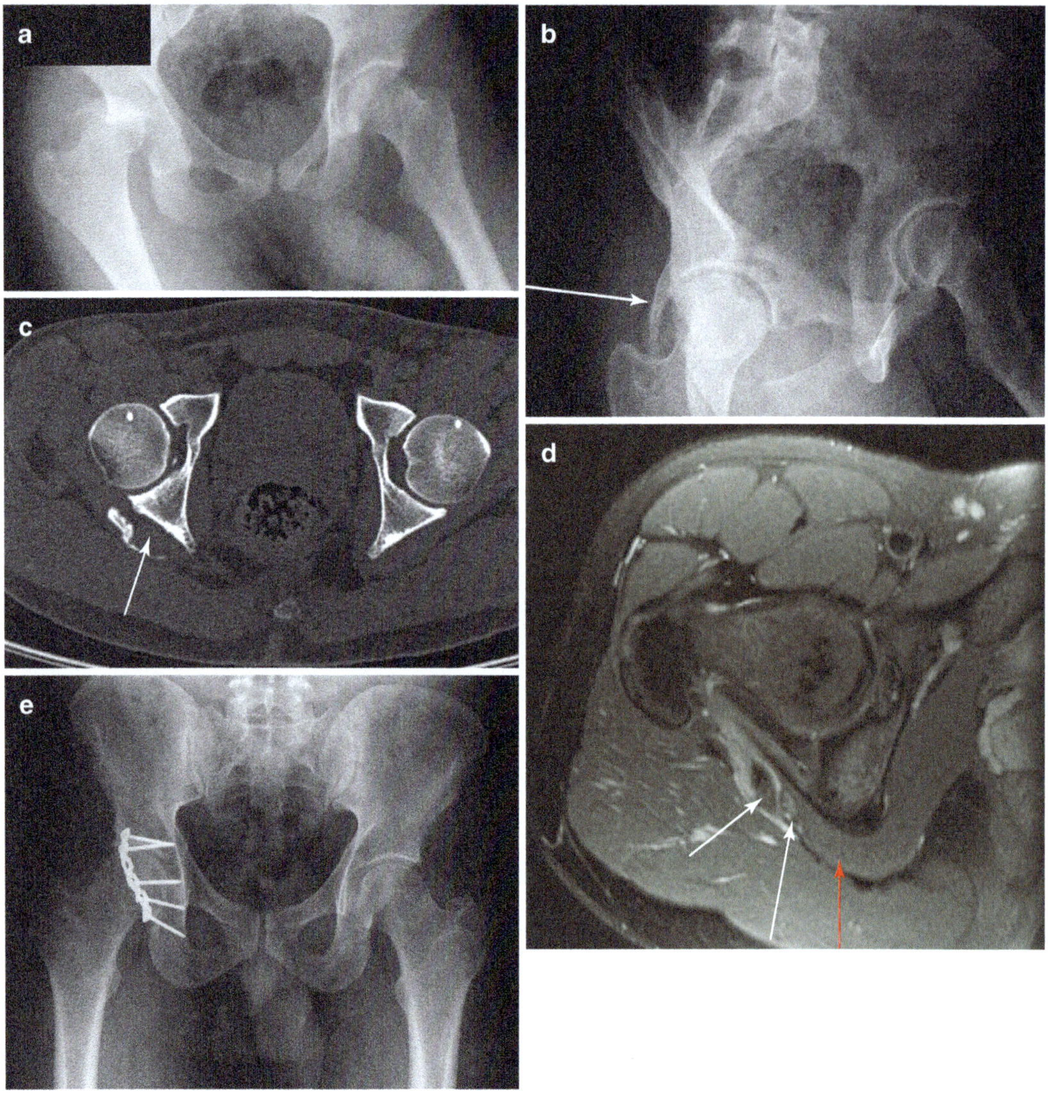

Fig. 14.1 (**a**) AP pelvis radiograph demonstrating right hip dislocation with posterior wall acetabular fracture. The patient declined admission and was subsequently lost to follow-up. He represented to our clinic 9 months later after a fall from standing onto his knees with subsequent feeling of right hip subluxation and instability. He had been noticing increasing pain and paresthesias in a distribution consistent with the right sciatic nerve for several months. Radiographs, CT scans, and MRI were obtained confirming right acetabular nonunion with the sciatic nerve entrapped within the fracture site. (**b**) Obturator oblique radiograph demonstrating heterotopic bone formation about the displaced posterior wall acetabular fragment (white arrow). (**c**) A representative axial CT image demonstrating the entrapped sciatic nerve (white arrow) within the right acetabular nonunion. (**d**) T2 fat-saturated weighted MRI showing the sciatic nerve (white arrow) and piriformis tendon (red arrow) entrapped within the nonunion. The posterior wall fragment (black arrow) is lateral to the nerve. The patient was subsequently taken to the operating room for exploration of the right sciatic nerve and ORIF of the right acetabular nonunion through a Kocher-Langenbeck approach. The sciatic nerve was identified and freed from the nonunion. A femoral distractor was used assist in direct visualization of the hip joint; grade 2 cartilage wear was noted on the femoral head. The posterior wall fragment was anatomically reduced and secured with a plate and screws. (**e**) Ten-year follow-up AP pelvis radiograph demonstrating intact fixation, preserved joint space with pain free range of motion without any activity limitations

Table 14.1 Algorithm for conversion THA after unsuccessful ORIF of femoral neck fractures or acetabular fracture

Indication	– Nonunion – Malunion – Avascular necrosis of the femoral head – Post-traumatic osteoarthritis of the hip			
Goals	– Confirm the absence of infection – Restore pelvis/acetabular stability to receive the THA – Stable hip postoperatively with restoration of hip center if possible – Functional, pain free ambulation and ROM			
Preoperative algorithm	*General*	*Radiograph*	*Acetabular bone stock*	*Femoral hardware*
	• Ensure appropriate indications for surgery • Preop. rule out of infection – Ruled out → proceed – If infected; then patient is not ready for THA, plan should be changed to appropriate treatment of infection – MRSA screen Positive: Povidone nasal swabs preoperatively and vancomycin intraoperatively Negative: Standard preoperative antibiotics • Critical evaluation of previous operative reports – Skin incision – Deep interval – Hardware applied and manufacturer identified, removal tools available	• Critical evaluation of imaging (XR and CT) • Acetabular hardware – Absent → proceed – Hardware present requires removal If accessible for primary removal through KL approach: KL approach with plan to remove minimal amount of hardware as necessary to complete THA If not accessible primarily, buried hardware will need to be removed from the acetabulum during the course of preparation	• Adequate or minimal loss: – Without nonunion: proceed – With nonunion: Hardware removal as necessary to allow for revision ORIF with bone grafting and restoration of stability prior to THA • Inadequate – Use AAOS or Paprosky classifications and principles for dealing with bone loss as in revision THA [45, 46] – Nonunion or Malunion Augmentation Trabecular metal augment to restore posterior wall and/or column support Multihole porous metal revision cup Cup/cage construct Maintains ability to place screws into ilium and ischium Bone graft (autograft ± allograft) with ORIF ± augment Type I (posterior wall deficiency): Buttress with femoral head or iliac crest Type II (contained cavitary): Morcelize and impact Type III (column/wall deficiency): Strut allograft ± femoral head or iliac crest	• Not present: proceed • Hardware present (compression hip screw, cannulated screws, cephalomedullary nail) – Surgically dislocate hip prior to hardware removal – Reduce hip and remove hardware

(continued)

Table 14.1 (continued)

Approach/ positioning	• KL in lateral decubitus position – Extensile – Can incorporate trochanteric slide osteotomy for improved visualization • Other approaches not recommended – Increased difficulty to address posterior wall and/or column deficiencies intraoperatively – Increased difficulty to address intraoperative femur fracture – Subsequent revision surgery is more challenging			
Intraoperative	*Surgical exposure*	*Culture/sonication*	*Stability*	*Closure*
	• KL approach and bone cut for removal of femoral head and neck • Identification and protection of sciatic nerve • Address femoral hardware if necessary • Address acetabular hardware if necessary • Hardware removal – Minimum necessary with stable bone stock – Buried: Metal- cutting burr and ultrasound gel	• Intraoperative rule out of infection • Minimum two cultures for gram stain, culture for anaerobes, aerobes • Native section for histology • Frozen section to pathology STAT – Less than 5 neutrophils per high power field: proceed – More than 5 neutrophils per high power field: convert to antibiotic articulating hip spacer or Gridlestone – Consider sonication and culture of hardware	• Revision acetabular ORIF with autograft ± structural allograft (if needed) • Fill contained cavitary bone defects with femoral head autograft ± allograft (if needed) • Ream for line to line sizing of the acetabular component • Application of acetabular hardware – Augments – Multihole revision cup – Cup/cage construct • Ensure stability of the acetabulum before proceeding to the femoral component • Stability adjuncts – Medialization of acetabulum to ensure host bony support – Additional screw fixation into ilium, ischium, pubis Awareness of safe zones is critical – Lipped liner (10–20°) – Lateralized liner in setting of medialized acetabular component – Dual mobility cup – Larger heads – Increased offset through increased neck length modularity • Femoral component stability – Press fit stem Younger patient with good bone quality – Cemented stem: Older patient Poor bone stock Previous instrumentation – Anteversion can be increased to improve stability	• Multiple layers • Drains as necessary

Post-operative	*Weight bearing*	*Mobility*	*Pain control*	*DVT prophylaxis/ antibiotics*
	• As tolerated – If preoperative bony stability verified • Toe touch weight bearing – If bony pelvis unstable preoperatively – If bony instability recognized intraoperatively – Advance weight bearing at 8 weeks	• Ambulation post-operative day 1 with assistive device • Daily physical therapy/occupational therapy for gait training, ROM, stairs • Posterior hip precautions – For 3 months post operatively – Limit flexion to 90° – Avoid internal rotation beyond neutral – Avoid adduction past neutral	• Multimodal oral medications preferred	• Per institutional protocol • Antibiotics × 24 h or drains removed

Case Example 2
A 23 year old male involved in a motor vehicle accident presents with right hip dislocation and comminuted posterior wall acetabular fracture with a nondisplaced transverse component. His hip was reduced in the emergency department under conscious sedation within 7 h of injury (after transfer from outside hospital where staff were unable to reduce his hip). His sciatic nerve function was preserved pre and post reduction (Figs. 14.2a–e).

14.2 Femoral Neck Fractures

14.2.1 Introduction

Femoral neck nonunion is the most common complication following surgical fixation of a displaced femoral neck fracture with recent studies reporting rates of 10–30% [47–49]. When combined with avascular necrosis of the femoral head, these two complications affect up to 20–50% of patients [47–49].

Femoral neck fractures have a bimodal distribution occurring primarily due to high-energy mechanisms in the young population and lower energy mechanisms in the elderly cohort [47, 50, 51]. However, they are uncommon in patients younger than age 50, encompassing only 3% of total hip fractures [51]. In contrast, their incidence rises substantially in the elderly, with 27.7 and 63.3 per 1000 patients for men and women, respectively [52]. They make up approximately half of the proximal femur fractures in the geriatric population after fall from standing height [51].

Displaced femoral neck fractures are associated with significant morbidity in the young patient cohort as they most commonly occur in the setting of a high energy mechanism [47, 53]. In these cases, there is often significant damage to the proximal femoral soft tissues and periosteum. The neck area is a watershed for blood supply where the main contribution from the medial femoral circumflex artery ascends posteriorly within the quadratus femoris. It stays ventral to the piriformis tendon and penetrates the hip capsule before arborizing within the periosteum of the superior femoral neck [54].

Femoral neck fractures are intracapsular and lack a periosteal blood supply thereby increasing the risk of nonunion even after stabilization. This challenging complication occurs even more frequently than malunion [49].

The morphology of the fracture also plays a significant role in the development of a nonunion. In young patients the high energy mechanism can generate fracture lines that tend to be more vertically oriented [50] and classified as Pauwels' type III (above 50°) [55]. The shearing forces seen across the fracture site predispose to varus angulation and nonunion rather than healing under compression [56]. Since the early characterizations of femoral neck fractures by Pauwels [55], the Garden classification has become commonly used and relies on the displacement of the femoral head relative to the neck [57]. Garden stages III and IV are considered displaced and are at higher risk for nonunion after fixation than stages I and II [57].

The recently published "fracture fixation in the operative management of hip fractures" (FAITH) trial compared the effect of using a sliding hip screw against cannulated screws for fixation of femoral neck fractures in the elderly population [58]. It did not find a difference in the nonunion rate between the different groups based on the Garden or Pauwels' classifications (though it was not specifically powered to identify this parameter). It also did not find a difference in reoperation rate between fixation methods [58].

14.2.2 Definition and Diagnosis

The absence of obvious radiographic union and a patient with ongoing pain and limp for several months after operative fixation should prompt the surgeon to have a high suspicion for femoral neck nonunion. The patient with progressive hardware failure on sequential radiographs, late fracture migration or femoral neck shortening should also be evaluated for nonunion [59]. The differential diagnosis should also include malunion, delayed union with inadequate fixation,

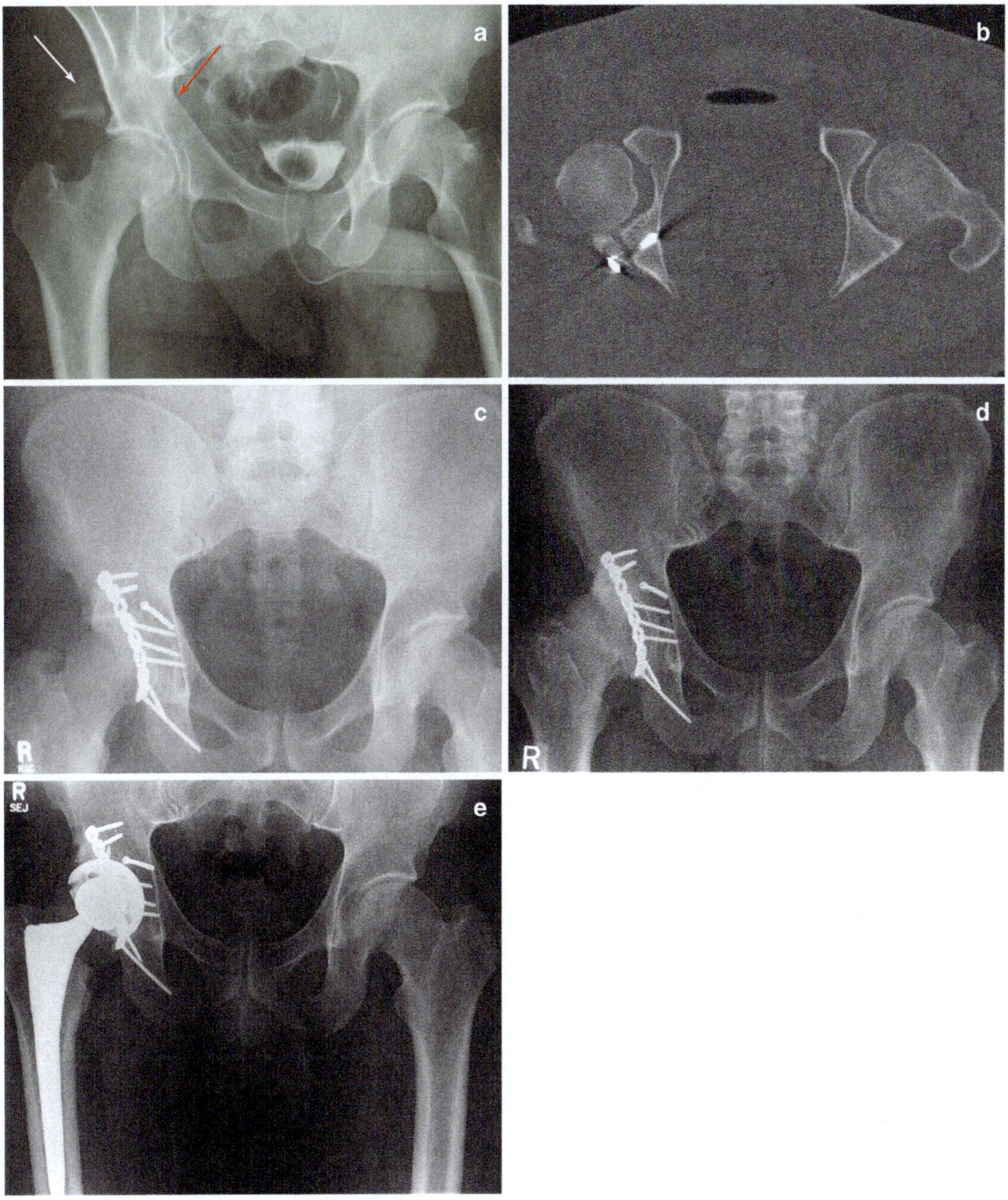

Fig. 14.2 (**a**) Obturator oblique view demonstrating the nondisplaced transverse fracture (red arrow). There are multiple posterior wall fragments. The largest measures approximately 35 × 35 mm (white arrow). (**b**) A Kocher-Langenbeck approach was used to treat the acetabular fracture. There was cartilage loss on the femoral head side and several non-viable pieces of comminuted posterior wall bone and cartilage were removed. Retroacetabular congruence was obtained under direct visualization and intraoperative fluoroscopy demonstrated a near anatomic reduction. A post-operative CT was taken demonstrating 5 mm of gapping at the fracture site related to the bone loss but without step-off. (**c**) AP pelvis radiograph showing concentric reduction. (**d**) AP pelvis radiograph 5 years later demonstrates complete joint space loss of the right hip with intact hardware. No evidence of hardware failure or displacement of the transverse posterior wall fractures was noted. There was sufficient retained posterior wall and no hardware expected within the area of expected acetabular reaming, therefore a CT scan was deferred. (**e**) AP pelvis radiograph 4 months after THA. Good bone stock was noted intraoperatively and no hardware was encountered with acetabular reaming. Multiple acetabular screws were placed and excellent purchase was noted. The patient has returned to work as a laborer and has hip range of motion equal to the uninjured side

and infection. Ultimately, the diagnosis of nonunion is multifactorial and takes into account the ongoing clinical findings, physical examination, and radiographic data.

The definition of a femoral neck nonunion can be challenging, in part due to the lack of consensus regarding imaging findings, time at which nonunion is declared and location of the fracture [17]. In 2013 the Radiographic Union Score for Hip (RUSH) was published as a validated scoring checklist system that for predicting radiographic hip fracture union [60–62]. It has shown improved intra- and interobserver reliability in accurately predicting union [62] and was recently used on a cohort of patients from the FAITH trial where it was able to accurately predict radiographic nonunion with 100% specificity and positive predictive values for a specific threshold scoring level [63].

Finally, computed tomography can be used to help diagnose nonunions but can have limited specificity (62%) even with 100% sensitivity [64].

14.2.3 Incidence of Femoral Neck Nonunion

14.2.3.1 Elderly Patients

In the physiologically elderly population, displaced femoral neck fractures (Garden III/IV) are usually treated with some form of arthroplasty whereas nondisplaced fractures (Garden I/II) are typically treated with cannulated hip screws or a sliding hip screw construct [58]. The definition of "elderly" is vague and is intentionally not defined here as a 45 year old with end stage renal disease on dialysis may receive a hemiarthoplasty and a healthy, active 60 year old may undergo ORIF for the same displaced femoral neck fracture.

Recent literature has suggested also that the nonunion rate in the elderly may vary according to the treatment methods with a 19% rate for cannulated screws and an 8% for a fixed angle device [65], though this was not supported by the FAITH trial with a 6% nonunion rate for both devices [58]. Since a significant portion of the fractures have been treated by methods (e.g., arthroplasty) other than open reduction internal fixation (ORIF), data regarding the rate of femoral neck nonunion in the elderly are more challenging to interpret than in the younger cohort.

14.2.3.2 Young Patients

In a recent meta-analysis, patients younger than age 50 had a nonunion rate of 8.9% after ORIF [47]. It does not appear to be higher if surgery is delayed more than 12 h (or even as many as 48 h) [66], although there are conflicting reports in a number of studies [47]. Displaced fractures at presentation are more likely to go on to nonunion after ORIF (compared to nondisplaced fractures) with rates between 6 and 33% [47, 67]. Femoral neck fractures fixed in varus angulation or those fixed with increasing fracture displacement are more likely to fail to unite compared to those with anatomical reductions [66]. This is of particular importance in the young population as these fractures most often present with significant posterior and inferior comminution (80%) and vertically oriented fracture lines in excess of 60° [50]. They are shortened and externally rotated with varus coronal alignment, and apex anterior axial fracture orientation [50]—precisely the orientation associated with increased rates of nonunion [66]. Regardless of open or closed reduction and the treatment method employed, better union rates are achieved after an anatomic reduction [68].

14.2.4 Management Principles: Non-operative Treatment

The work-up of any suspected nonunion begins with the history and physical exam. A patient with a femoral neck nonunion will often present with ongoing deep groin pain and difficulty ambulating without an assistive device [59, 69]. They will also often fail to progress with physical therapy and can have difficulty weaning from narcotic medications. A cause for the nonunion can likely be related to patient or surgeon-controlled factors, however infection and systemic causes should be considered.

Infection should be ruled out early during the work-up as discussed in Sect. 14.1.7.

Smoking cessation and discontinuation of anti-inflammatory medications should be encouraged as nicotine and NSAIDs have been associated with increased rates of nonunion, revision surgery, and decreased patient outcomes [38, 53].

Diabetes is a common and potentially modifiable risk factor and is associated with increased risk of infection, as well as delayed fracture healing and nonunion [70]. In the absence of obviously modifiable risk factors referral to an endocrine clinic may be of significant benefit. As discussed in Sect. 14.1.7, evaluation of the other metabolic components of nonunion can be of significant value in non-operative management.

Radiographs may not clearly demonstrate a nonunion of the femoral neck but can be used to easily determine angulation of the femoral neck and hardware failure. Other radiographic factors associated with poor outcomes in these patients include varus angulation of the fracture and calcar comminution [71]. Computed tomographic imaging can demonstrate progressive failure of hardware or sclerosis at the level of the previous fracture with variable amounts of femoral head avascular necrosis [59] (see Case Example 3).

Unlike long-bone nonunions, treatment options for a femoral neck nonunion are more limited. The blood supply to the femoral head is retrograde and the nonunion site is intra-articular with synovial fluid disrupting bone graft healing. The femoral neck is also difficult to address using conventional techniques used for long-bone nonunions due to limited bone on either side of the nonunion inhibiting stable fixation.

14.2.5 Management Principles: Operative Treatment

14.2.5.1 Elderly Patient

The decision making regarding operative versus non-operative treatment of a geriatric femoral neck nonunion is simplified due to the superior results that can be achieved with hip arthroplasty relative to ORIF [72]. Generally, older patients with nonunion can expect good long-term outcomes when treated with total hip arthroplasty (THA). Dislocation rates at 25 years follow-up are approximately 7% with females, patients treated for acute fracture or nonunion, and patients older than 70 being more likely to dislocate than patients receiving THA for osteoarthritis [73].

Total hip arthroplasty has been associated with higher rates of dislocation than hemiarthroplasty after femoral neck fracture but provides a more durable long-term solution with lower overall reoperation rate and better functional outcomes [74].

Removal of the femoral hardware is best addressed in a step-wise fashion to prevent unnecessary complications. This process begins with a review of the previous operative report(s), knowledge of the previous implant system, and appropriate removal tools. A careful review of imaging is also important to confirm the diagnosis with radiographs and CT as needed. However, a nonunion should be suspected from the clinical history, absence of clear bony union on AP and lateral radiographs, and progressive hardware failure [59]. It is also important to radiographically examine the integrity of the greater trochanter and clinically evaluate the function of the hip abductors.

Conversion to Total Hip Arthroplasty

Abductor damage is more important in the femoral neck nonunion patient initially treated with a cephalomedullary nail (CMN) than one treated with a sliding hip screw or cannulated screws. The starting point for the CMN is frequently a trochanteric entry location and involves the creation of a 15 mm hole through the insertion of the gluteus medius and greater trochanter. Patients with previous CMN and femoral neck nonunion may require some degree of abductor repair at the time of revision surgery. In addition to hip abductor damage, the entry reamer creates a stress riser in the greater trochanter increasing the risk of its fracture during revision surgery.

Most implants used to treat the initial femoral neck fracture are placed through a laterally based incision. Therefore, to readily access this hardware and allow for extensile visualization to the proximal femur, a posterior approach to the hip is preferred. Following the surgical approach, the hip should be dislocated then reduced with the hardware left in situ. If the proximal femoral hardware is removed before the dislocation, then an iatrogenic fracture may occur through the newly exposed screw hole(s). After the hardware has been removed, prophylactic cabling of the proximal femoral shaft can be performed (if indicated). The proximal femur is then re-dislocated in preparation for the femoral neck cut.

Occasionally a patient will have femoral hardware cut out and an associated acetabular defect. Cemented acetabular components can still be used in primary and revision arthroplasty with good long-term outcomes [22]. However, these have been increasingly replaced by bone-stock preserving, noncemented metal backed acetabular components with improving outcome superiority since the mid-1990s [17]. The noncemented acetabular components have excellent track records with higher retention rates in primary THA than cemented acetabular components at 10-year follow up (94% vs. 85%) [75].

The author's preferred choice for the femoral component is a cemented stem, which is backed by good results with cementation of the femoral component in primary hip arthroplasty and in the setting of femoral neck fracture [76]. The cemented femoral stem also has the benefit of increased flexibility to adjust femoral anteversion compared to press fit systems. Bearing surface selection for the conversion THA is a controversial topic and should be evaluated by the surgeon on a case by case basis.

The decision to convert a femoral neck nonunion to a THA or hemiarthroplasty is multifactorial. Patients with a femoral neck nonunion have additional deconditioning due to their inability to return to preambulatory function. Although no studies exist directly comparing hemiarthroplasty with THA for the treatment of a femoral neck nonunion, it is reasonable to use the acute geriatric femoral neck fracture population instead.

Case Example 3

A 70 year old male fell from ground level onto his right hip and sustained a subcapital femoral neck fracture. He ambulates independently and his medical history is significant for diabetes (HbA1c of 8.1), hypothyroidism, and hypertension (Figs. 14.3a–e).

14.2.5.2 Young Patient

The evaluation of a femoral neck nonunion is more complicated in the young patient compared to the elderly, as joint preservation in the former remains the priority. Though the upper limit of when patients are considered as "young" continues to decrease as long-term arthroplasty options improve, most do not consider a patient for an arthroplasty over a salvage procedure under the 40- 50-year-old age range [69]. This was recently supported by Swart et al. who found it more cost effective to perform a THA than an ORIF for a patient with a femoral neck fracture between the ages of 45–65 [77]. Those with increased comorbidities and increased risk of fixation failure would also benefit from THA at a younger ages compared with age adjusted healthy patients [77]. Joint preservation seeks to primarily address the lack of a proper biomechanical loading environment through reorientation of loading vectors [69].

Mechanical Environment and Results of Valgus Intertrochanteric Osteotomy

The shearing forces produced with ambulation on a vertically oriented femoral neck fracture are believed to be one of the primary causes of femoral neck nonunion. The inability to control these forces biomechanically with current fixation methods results in hardware failures which occur more often in the setting of a high Pauwels' angle fracture [65]. A valgus producing intertrochanteric osteotomy as originally described by Pauwels and subsequently modified by Muller is selected and functions by conversion of shearing into compression forces to promote bony union [55, 56].

Retention of the fibrous tissue and compression through the nonunion can achieve union and is used effectively in other locations of the body [78]. The valgus intertrochanteric osteotomy has reliable outcomes without removal of the intervening fibrous tissue when treated appropriately with extensive preoperative planning and a fixed angle device such as a blade plate [79]. These osteotomies have success rates approaching 90%, but are technically demanding [80].

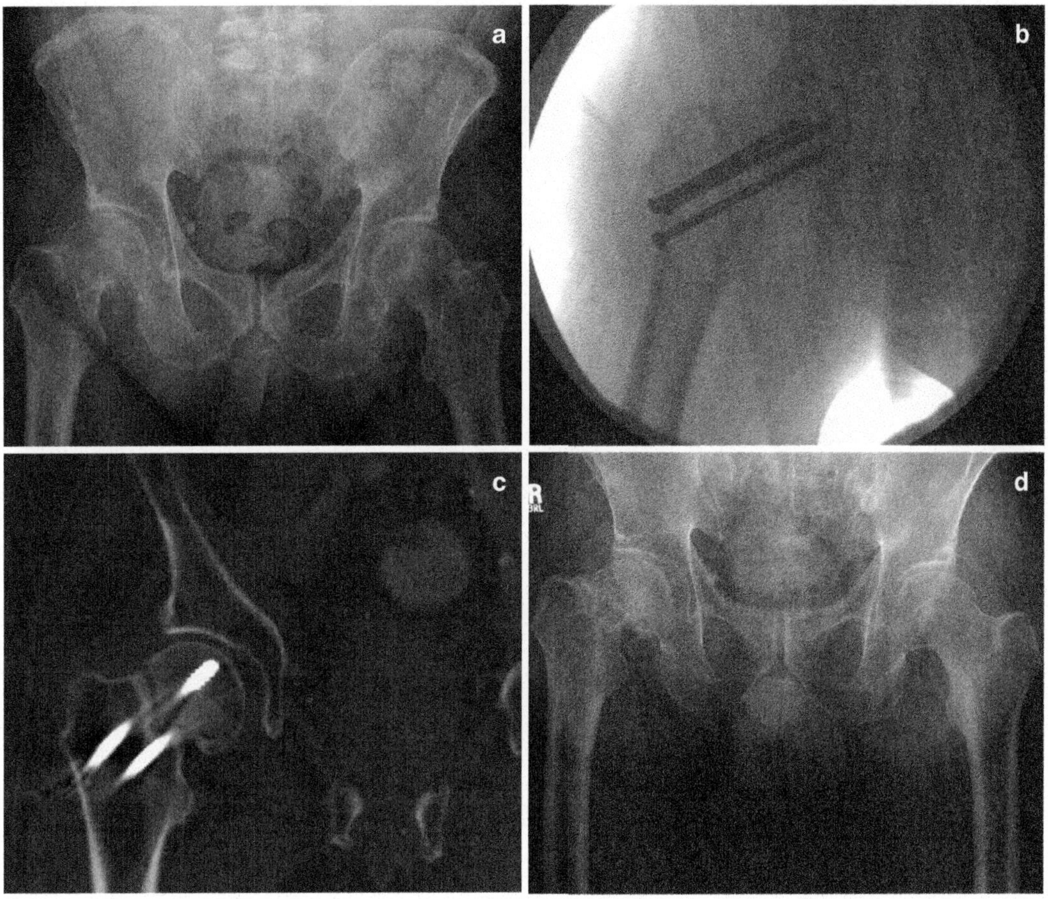

Fig. 14.3 (**a**) AP pelvis radiograph demonstrating a right subcapital femoral neck fracture. The patient was subsequently treated with three partially threaded 7.3 mm cannulated screws in an inverted triangle configuration. (**b**) AP intraoperative fluoroscopic image demonstrating final hardware placement. The patient eventually returned to independent ambulation with a cane. However, he had continued right hip pain, which was attributed to trochanteric bursitis from screw prominence. Sixteen months later the patient received a CT scan for evaluation of abdominal pain that noted an "incompletely healed femoral neck fracture". (**c**) Coronal CT image 16 months after initial fixation. A vertically oriented nonunion with sclerotic margins is present. The patient was taken to surgery 1 month later for removal of his "symptomatic hardware" in the setting of presumed trochanteric bursitis. The treating physician was unaware of the CT scan demonstrating nonunion. A metabolic work-up was not obtained prior to his second right hip surgery. The patient followed up in clinic 1 week later where he was noted to have significant displacement of his femoral neck nonunion. (**d**) AP radiograph demonstrating a displaced varus femoral neck nonunion after removal of the cannulated hip screws. Treatment with total hip arthroplasty was recommended. During surgery, the acetabulum was initially reamed for a 56 mm diameter multihole uncemented component and secured with 4 acetabular screws. The acetabular bone stock was osteoporotic and the screws had poor purchase. During subsequent trialing of the femoral neck length, the metal acetabular component displaced and was removed with subsequent revision to a cemented all-polyethylene acetabular component. This intraoperative challenge might have been anticipated by considering that the patient had been using an assistive device to unload his painful right hip. To some degree, this likely produced a functional disuse osteopenia of the subchondral bone about the acetabulum. The patient made a full recovery and three-year follow-up radiographs were taken in clinic without change in femoral or acetabular component location. The patient has pain free range of motion, ambulates without assistive device and has returned to all activities. (**e**) AP radiograph demonstrating cemented acetabular and femoral components with restoration of offset and leg length

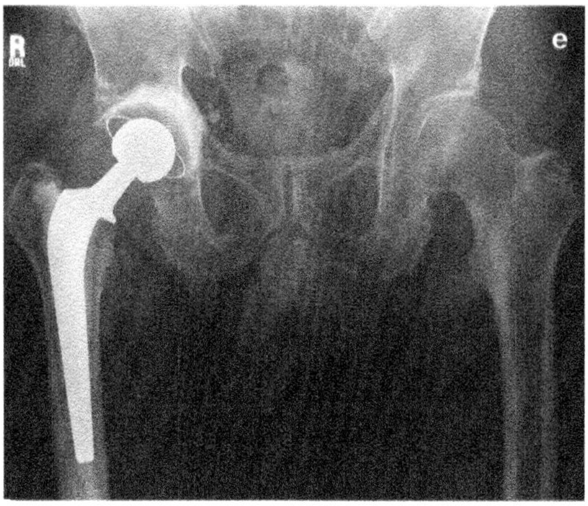

Fig. 14.3 (continued)

The advantages of more normal hip joint biomechanics through restoration of femoral offset and leg length must be weighed against the benefits of preserving the native femoral and acetabular articulation. Femoral neck nonunion patients typically exhibit abnormal hip biomechanics in addition to pain due to significant amounts of femoral neck shortening [69]. However, while a successful valgus intertrochanteric osteotomy can eliminate the painful nonunion and potentially increase leg length, it cannot improve femoral offset and patients are left with an altered gait [69]. A successful valgus intertrochanteric osteotomy is generally accepted as "in most cases, moderately suboptimal hip biomechanics are accepted as the trade-off to gain good bone apposition in a stable position and fracture union" [69]. Subsequent conversion to THA after a joint preserving osteotomy is more challenging (due to the altered proximal femoral anatomy and in situ hardware) though this should not preclude an attempt at a joint salvage procedure in a young patient.

The technique for a valgus intertrochanteric osteotomy is classically described by Muller [56] and Marti [79] and more recently updated by Mayo [81]. It begins with thorough preoperative planning beginning with comparing the injured and uninjured sides in both the coronal and sagittal planes to quantify the deformity [81]. Based on the initial measurements an osteotomy is planned to reorient the femoral neck nonunion angle while appreciating how this selection will affect osteotomy stability and limb length [81]. An appropriately selected fixed angle device is then templated and applied to allow restoration of a more normal femoral neck shaft angle while gaining compression across the osteotomy site [56, 79, 81].

Results of Total Hip Arthroplasty in the Young Patient

Although no epidemiologic study of young patients with a femoral neck nonunion exists, most patients are presumed to be treated with valgus intertrochanteric osteotomy. Native articular cartilage and an altered gait are generally considered preferable to the relative activity restrictions and higher risks of future revision surgery accompanying THA. This may change as THA becomes a more cost-effective option with immediate weight bearing as both revision and primary results continue to improve [77].

Young patients requiring conversion to THA resemble the younger population with AVN requiring primary THA. Should THA be selected, management of pre-existing femoral hardware should be addressed similar to that previously described for elderly patients. The use of prophylactic cerclage wiring should be considered in the setting of a press fit stem in this situation given the hoop stresses that will be imparted during the seating of the final implant. Cemented femoral fixation is used frequently in Europe for primary arthroplasty with an excellent track record [75]. It is less frequently used in the USA for primary arthroplasty, but could be considered in the revision setting given the added benefits of antibiotic delivery, improved anteversion control, and improved management of the stress risers from previous fixation efforts.

References

1. Letournel E. Acetabulum fractures: classification and management. Clin Orthop Relat Res. 1980;151:81–106.
2. Matta JM. Fractures of the acetabulum: accuracy of reduction and clinical results in patients managed operatively within three weeks after the injury. J Bone Joint Surg Am. 1996;78:1632–45.

3. Mayo KA. Open reduction and internal fixation of fractures of the acetabulum. Results in 163 fractures. Clin Orthop Relat Res. 1994;305:31–7.
4. Mears DC, Velyvis JH, Chang CP. Displaced acetabular fractures managed operatively: indicators of outcome. Clin Orthop Relat Res. 2003;407:173–86.
5. Mohanty K, Taha W, Powell JN. Non-union of acetabular fractures. Injury. 2004;35:787–90.
6. Briffa N, Pearce R, Hill AM, et al. Outcomes of acetabular fracture fixation with ten years' follow-up. J Bone Joint Surg Br. 2011;93:229–36.
7. Hull JB, Raza SA, Stockley I, et al. Surgical management of fractures of the acetabulum: the Sheffield experience 1976-1994. Injury. 1997;28:35–40.
8. Matta JM. Operative treatment of acetabular fractures through the ilioinguinal approach. A 10-year perspective. Clin Orthop Relat Res. 1994;305:10–9.
9. Moed BR, Willsoncarr SE, Watson JT. Results of operative treatment of fractures of the posterior wall of the acetabulum. J Bone Joint Surg Am. 2002;84-A:752–8.
10. Murphy D, Kaliszer M, Rice J, et al. Outcome after acetabular fracture. Prognostic factors and their inter-relationships. Injury. 2003;34:512–7.
11. Saterbak AM, Marsh JL, Nepola JV, et al. Clinical failure after posterior wall acetabular fractures: the influence of initial fracture patterns. J Orthop Trauma. 2000;14:230–7.
12. Starr AJ, Watson JT, Reinert CM, et al. Complications following the "T extensile" approach: a modified extensile approach for acetabular fracture surgery-report of forty-three patients. J Orthop Trauma. 2002;16:535–42.
13. Stockle U, Hoffmann R, Sudkamp NP, et al. Treatment of complex acetabular fractures through a modified extended iliofemoral approach. J Orthop Trauma. 2002;16:220–30.
14. Wright R, Barrett K, Christie MJ, et al. Acetabular fractures: long-term follow-up of open reduction and internal fixation. J Orthop Trauma. 1994;8:397–403.
15. Judet R, Judet J, Letournel E. Fractures of the acetabulum: classification and surgical approaches for open reduction. Preliminary report. J Bone Joint Surg Am. 1964;46:1615–46.
16. Johnson EE, Matta JM, Mast JW, et al. Delayed reconstruction of acetabular fractures 21-120 days following injury. Clin Orthop Relat Res. 1994;305:20–30.
17. Morshed S. Current options for determining fracture union. Adv Med. 2014;2014:708574.
18. Giannoudis PV, Grotz MR, Papakostidis C, et al. Operative treatment of displaced fractures of the acetabulum. A meta-analysis. J Bone Joint Surg Br. 2005;87:2–9.
19. Tannast M, Najibi S, Matta JM. Two to twenty-year survivorship of the hip in 810 patients with operatively treated acetabular fractures. J Bone Joint Surg Am. 2012;94:1559–67.
20. Sagi HC, Jordan CJ, Barei DP, et al. Indomethacin prophylaxis for heterotopic ossification after acetabular fracture surgery increases the risk for nonunion of the posterior wall. J Orthop Trauma. 2014;28:377–83.
21. Berry DJ, Halasy M. Uncemented acetabular components for arthritis after acetabular fracture. Clin Orthop Relat Res. 2002;405:164–7.
22. Schreurs BW, Zengerink M, Welten ML, et al. Bone impaction grafting and a cemented cup after acetabular fracture at 3-18 years. Clin Orthop Relat Res. 2005;437:145–51.
23. Sen RK, Veerappa LA. Long-term outcome of conservatively managed displaced acetabular fractures. J Trauma. 2009;67:155–9.
24. Mcnamara AR, Boudreau JA, Moed BR. Nonoperative treatment of posterior wall acetabular fractures after dynamic stress examination under anesthesia: revisited. J Orthop Trauma. 2015;29:359–64.
25. Clarke-Jenssen J, Wikeroy AK, Roise O, et al. Long-term survival of the native hip after a minimally displaced, nonoperatively treated acetabular fracture. J Bone Joint Surg Am. 2016;98:1392–9.
26. Carroll EA, Huber FG, Goldman AT, et al. Treatment of acetabular fractures in an older population. J Orthop Trauma. 2010;24:637–44.
27. Mayo KA, Letournel E, Matta JM, et al. Surgical revision of malreduced acetabular fractures. Clin Orthop Relat Res. 1994;305:47–52.
28. Bellabarba C, Berger RA, Bentley CD, et al. Cementless acetabular reconstruction after acetabular fracture. J Bone Joint Surg Am. 2001;83-A:868–76.
29. Makridis KG, Obakponovwe O, Bobak P, et al. Total hip arthroplasty after acetabular fracture: incidence of complications, reoperation rates and functional outcomes: evidence today. J Arthroplast. 2014;29:1983–90.
30. Weber M, Berry DJ, Harmsen WS. Total hip arthroplasty after operative treatment of an acetabular fracture. J Bone Joint Surg Am. 1998;80:1295–305.
31. Lizaur-Utrilla A, Sanz-Reig J, Serna-Berna R. Cementless acetabular reconstruction after acetabular fracture: a prospective, matched-cohort study. J Trauma Acute Care Surg. 2012;73:232–8.
32. Salama W, Ditto P, Mousa S, et al. Cementless total hip arthroplasty in the treatment after acetabular fractures. Eur J Orthop Surg Traumatol. 2017;28:59.
33. Sermon A, Broos P, Vanderschot P. Total hip replacement for acetabular fractures. Results in 121 patients operated between 1983 and 2003. Injury. 2008;39:914–21.
34. Von Roth P, Abdel MP, Harmsen WS, et al. Total hip arthroplasty after operatively treated acetabular fracture: a concise follow-up, at a mean of twenty years, of a previous report. J Bone Joint Surg Am. 2015;97:288–91.
35. Morison Z, Moojen DJ, Nauth A, et al. Total hip arthroplasty after acetabular fracture is associated with lower survivorship and more complications. Clin Orthop Relat Res. 2016;474:392–8.
36. O'toole RV, Hui E, Chandra A, et al. How often does open reduction and internal fixation of geriatric ace-

tabular fractures lead to hip arthroplasty? J Orthop Trauma. 2014;28:148–53.
37. Brinker MR, O'connor DP, Monla YT, et al. Metabolic and endocrine abnormalities in patients with nonunions. J Orthop Trauma. 2007;21:557–70.
38. Lindstrom D, Sadr Azodi O, Wladis A, et al. Effects of a perioperative smoking cessation intervention on postoperative complications: a randomized trial. Ann Surg. 2008;248:739–45.
39. Paprosky WG, O'rourke M, Sporer SM. The treatment of acetabular bone defects with an associated pelvic discontinuity. Clin Orthop Relat Res. 2005;441:216–20.
40. Paprosky WG, Perona PG, Lawrence JM. Acetabular defect classification and surgical reconstruction in revision arthroplasty. A 6-year follow-up evaluation. J Arthroplast. 1994;9:33–44.
41. Solomon LB, Studer P, Abrahams JM, et al. Does cup-cage reconstruction with oversized cups provide initial stability in THA for osteoporotic acetabular fractures? Clin Orthop Relat Res. 2015;473:3811–9.
42. Sternheim A, Backstein D, Kuzyk PR, et al. Porous metal revision shells for management of contained acetabular bone defects at a mean follow-up of six years: a comparison between up to 50% bleeding host bone contact and more than 50% contact. J Bone Joint Surg Br. 2012;94:158–62.
43. Veerappa LA, Tripathy SK, Sen RK. Management of neglected acetabular fractures. Eur J Trauma Emerg Surg. 2015;41:343–8.
44. Mcgrory AC, Replogle L, Endrizzi D. Ultrasound gel minimizes third body debris with partial hardware removal in joint arthroplasty. Arthroplast Today. 2017;3:29–31.
45. Paprosky WG, O'Rourke M, Sporer SM. The treatment of acetabular bone defects with an associated pelvic discontinuity. Clin Orthop Relat Res. 2005;441:216–20.
46. D'Antonio JA. Periprosthetic bone loss of the acetabulum. Classification and management. Orthop Clin North Am. 1992;23(2):279–90.
47. Damany DS, Parker MJ, Chojnowski A. Complications after intracapsular hip fractures in young adults. A meta-analysis of 18 published studies involving 564 fractures. Injury. 2005;36:131–41.
48. Slobogean GP, Sprague SA, Scott T, et al. Complications following young femoral neck fractures. Injury. 2015;46:484–91.
49. Slobogean GP, Stockton DJ, Zeng B, et al. Femoral neck fractures in adults treated with internal fixation: a prospective multicenter Chinese cohort. J Am Acad Orthop Surg. 2017;25:297–303.
50. Collinge CA, Mir H, Reddix R. Fracture morphology of high shear angle "vertical" femoral neck fractures in young adult patients. J Orthop Trauma. 2014;28:270–5.
51. Thorngren KG, Hommel A, Norrman PO, et al. Epidemiology of femoral neck fractures. Injury. 2002;33(Suppl 3):C1–7.
52. Egol KA, Koval KJ, Zuckerman JD. Handbook of fractures. Philadelphia: Wolters Kluwer Health; 2015.
53. Haidukewych GJ, Rothwell WS, Jacofsky DJ, et al. Operative treatment of femoral neck fractures in patients between the ages of fifteen and fifty years. J Bone Joint Surg Am. 2004;86-A:1711–6.
54. Seeley MA, Georgiadis AG, Sankar WN. Hip vascularity: a review of the anatomy and clinical implications. J Am Acad Orthop Surg. 2016;24:515–26.
55. Pauwels F. Der Schenkelhalsbruch. Ein mechaizisches problem: Grundagen des Heilungsvorganges Prognose und kausale Therapie. Beilagheft Z. Orthop. Chir. 63 Stuttgart, Enke. 1935.
56. Muller M. Intertrochanteric osteotomy: indications, preoperative planning, technique. In: Schatzker J, editor. The trochanteric osteotomy. Berlin: Springer; 1984.
57. Garden R. Low-angle fixation in fractures of the femoral neck. J Bone Joint Surg Br. 1961;48-B:647–63.
58. Fixation Using Alternative Implants for the Treatment of Hip Fractures Investigators. Fracture fixation in the operative management of hip fractures (FAITH): an international, multicentre, randomised controlled trial. Lancet. 2017;389:1519–27.
59. Stockton DJ, Lefaivre KA, Deakin DE, et al. Incidence, magnitude, and predictors of shortening in young femoral neck fractures. J Orthop Trauma. 2015;29:e293–8.
60. Bhandari M, Chiavaras M, Ayeni O, et al. Assessment of radiographic fracture healing in patients with operatively treated femoral neck fractures. J Orthop Trauma. 2013;27:e213–9.
61. Bhandari M, Chiavaras MM, Parasu N, et al. Radiographic union score for hip substantially improves agreement between surgeons and radiologists. BMC Musculoskelet Disord. 2013;14:70.
62. Chiavaras MM, Bains S, Choudur H, et al. The Radiographic Union Score for Hip (RUSH): the use of a checklist to evaluate hip fracture healing improves agreement between radiologists and orthopedic surgeons. Skelet Radiol. 2013;42:1079–88.
63. Frank T, Osterhoff G, Sprague S, et al. The Radiographic Union Score for Hip (RUSH) identifies radiographic nonunion of femoral neck fractures. Clin Orthop Relat Res. 2016;474:1396–404.
64. Bhattacharyya T, Bouchard KA, Phadke A, et al. The accuracy of computed tomography for the diagnosis of tibial nonunion. J Bone Joint Surg Am. 2006;88:692–7.
65. Liporace F, Gaines R, Collinge C, et al. Results of internal fixation of Pauwels type-3 vertical femoral neck fractures. J Bone Joint Surg Am. 2008;90:1654–9.
66. Upadhyay A, Jain P, Mishra P, et al. Delayed internal fixation of fractures of the neck of the femur in young adults. A prospective, randomised study comparing closed and open reduction. J Bone Joint Surg Br. 2004;86:1035–40.
67. Lu-Yao GL, Keller RB, Littenberg B, et al. Outcomes after displaced fractures of the femoral neck. A meta-

analysis of one hundred and six published reports. J Bone Joint Surg Am. 1994;76:15–25.
68. Swiontkowski MF. Intracapsular fractures of the hip. J Bone Joint Surg Am. 1994;76:129–38.
69. Haidukewych GJ, Berry DJ. Salvage of failed treatment of hip fractures. J Am Acad Orthop Surg. 2005;13:101–9.
70. Beam HA, Parsons JR, Lin SS. The effects of blood glucose control upon fracture healing in the BB Wistar rat with diabetes mellitus. J Orthop Res. 2002;20:1210–6.
71. Alho A, Benterud JG, Ronningen H, et al. Prediction of disturbed healing in femoral neck fracture. Radiographic analysis of 149 cases. Acta Orthop Scand. 1992;63:639–44.
72. Blomfeldt R, Tornkvist H, Ponzer S, et al. Comparison of internal fixation with total hip replacement for displaced femoral neck fractures. Randomized, controlled trial performed at four years. J Bone Joint Surg Am. 2005;87:1680–8.
73. Berry DJ, Von Knoch M, Schleck CD, et al. The cumulative long-term risk of dislocation after primary Charnley total hip arthroplasty. J Bone Joint Surg Am. 2004;86-A:9–14.
74. Burgers PT, Van Geene AR, Van Den Bekerom MP, et al. Total hip arthroplasty versus hemiarthroplasty for displaced femoral neck fractures in the healthy elderly: a meta-analysis and systematic review of randomized trials. Int Orthop. 2012;36:1549–60.
75. Hailer NP, Garellick G, Karrholm J. Uncemented and cemented primary total hip arthroplasty in the Swedish Hip Arthroplasty Register. Acta Orthop. 2010;81:34–41.
76. Parker MI, Pryor G, Gurusamy K. Cemented versus uncemented hemiarthroplasty for intracapsular hip fractures: a randomised controlled trial in 400 patients. J Bone Joint Surg Br. 2010;92:116–22.
77. Swart E, Roulette P, Leas D, et al. ORIF or arthroplasty for displaced femoral neck fractures in patients younger than 65 years old: an economic decision analysis. J Bone Joint Surg Am. 2017;99:65–75.
78. Rodriguez-Merchan EC, Gomez-Castresana F. Internal fixation of nonunions. Clin Orthop Relat Res. 2004;419:13–20.
79. Marti RK, Schuller HM, Raaymakers EL. Intertrochanteric osteotomy for non-union of the femoral neck. J Bone Joint Surg Br. 1989;71:782–7.
80. Magu NK, Singla R, Rohilla R, et al. Modified Pauwels' intertrochanteric osteotomy in the management of nonunion of a femoral neck fracture following failed osteosynthesis. Bone Joint J. 2014;96-B:1198–201.
81. Mayo K, Kuldjanov D. Generic preoperative planning for proximal femoral osteotomy in the treatment of nonunion of the femoral neck. J Orthop Trauma. 2018;32(Suppl 1):S46–54.

The Use of Hip Arthroscopy in Trauma of the Hip

15

Alessandro Aprato, Federico Bertolo, Alessandro Bistolfi, Luigi Sabatini, and Alessandro Massè

Abstract

Hip arthroscopy may be used to treat selected intra-articular lesions even in trauma cases. Although most of the published studies are small case series, results are encouraging. On the other hand, there is consensus about the importance of surgeon's experience in hip arthroscopy and about the limitations of this technique. Intra-articular injuries are not limited to hip dislocations only, but can be associated with femur head fractures, acetabular fractures, and even soft tissue injuries not associated with a fracture. During arthroscopic treatment of these affections care must be taken in mobilizing, translating, and reducing fracture fragment(s), considering fluoroscopic guidance and the use of chopstick technique where indicated. Allowing early mobilization of hip and protected weight bearing as well as performing interval postoperative radiographic assessment is mandatory.

Arthroscopic treatment of traumatic events is conditioned to the amount of articular damage suffered and to the time the hip has been dislocated before reduction. Complications directly related to the performance of hip arthroscopy such as fluid extravasation into the gluteal compartment, scrotal or perineal pressure wounds, nerve injuries, iatrogenic cartilage injury, and cardiac arrest resulting from abdominal compartment syndrome are rare.

In this chapter we review the indications for hip arthroscopy in trauma cases and the current evidence for these arthroscopic techniques.

Keywords

Hip arthroscopy · Loose bodies · Traumatic hip dislocation · Arthroscopic reduction · Hip fractures

15.1 Introduction

Hip arthroscopy permits a direct visualization of hip articular surface (femoral head and acetabulum) without the tissues disruption of the open surgery techniques [1] and has gained considerable popularity in the past decade. Although at present non-traumatic pathologies are the most common indications for hip arthroscopy, several traumatic intra-articular conditions are also treated. Indications for arthroscopy in hip trauma cases are acetabular fractures, hip dislocation, and femoral head fractures and their sequelae, although only selected cases may be treated without concomitant open procedures.

A. Aprato (✉) · F. Bertolo · A. Bistolfi · L. Sabatini · A. Massè
University of Turin, Turin, Italy
e-mail: alessandro.aprato@unito.it

L. Büchler, M. J.B. Keel (eds.), *Fractures of the Hip*, Fracture Management Joint by Joint,
https://doi.org/10.1007/978-3-030-18838-2_15

Initially only extraction of loose bodies or small intra-articular fragments after hip fracture dislocation and bullet extraction have been described; with the advances in arthroscopic techniques, reduction and fixation of femoral head or posterior wall fractures have been reported in literature. Furthermore labral suture, chondral injuries fixation, and capsulorrhaphy in traumatic hip dislocation sequelae have been described. Finally, arthroscopic cam resection in neck fracture sequelae is now a standard treatment.

Standard arthroscopic principles have been applied to facilitate visualization and navigation within the hip joint for these traumatic cases incorporating infusion pumps, specific hip portals with multiple cannulas and leg traction. On the other hand, the advantage of arthroscopic techniques should always be balanced with the possible complications: They include fluid extravasation into the gluteal compartment; scrotal or perineal pressure wounds; lateral femoral cutaneous nerve injury; traction nerve palsies of the peroneal, pudendal, sciatic, and femoral nerves; iatrogenic cartilage injury caused by instruments and cardiac arrest resulting from abdominal compartment syndrome. Although these complications are described as rare, surgeon should be familiar with hip arthroscopy in non-traumatic patients in order to minimize them.

Hereby we described the most common trauma related indications and their treatment techniques.

15.2 Removal of Loose Bodies or Foreign Objects

Loose body removal is one of the primary indications for hip arthroscopy (Fig. 15.1). During a traumatic event involving the hip joint such as hip dislocation or hip fracture-dislocation, loose bodies originate by the femoral head shearing against the acetabular lip. The incidence of loose body formation however is unknown [2].

Epstein et al. first described the importance of removal of loose bodies. According to Epstein, loose bodies were so common that all hip fracture-dislocation should be treated with open debridement. Even in simple hip dislocations, traumatic arthritis is a common complication (prevalence rate of 24%), probably because of unrecognized intra-articular loose bodies [3, 4]. The prevalence rate rises as high as 54% when there's evidence of more complex injuries, such as fracture-dislocations [5–7]. In these cases the increased rate of traumatic arthritis would be attributed mainly to the femoral and/or acetabular fracture instead of the presence of loose bodies.

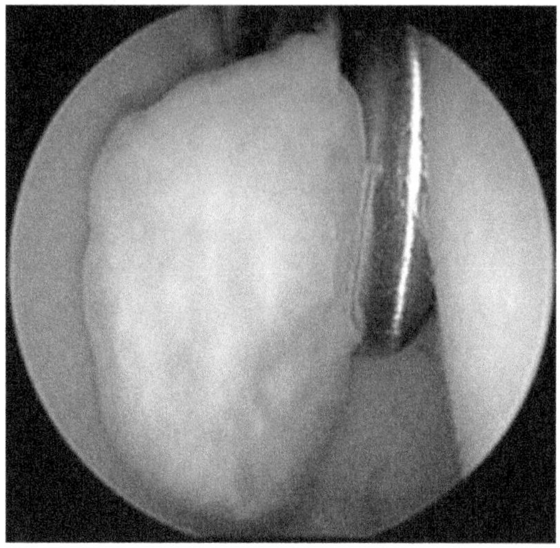

Fig. 15.1 Intra-operative image of a loose osteochondral fragment in a right hip joint: view from the mid anterior portal toward the fovea

Retained loose bodies can cause damage to the articular surface through a third-body wear mechanism, leading to premature degenerative changes and chronic synovitis.

It's important to obtain standard radiographs after hip dislocation, including AP pelvis and CT scans (not only axial scans but also sagittal and coronal scans), in order to evaluate the three-dimensional nature of the osteochondral injury and the degree of articular surface involvement.

Sometimes it can be difficult to recognize intra-articular loose bodies, especially if they consist of cartilaginous tissue. Presence of intra-articular unrecognized loose bodies can cause an incomplete or non-concentric reduction.

Although non-concentric reduction and presence of osteochondral fragments in the weight-bearing area of the acetabulum are absolute indications for removal of loose bodies, there is less general consensus regarding the necessity of loose bodies removal in concentric reductions, specially if loose bodies are located in or below the fovea [8].

According to authors' personal experience, loose bodies' removal may be easily performed in arthroscopy and may be performed either in supine or in lateral decubitus. Authors' personal choice is lateral position because floating bodies usually fall in the fovea and are easily removed.

Hip arthroscopy can be useful to remove intra-articular bullets too (Fig. 15.2). Singleton et al. have recently proposed a safe and useful method to remove bullets from hip joint by using a threaded pin. Instead of risking further trauma to the articular surface by removing with osteotomes or using curettes, the bullet is engaged end-on with a 3.2-mm threaded tipped guide pin from the dynamic hip screw set, that is inserted through the anterior portal. Then the pin is advanced into the bullet under fluoroscopic guidance and when is firmly seated is simply pulled out through the anterior portal [9].

15.3 Fixation of Posterior Wall Fractures

Arthroscopic-assisted percutaneous osteosynthesis has facilitated the surgeon's ability to closely observe the fracture site, helping in the reduction and to diagnose and treat associated chondral injuries. Although arthroscopic-assisted percutaneous osteosynthesis are well documented in tibia plateau fractures and ankle disorders, only small case series of acetabular fractures treatment are reported. That said, several authors have described either arthroscopic removal of small fragment of posterior wall (Fig. 15.3) or arthroscopic treatment for traumatic hip fracture-dislocations [2, 10–14]. The first successful percutaneous fixation of acetabular fracture was carried out by Gay et al. by using CT guidance [15]. Yamamoto et al. reported reduction and percutaneous fixation in patients with acetabular fracture [12]; Yang et al. reported arthroscopic guided percutaneous screw fixation of minimal displaced acetabular fractures [13]. In these cases, percutaneous screw fixation of the anterior column of the acetabulum was performed under guidance of hip arthroscopy to enable direct

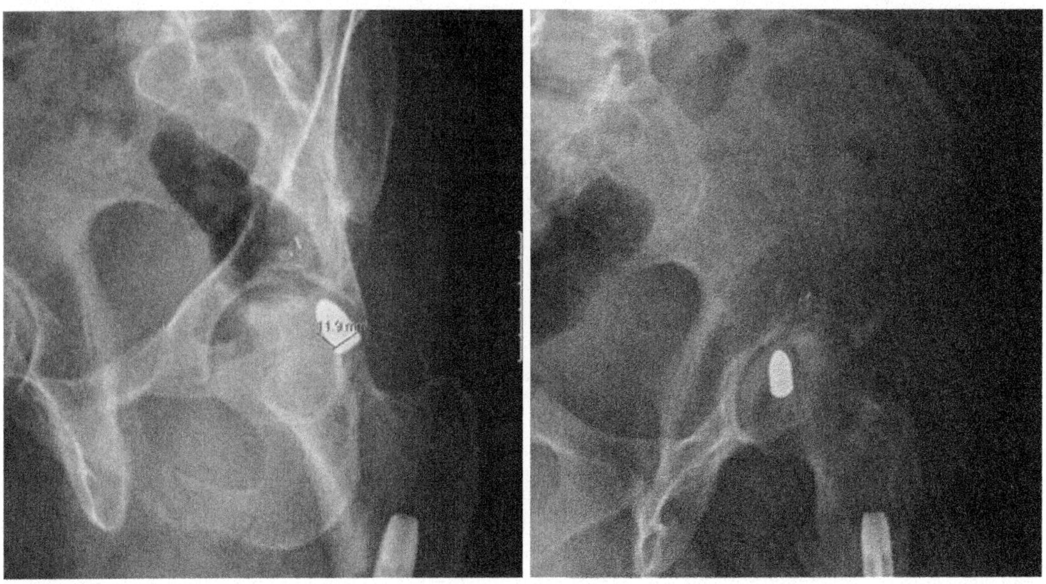

Fig. 15.2 X-rays showing a bullet inside the hip joint

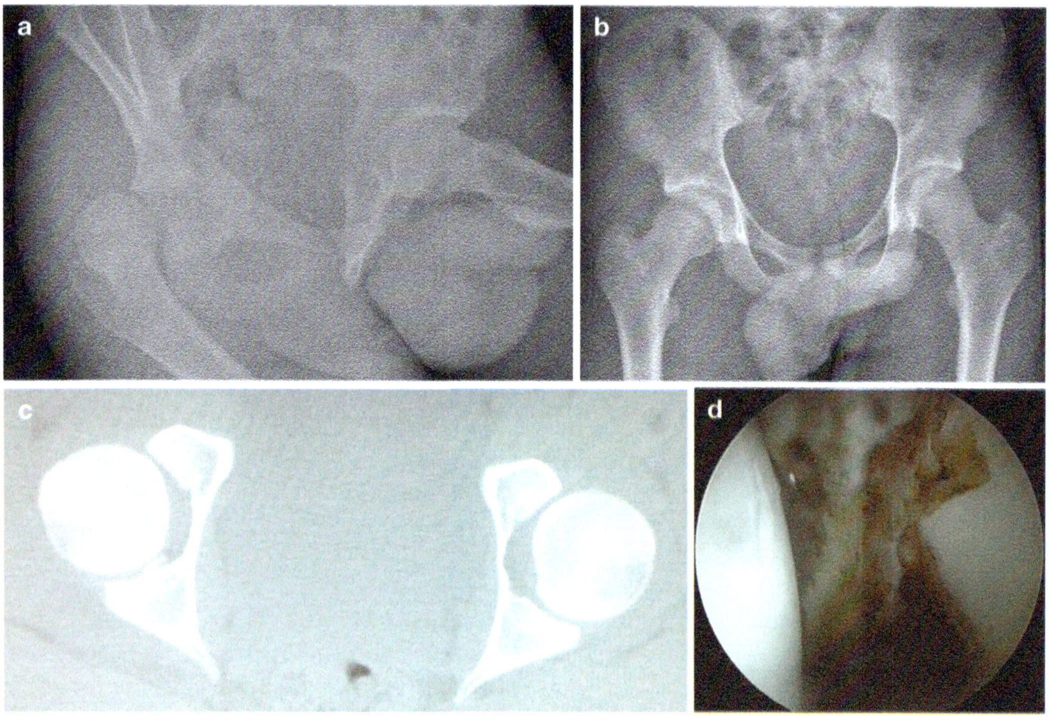

Fig. 15.3 (**a**) AP-pelvis x-ray showing a posterior hip dislocation. (**b**) X-ray of the same patient after reduction. (**c**) CT scan of the same patient showing an intra-articular fragment of the posterior wall. (**d**) intra-operative view of the fragment from the mid anterior portal

visual confirmation of the quality of the reduction and avoid any violation of the medial wall of the acetabulum with the screws.

Recently Kim et al. [14] have described two cases of arthroscopic reduction and internal fixation of acetabular fractures. In particular one of these was a displaced posterior wall fracture of the acetabulum: in this case hip arthroscopy was performed with the affected limb in traction to obtain a sufficient distraction of 10–12 mm. Access was through an antero-lateral, anterior and postero-lateral portal; after hematoma evacuation and detection of the bony fragment, they reduced anatomically and temporarily fixed the fragment with two K wires. Finally they used two 4.0-mm-diameter cannulated screws to fix the fragment under direct arthroscopic visualization.

On the other hand, the indications for arthroscopically assisted percutaneous fixation of acetabular fractures are limited and this technique has to be performed only in cases with minimal and moderate displaced fractures.

15.4 Fixation of Pipkin Fractures

Femoral head fractures are relatively uncommon injuries and occur in 5–15% of traumatic hip dislocations and are more common in posterior dislocations than anterior dislocations [4, 16–19]. Pipkin classified these fractures according to the morphology of the fracture and their occurrence in conjunction with femoral neck or acetabular fractures [20]. Arthroscopically assisted treatment of Pipkin Type 1 fractures, caudal to the fovea, has been reported; Lansford et al. described two cases of displaced Pipkin type 1 fractures, caused both by posterior hip dislocation, treated with excision of the fragments and debriding of the fracture bed [21]. Recently, Park et al. described some cases of displaced infra-foveal Pipkin Type 1 fractures, treated 7 days after the trauma with arthroscopically assisted percutaneous fixation through temporary K-wires fixation and then definitive 3.5-mm cortical screw fixation. They performed an accessory distal anterior portal and a T-shaped capsulotomy; they used metallic screws instead of bio-absorbable screws because the metallic screws are more easily visualized on radiographic images and decrease the risk of implant breakage [22, 23].

Matsuda [11] recently reported a case of supra-foveal fracture (Pipkin type II) with distally displaced osteochondral fracture fragment and no evidence of hip dislocation; once the fragment was identified through direct arthroscopic view, it was translated toward the fracture site. Using an additional anterior portal, the surgeon was able to use two thin guide pins in a chopstick manner to de-rotate the fragment and reduce the fracture; then he used a cannulated Herbert screw to fixate the central portion of the fragment and a mini-Herbert screw to fixate the proximal pole.

According to the literature [4, 6, 11, 16, 17], surgical indications for hip arthroscopy in femoral head fractures are: (1) displaced, large femoral head fracture configuration, (2) severely limited range of motion and impingement signs following conservative treatment, and (3) femoral head fracture associated with intra-articular lesions, such as loose bodies, labral tears, or ligamentum teres injury. Possible contraindications to arthroscopic surgery for femoral head fractures include: (1) hip instability with recurrent dislocation following closed reduction and (2) acetabular fractures with column fractures that can cause fluid extravasation during hip arthroscopy. If the femoral head fractures can't be reduced by arthroscopic methods, open reduction and internal fixation may be the most appropriate approach to achieve anatomic femoral head contours [11]. Unfortunately the decision regarding whether fragments should be internally fixed or simply excised remains controversial [24].

In conclusion the cornerstones for arthroscopic reduction and internal fixation of femoral head fractures are:

- Perform accurate preoperative fracture assessment
- Perform accurate preoperative self-assessment of surgical experience and arthroscopic skills
- Be willing to perform possible open reduction–internal fixation (rather than arthroscopic fragment removal) if arthroscopic method fails
- Consider fluoroscopic templating technique to standardize pelvic position under hip distraction
- Pay careful attention to safe portal placement (may require several accessory portals), capsulotomies, intra-articular fluid pressure, and distraction amount and time in order to avoid side effects like nerve injuries or fluid extravasation
- Mobilize, translate, and reduce fracture fragment(s); consider use of chopstick technique where indicated
- Consider arthroscopic fixation using radiopaque screw(s) or pin(s) visible under intermittent fluoroscopic guidance, instead of bio-absorbable implants
- Consider removal of osteochondral bone not essential to weight bearing or structural integrity of fracture construct
- Confirm accurate reduction and stable fixation by arthroscopic and fluoroscopic dynamic testing (such as anterior impingement test and Patrick test)
- Allow early mobilization of hip and protected weight bearing commensurate with assessed fracture fixation.
- Perform postoperative radiographic progressive investigations, with special attention to joint space narrowing and/or hardware migration/violation of hip joint [11]

15.5 Capsular Re-tension After Traumatic Instability

Traumatic hip instability can be due to frank dislocations following major trauma, hip subluxation from more minor trauma, and microtrauma following repetitive impinging movements [25].

Recognizing the various patterns of hip instability after trauma is complicated, and therefore management and outcome of these disorders are quite variable.

The evaluation of hip instability is important, especially if it is associated with evidence of generalized ligament laxity. This can be associated with bone-collagen type disorders, including Ehlers-Danlos syndrome, Down syndrome, arthrochalasis multiplex congenita, developmental dysplastic hip, and idiopathic type. As published by Bellabarba et al. [26], capsular laxity may be the underlying cause of dynamic hip instability. While previously managed by thermal capsulorrhaphy, capsular laxity is currently addressed through suture-based plication techniques [27].

There are several different techniques to incise, repair, or remove the capsule during hip arthroscopy; Capsulectomy, extensile interportal capsulotomy with or without repair, or a T-capsulotomy with partial or complete repair. Capsular plication (capsulorrhaphy) can limit capsular redundancy; it's performed with the hip in 45° flexion, so that side-to-side stitches take larger bites to reduce extraneous capsular tissue and decrease capsular volume [28].

Arthroscopic thermal modification of collagen in the hip capsular tissue appears to be a treatment option for patients with hip instability. The hip joint capsule is predominantly type 1 collagen, and the mechanism of tissue shrinkage through type 1 collagen alteration is well documented in the literature [29]. Short-term results appear promising. However, more studies are required to determine the long-term efficacy of this procedure in the treatment of this challenging disorder.

15.6 Cam Deformity in Neck Fracture Sequelae

Posttraumatic femoroacetabular impingement (FAI) can be a cause of hip pain in patients who sustained a fracture of the neck of the femur [30]. Impingement can develop when the head heals in retrotorsion or varus position. Retrotorsion of the head is a position often seen after cervical fractures. In these malpositions, the head–neck junction comes in contact with the acetabular rim on flexing the hip within normal range, especially when the leg is rotated internally. With further motion of the hip, the flat head–neck junction is jammed against the anterior acetabular cavity, causing damage not only to the undersurface of the labrum, but also to the anterior acetabular cartilage [31]. Anteroposterior hip or pelvic radiographs are indicative of impingement only when the fracture has healed in varus. Axial radiographs and MRI scans may show retrotorsion and the lack of offset on the anterior part of the femoral head and neck contour. MRI is also helpful in showing the sequelae of chronic impingement: degeneration and tearing of the labrum and defects of the adjacent acetabular cartilage.

Although osteotomies and arthroplasties play a major role in the treatment of those posttraumatic deformations, in slight to moderate deformity cases resection osteoplasty of the femoral head and neck junction may be performed arthroscopically (Fig. 15.4). The aim of this procedure is to improve the anterior head–neck offset in order to improve the clearance of the joint. The technique is similar to a standard cam resection. To confirm impingement, performing an extended anterior capsulotomy allows full visualization of the joint and testing for impingement. Creation of an improved femoral head–neck off set is performed by resection osteoplasty of the femoral neck. Damage to the cartilage cannot be reversed; this explains why most of patients complain of some persisting groin pain especially with the impingement test. The mean goal of treatment must therefore be early diagnosis and treatment of impingement to prevent further damage to the cartilage and subsequent osteoarthrosis. Prevention of impingement is possible by initial anatomic reduction, not only in the anteroposterior plane, but also in the axial plane. This may be difficult to achieve with closed or semi-open techniques and is much easier with open techniques [32].

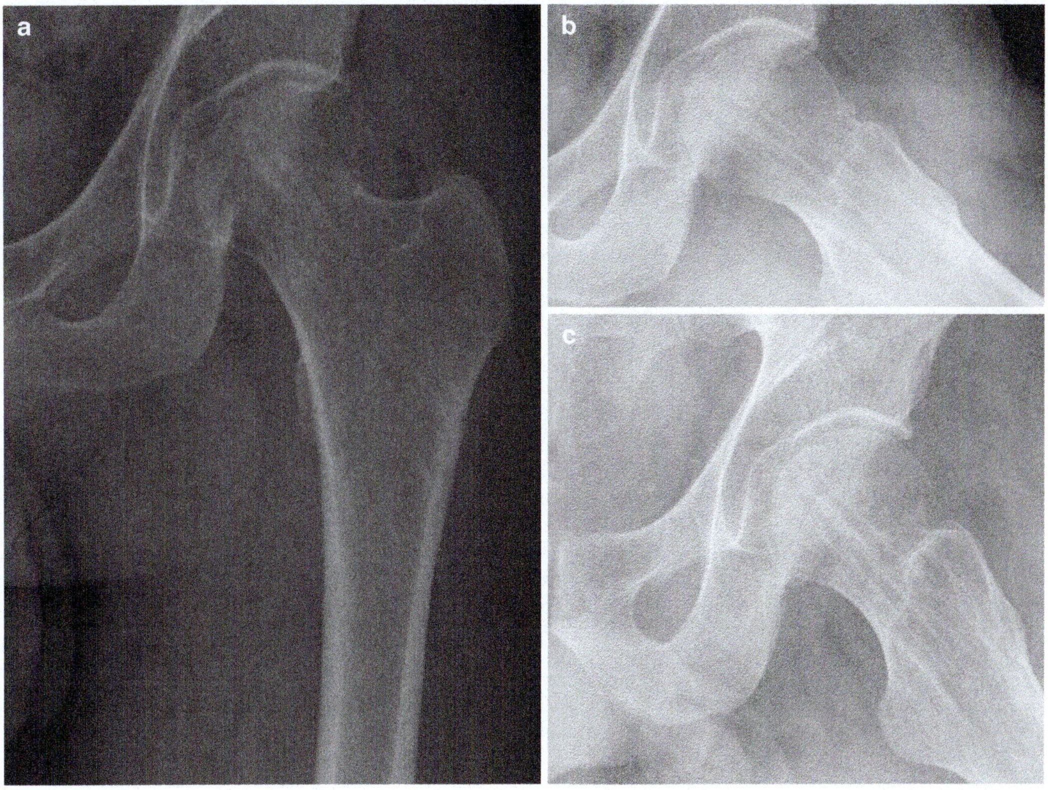

Fig. 15.4 (**a**) X-ray showing a consolidated subcapital neck femur fracture 2 years after the fracture and 1 year after screws' removal. (**b**) X-ray showing an excessive bone callus in a consolidated neck fracture. (**c**) X-ray showing the result of arthroscopic resection of the callus

References

1. Burman MS. Arthroscopy for direct visualization of joints. J Bone Joint Surg. 1931;13:669–95.
2. Mullis BH, Dahners LE. Hip arthroscopy to remove loose bodies after traumatic dislocation. J Orthop Trauma. 2006;20(1):22–6.
3. Hc E. Posterior fracture dislocations of the hip. J Bone Joint Surg Am. 1974;56:1103–27.
4. Epstein HC, Wiss d, Cozen L. Posterior fracture dislocation of the hip with fractures of the femoral head. Clin Orthop. 1985;201:9–17.
5. Armstrong JR. Traumatic dislocation of the hip joint: review of 101 dislocations. J Bone Joint Surg Br. 1948;30:430–5.
6. Steward MJ, McCarroll HR Jr, Mulhollan JS. Fracture-dislocation of the hip. Acta Orthop Scand. 1975;46:507–25.
7. Brav CE. Traumatic dislocation of the hip. J Bone Joint Surg Am. 1962;44:1115–34.
8. Svoboda SJ, Williams DM, Murphy KP. Hip arthroscopy for osteochondral loose body removal after a posterior hip dislocation. Arthroscopy. 2003;19(7):777–81.
9. Singleton SB, Joshi A, Schwartz MA, Collinge CA. Arthroscopic bullet removal from the acetabulum. Arthroscopy. 2005;21(3):360–4.
10. Ilizaliturri VM Jr, Gonzalez-Gutierrez B, Gonzalez-Ugalde H, Camacho-Galindo J. Hip arthroscopy after traumatic hip dislocation. Am J Sports Med. 2011;39(Suppl):50S–7S.
11. Matsuda DK. A rare fracture, an even rarer treatment: the arthroscopic reduction and internal fixation of an isolated femoral head fracture. Arthroscopy. 2009;25(4):408–12. https://doi.org/10.1016/j.arthro.2009.01.011.
12. Yamamoto Y, Ide T, Ono T, Hamada Y. Usefulness of arthroscopic surgery in hip trauma cases. Arthroscopy. 2003;19:269–73.
13. Yang JH, Chouhan DK, Oh KJ. Percutaneous screw fixation of acetabular fractures: applicability of hip

arthroscopy. Arthroscopy. 2010;26(11):1556–61. https://doi.org/10.1016/j.arthro.2010.04.068.
14. Kim H, Baek JH, Park SM, Ha YC. Arthroscopic reduction and internal fixation of acetabular fractures. Knee Surg Sports Traumatol Arthrosc. 2014;22(4):867–70. https://doi.org/10.1007/s00167-013-2799-y.
15. Gay SB, Sistrom C, Wang GJ, et al. Percutaneous screw fixation of acetabular fractures with CT guidance: preliminary results of a new technique. AJR Am J Roentgenol. 1992;158:819–22.
16. Hougaard K, Thomsen PB. Traumatic posterior fracture-dislocation of the hip with fracture of the femoral head or neck, or both. J Bone Joint Surg Am. 1988;70:233–9.
17. Roeder LF, Delee JC. Femoral head fractures associated with posterior hip dislocation. Clin Orthop Relat Res. 1980;147:121–30.
18. Sahin V, Karankas ES, Aksu S, et al. Traumatic hip dislocation and fracture-dislocation of the hip. A long term follow up study. J Trauma. 2003;54:520–9.
19. Gillespie P, Aprato A, Bircher M. Hip dislocation and femoral head fractures. In: Bentley G, editor. European surgical orthopaedics and traumatology. Berlin: Springer; 2014. p. 2179–202. https://doi.org/10.1007/978-3-642-34746-7_114.
20. Pipkin G. Treatment of grade IV fracture dislocation of the hip. J Bone Joint Surg Am. 1957;39:1027–42.
21. Lansford T, Munns SW. Arthroscopic treatment of Pipkin type I femoral head fractures: a report of 2 cases. J Orthop Trauma. 2012;26(7):e94–6. https://doi.org/10.1097/BOT.0b013e3182323f4f.
22. Park MS, Her IS, Cho HM, Chung YY. Internal fixation of femoral head fractures (Pipkin I) using hip arthroscopy. Knee Surg Sports Traumatol Arthrosc. 2014;22(4):898–901. https://doi.org/10.1007/s00167-013-2821-4.
23. Park MS, Yoon SJ, Choi SM. Arthroscopic reduction and internal fixation of femoral head fractures. J Orthop Trauma. 2014;28(7):e164–8. https://doi.org/10.1097/BOT.0000000000000048.
24. Ross JR, Gardner MJ. Femoral head fractures. Curr Rev Musculoskelet Med. 2012;5:199–205.
25. Boykin RE, Anz AW, Bushnell BD, Kocher MS, Stubbs AJ, Philippon MJ. Hip Instability. J Am Acad Orthop Surg. 2011;19(6):340–9.
26. Bellabarba C, Sheinkop MB, Kuo KN. Idiopathic hip instability. An unrecognized cause of coxa saltans in the adult. Clin Orthop Relat Res. 1998;355:261–71.
27. Bedi A, Galano G, Walsh C, Kelly BT. Capsular management during hip arthroscopy: from femoroacetabular impingement to instability. Arthroscopy. 2011;27(12):1720–31. https://doi.org/10.1016/j.arthro.2011.08.288.
28. Kuhns BD, Weber AE, Levy DM, Bedi A, Mather RC 3rd, Salata MJ, Nho SJ. Capsular management in hip arthroscopy: an anatomic, biomechanical and technical review. Front Surg. 2016;3:13. https://doi.org/10.3389/fsurg.2016.00013.
29. Philippon MJ. The role of arthroscopic thermal capsulorrhaphy in the hip. Clin Sports Med. 2001;20(4):817–29. Review.
30. Ganz R, Bamert P, Hausner P, et al. Zervikoazetabuläres Impingement nach Schenkelhalsfraktur. Unfallchirurg. 1991;94:172–5.
31. Klaue K, Durnin C, Ganz R. The acetabular rim syndrome. A clinical presentation of dysplasia of the hip. J Bone Joint Surg Br. 1991;73:423–9.
32. Eijer H, Myers SR, Ganz R. Anterior femoroacetabular impingement after femoral neck fractures. J Orthop Trauma. 2001;15(7):475–81.

The manufacturer's authorised representative in the EU is Springer Nature Customer Service Centre GmbH, Europaplatz 3, 69115 Heidelberg, Germany. If you have any concerns regarding our products, please contact ProductSafety@springernature.com

Printed and bound by CPI Group (UK) Ltd, Croydon, CR0 4YY
13/08/2026
02195497-0005